DIET and NUTRITION SOURCEBOOK

Health Reference Series

Volume Fifteen

DIET and NUTRITION SOURCEBOOK

Basic Information about Nutrition, Including the Dietary Guidelines for Americans, the Food Guide Pyramid, and Their Applications in Daily Diet, Nutritional Advice for Specific Age Groups, Current Nutritional Issues and Controversies, the New Food Label and How to Use It to Promote Healthy Eating, and Recent Developments in Nutritional Research

Edited by
Dan R. Harris

Omnigraphics, Inc.

Penobscot Building / Detroit, MI 48226

BIBLIOGRAPHIC NOTE

This volume contains individual publications issued by the Food and Drug Administration (FDA), Department of Health and Human Services (DHHS) of the FDA, Human Nutrition Information Service (HNIC) of the U.S. Department of Agriculture (USDA), and the Agricultural Marketing Service (AMS) of the USDA. Selected articles from *FDA Consumer* and *Nutrition: Eating for Good Health*, USDA Agricultural Information Bulletin 685 are also included. Document numbers where applicable and specific source citations are listed on the first page of each chapter.

Edited by Dan R. Harris

Karen Bellenir, Series Editor, *Health Reference Series*

Peter D. Dresser, Managing Editor, *Health Reference Series*

Omnigraphics

Matthew P. Barbour, *Production Manager*
Laurie Lanzen Harris, *Vice President, Editorial*
Peter E. Ruffner, *Vice President, Administration*
James A. Sellgren, *Vice President, Operations and Finance*
Jane J. Steele, *Vice President, Research*

Frederick G. Ruffner, Jr., *Publisher*

Copyright © 1996, Omnigraphics

Library of Congress Cataloging-in-Publication Data

Diet & nutrition sourcebook : basic information about nutrition,
   including the dietary guidelines for Americans,
   . . . / edited by Dan R. Harris.
      p.   cm. — (Health reference series)
   Includes bibliographical references and index.
   ISBN 0-7808-0084-2 (lib. bdg. : alk. paper)
   1. Nutrition.   I. Harris, Dan R.   II. Series.
RA784.D534   1996
613.2—dc20   96-9512
                                                                        CIP

∞

This book is printed on acid-free paper meeting the ANSI Z39.48 standard. The infinity symbol that appears above indicates that the paper in this book meets that standard.

Printed in the United States

Contents

Part III: Current Issues in Nutrition

Part IV: The Food Label

Part V: Recent Developments in Nutritional Research

Part VI: Nutrition in Public Health

Appendix A: Advice on Purchasing Foods

Appendix B: Advice on Safe Food Handling and Preparation

Appendix C: Sources of Additional Information

Index

Preface

About This Book

Today more and more Americans are obsessed with diet. At any time, 1 in 3 men claim to be on a diet; for women, the figure is 1 in 2. Yet at the same time, 30% of the adult population in the U.S. is obese. The contemporary American lifestyle has led to one in five meals eaten outside the home, and four out of seven of those meals is eaten in a fast food restaurant. It is not surprising, therefore, that there has been a general reappraisal of nutritional practices.

This book contains information about nutrition and healthy dietary practices. It consists of numerous individual documents produced by several government agencies including the Food and Drug Administration (FDA), the Department of Health and Human Services (DHHS), the United States Department of Agriculture (USDA), the Human Nutrition Information Service (HNIS), and subagencies of the National Institutes of Health (NIH). The documents selected for inclusion were chosen to help the general reader learn about food values; current nutritional issues and concerns which affect the general public, specific demographic groups, and people with various medical conditions; recent findings in nutritional research; and how to use the new Food Label, established by the FDA in 1993, to promote healthy dietary practices. All of the pamphlets and bulletins included represent the most recent published information available that has been verified by government agencies. They do not include current news reports of preliminary and unverified research findings. The Dietary Guidelines of Americans, published by the United States Department of Agriculture and the Department of Health and Human Services, provide the basic framework for the contents of this volume. These guidelines are as follows:

- Eat a variety of foods.

- Maintain healthy weight.

- Choose a diet low in fat, saturated fat, and cholesterol.

- Choose a diet with plenty of vegetables, fruits, and grain.

- Use sugars only in moderation.

- Use salt and sodium only in moderation.

- If you drink alcoholic beverages, do so in moderation.

References to these guidelines, as well as the Food Pyramid will be found throughout the various chapters of the book.

How to Use This Book

This book is divided into parts, chapters, and appendices. Parts focus on broad areas of interest. Chapters are devoted to single topics within a part.

Part I: The Foundations of Good Nutrition outlines the Dietary Guidelines for Americans developed by the USDA and DHHS, and shows how to implement them in the daily diet. Also included is a chapter on the new Food Guide Pyramid which was designed to help plan meals in accordance with the Dietary Guidelines. The concluding chapter covers the sources and functions of vitamins in the diet.

Part II: Applying the Dietary Guidelines contains information on how the Dietary Guidelines are applied to special situations. Chapters 4 through 9 provide nutritional information for each stage of life: infants, children, teenagers, pregnant women, and the elderly. The concluding chapter shows how to follow the Dietary Guidelines when eating out.

Part III: Current Issues in Nutrition focuses on some of the most popular and controversial topics in nutrition today. Chapters on fats, fiber, MSG, artificial sweeteners, calcium and osteoporosis, vegetarianism, and the use of dietary supplements are included in this section.

Part IV: The Food Label outlines the new product food labels now mandated by federal law and how to use them to make wise eating choices. Special chapters focus on how to use the food label to cope with the special dietary needs of people with high blood pressure, diabetes, cancer and heart disease, as well as how to use the label to lose weight and plan nutritious meals for children.

Part VII: Recent Developments in Nutritional Research offers chapters on the latest research concerning how the body uses food, with special focus on the immune system, nutrition and the brain, how the body makes food into energy, nutritional concerns of mothers and infants, and nutritional needs of adolescents.

Part VIII: Nutrition in Public Health presents information on the food and nutrition programs offered by the federal government for citizens in need.

The *Appendices* provide helpful information for all consumers in buying food for optimum nutrition and for safe handling and preparation of foods at home. The Appendix concludes with a list of government agencies and other organizations with addresses so that consumers may write for further information on the topics covered in this volume.

The book concludes with a general and key word *Index*.

Acknowledgments

The editor wishes to thank researcher Margaret Mary Missar for her perseverance in locating and obtaining all the documents included in this volume; and Karen Bellenir and Pete Dresser for generously sharing their knowledge and experience, which greatly aided the development of this series.

Note from the Editor

This book is part of Omnigraphic's *Health Reference Series.* The series provides basic information about a broad range of medical concerns. Although some of the information contained in this volume discusses the effect of diet and nutrition on various medical conditions, it is not intended to serve as a tool for diagnosing illness, in prescribing treatments, or as a substitute for the physician/patient relationship. All persons concerned about medical symptoms or the possibility of disease are encouraged to seek professional care from an appropriate health care provider.

Part One

The Foundations of Good Nutrition

Chapter 1

Nutrition and Your Health: Dietary Guidelines for Americans

Dietary Guidelines for Americans

- Eat a variety of foods

- Balance the food you eat with physical activity—maintain or improve your weight

- Choose a diet with plenty of grain products, vegetables, and fruits

- Choose a diet low in fat, saturated fat, and cholesterol

- Choose a diet moderate in sugars

- Choose a diet moderate in salt and sodium

- If you drink alcoholic beverages, do so in moderation

What should Americans eat to stay healthy?

These guidelines are designed to help answer this question. They provide advice for healthy Americans age 2 years and over about food choices that promote health and prevent disease. To meet the Dietary Guidelines for Americans, choose a diet with most of the calories from grain products, vegetables, fruits, lowfat milk products, lean meats, fish, poultry, and dry beans. Choose fewer calories from fats and sweets.

Home and Garden Bulletin No. 232

Eating is one of life's greatest pleasures

Food choices depend on history, culture, and environment, as well as on energy and nutrient needs. People also eat foods for enjoyment. Family, friends, and beliefs play a major role in the ways people select foods and plan meals. This booklet describes some of the many different and pleasurable ways to combine foods to make healthful diets.

Diet is important to health at all stages of life

Many genetic, environmental, behavioral, and cultural factors can affect health. Understanding family history of disease or risk factors—body weight and fat distribution, blood pressure, and blood cholesterol, for example—can help people make more informed decisions about actions that can improve health prospects. Food choices are among the most pleasurable and effective of these actions.

Healthful diets help children grow, develop, and do well in school. They enable people of all ages to work productively and feel their best. Food choices also can help to reduce the risk for chronic diseases, such as heart disease, certain cancers, diabetes, stroke, and osteoporosis, that are leading causes of death and disability among Americans. Good diets can reduce major risk factors for chronic diseases—factors such as obesity, high blood pressure, and high blood cholesterol.

Foods contain energy, nutrients, and other components that affect health

People require energy and certain other essential nutrients. These nutrients are essential because the body cannot make them and must obtain them from food. Essential nutrients include vitamins, minerals, certain amino acids, and certain fatty acids. Foods also contain other components such as fiber that are important for health. Although each of these food components has a specific function in the body, all of them together are required for overall health. People need calcium to build and maintain strong bones, for example, but many other nutrients also are involved.

The carbohydrates, fats, and proteins in food supply energy, which is measured in calories. Carbohydrates and proteins provide about 4 calories per gram. Fat contributes more than twice as much—about 9 calories per gram. Alcohol, although not a nutrient, also supplies energy—about 7 calories per gram. Foods that are high in fat are also high in calories. However, many lowfat or nonfat foods can also be high in calories.

Physical activity fosters a healthful diet

Calorie needs vary by age and level of activity. Many older adults need less food, in part due to decreased activity, relative to younger, more active individuals. People who are trying to lose weight and eating little food may need to select more nutrient-dense foods in order to meet their nutrient needs in a satisfying diet. Nearly all Americans need to be more active, because a sedentary lifestyle is unhealthful. Increasing the calories spent in daily activities helps to maintain health and allows people to eat a nutritious and enjoyable diet.

What is a healthful diet?

Healthful diets contain the amounts of essential nutrients and calories needed to prevent nutritional deficiencies and excesses. Healthful diets also provide the right balance of carbohydrate, fat, and protein to reduce risks for chronic diseases, and are a part of a full and productive lifestyle. Such diets are obtained from a variety of foods that are available, affordable, and enjoyable.

The Recommended Dietary Allowances refer to nutrients

Recommended Dietary Allowances (RDAs) represent the amounts of nutrients that are adequate to meet the needs of most healthy people. Although people with average nutrient requirements likely eat adequately at levels below the RDAs, diets that meet RDAs are almost certain to ensure intake of enough essential nutrients by most healthy people. The Dietary Guidelines describe food choices that will help you meet these recommendations. Like the RDAs, the Dietary Guidelines apply to diets consumed over several days and not to single meals or foods.

The Dietary Guidelines describe food choices that promote good health

The Dietary Guidelines are designed to help Americans choose diets that will meet nutrient requirements, promote health, support active lives, and reduce chronic disease risks. Research has shown that certain diets raise risks for chronic diseases. Such diets are high in fat, saturated fat, cholesterol, and salt and they contain more calories than the body uses. They are also low in grain products, vegetables, fruit, and fiber. This bulletin helps you choose foods, meals, and diets that can reduce chronic disease risks.

Food labels and the Food Guide Pyramid are tools to help you make food choices

The Food Guide Pyramid and the Nutrition Facts Label serve as educational tools to put the Dietary Guidelines into practice. The Pyramid translates the RDAs and the Dietary Guidelines into the kinds and amounts of food to eat each day. The Nutrition Facts Label is designed to help you select foods for a diet that will meet the Dietary Guidelines. Most processed foods now include nutrition information. However, nutrition labels are not required for foods like coffee and tea (which contain no significant amounts of nutrients), certain ready-to-eat foods like unpackaged deli and bakery items, and restaurant food. Labels are also voluntary for many raw foods—your grocer may supply this information for the fish, meat, poultry, and raw fruits and vegetables that are consumed most frequently. Use the Nutrition Facts Label to choose a healthful diet.

Eat a Variety of Foods

To obtain the nutrients and other substances needed for good health, vary the foods you eat

Foods contain combinations of nutrients and other healthful substances. No single food can supply all nutrients in the amounts you need. For example, oranges provide vitamin C but no vitamin B_{12}; cheese provides vitamin B_{12} but no vitamin C. To make sure you get all of the nutrients and other substances needed for health, choose the recommended number of daily servings from each of the five major food groups displayed in the Food Guide Pyramid (Figure 1).

Figure 1

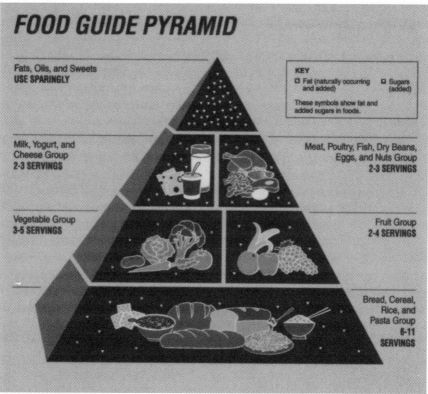

Use foods from the base of the Food Guide Pyramid as the foundation of your meals

Americans do choose a wide variety of foods. However, people often choose higher or lower amounts from some food groups than suggested in the Food Guide Pyramid. The Pyramid shows that foods from the grain products group, along with vegetables and fruits, are the basis of healthful diets. Enjoy meals that have rice, pasta, potatoes, or bread at the center of the plate, accompanied by other vegetables and fruit, and lean and lowfat foods from the other groups. Limit fats and sugars added in food preparation and at the table. Compare the recommended number of servings in Box 1 with what you usually eat.

Box 1

CHOOSE FOODS FROM EACH OF FIVE FOOD GROUPS

The Food Guide Pyramid illustrates the importance of balance among food groups in a daily eating pattern. Most of the daily servings of food should be selected from the food groups that are the largest in the picture and closest to the base of the Pyramid.

- Choose most of your foods from the grain products group (6-11 servings), the vegetable group (3-5 servings), and the fruit group (2-4 servings).

- Eat moderate amounts of foods from the milk group (2-3 servings) and the meat and beans group (2-3 servings).

- Choose sparingly foods that provide few nutrients and are high in fat and sugars.

Note: A range of servings is given for each food group. The smaller number is for people who consume about 1,600 calories a day, such as many sedentary women. The larger number is for those who consume about 2,800 calories a day, such as active men.

What counts as a "serving"?

See box 2 for suggested serving sizes in the Food Guide Pyramid food groups. Notice that some of the serving sizes are smaller than what you might usually eat. For example, many people eat a cup or more of pasta in a meal, which equals two or more servings. So, it is easy to eat the number of servings recommended.

Choose different foods within each food group

You can achieve a healthful, nutritious eating pattern with many combinations of foods from the five major food groups. Choosing a variety of foods within and across food groups improves dietary patterns because foods within the same group have different combinations of nutrients and other beneficial substances. For example, some vegetables and fruits are good sources of vitamin C or vitamin A, while others are high in folate (page 20); still others are good sources of calcium or iron. Choosing a variety of foods within each group also helps to make your meals more interesting from day to day.

Box 2

WHAT COUNTS AS A SERVING?*

Grain Products Group (bread, cereal rice, and pasta)

- 1 slice of bread
- 1 ounce of ready-to-eat cereal
- ½ cup of cooked cereal, rice, or pasta

Vegetable Group

- 1 cup of raw leafy vegetables
- ½ cup of other vegetables—cooked or chopped raw
- ¾ cup of vegetable juice

Fruit Group

- 1 medium apple, banana, orange
- ½ cup of chopped, cooked, or canned fruit
- ¾ cup of fruit juice

Milk Group (milk, yogurt, and cheese)

- 1 cup of milk or yogurt
- 1½ ounces of natural cheese
- 2 ounces of processed cheese

Meat and Beans Group (meat, poultry, fish, dry beans, eggs, and nuts)

- 2-3 ounces of cooked lean meat, poultry, or fish
- ½ cup of cooked dry beans or 1 egg counts as 1 ounce of lean meat. Two tablespoons of peanut butter or 1/3 cup of nuts count as 1 ounce of meat.

*Some foods fit into more than one group.
Dry beans, peas, and lentils can be counted as servings in either the meat and beans group or vegetable group. These "cross over" foods can be counted as servings from either one or the other group, but not both. Serving sizes indi-

cated here are those used in the Food Guide Pyramid and based on both suggested and usually consumed portions necessary to achieve adequate nutrient
intake. They differ from serving sizes on the Nutrition Facts Label, which reflect
portions usually consumed.

What about vegetarian diets?

Some Americans eat vegetarian diets for reasons of culture, belief,
or health. Most vegetarians eat milk products and eggs, and as a
group, these lacto-ovo-vegetarians enjoy excellent health. Vegetarian
diets are consistent with the Dietary Guidelines for Americans and
can meet Recommended Dietary Allowances for nutrients. You can get
enough protein from a vegetarian diet as long as the variety and
amounts of foods consumed are adequate. Meat, fish, and poultry are
major contributors of iron, zinc, and B vitamins in most American
diets, and vegetarians should pay special attention to these nutrients.

Vegans eat only food of plant origin. Because animal products are
the only food sources of vitamin B_{12}, vegans must supplement their
diets with a source of this vitamin. In addition, vegan diets, particularly those of children, require care to ensure adequacy of vitamin D
and calcium, which most Americans obtain from milk products.

Foods vary in their amounts of calories and nutrients

Some foods such as grain products, vegetables, and fruits have
many nutrients and other healthful substances but are relatively low
in calories. Fat and alcohol are high in calories. Foods high in both
sugars and fat contain many calories but often are low in vitamins,
minerals, or fiber.

People who do not need many calories or who must restrict their
food intake need to choose nutrient-rich foods from the five major food
groups with special care. They should obtain most of their calories
from foods that contain a high proportion of essential nutrients and
fiber.

Growing children, teenage girls, and women have higher needs for some nutrients

Many women and adolescent girls need to eat more calcium-rich
foods to get the calcium needed for healthy bones throughout life. By

---

Box 3

SOME GOOD SOURCES OF CALCIUM*

* Most foods in the milk group†

    –milk and dishes made with milk, such as puddings and soups made with milk

    –cheeses such as Mozzarella, Cheddar, Swiss, and Parmesan

    –yogurt

* Canned fish with soft bones such as sardines, anchovies, and salmon†

* Dark-green leafy vegetables, such as kale, mustard greens, and turnip greens, and pak-choi

* Tofu, if processed with calcium sulfate. Read the labels.

* Tortillas made from lime-processed corn. Read the labels.

*Does not include complete list of examples. You can obtain additional information from "Good Sources of Nutrients," USDA, January 1990. Also read food labels for brand-specific information.

†Some foods in this group are high in fat, cholesterol, or both. Choose lower fat, lower cholesterol foods most often. Read the labels.

---

selecting lowfat or fat-free milk products and other lowfat calcium sources, they can obtain adequate calcium and keep fat intake from being too high (box 3). Young children, teenage girls, and women of childbearing age should also eat enough iron-rich foods, such as lean meats and whole-grain or enriched white bread, to keep the body's iron stores at adequate levels (box 4).

Enriched and fortified foods have essential nutrients added to them

National policy requires that specified amounts of nutrients be added to enrich some foods. For example, enriched flour and bread contain added thiamin, riboflavin, niacin, and iron; skim milk, lowfat milk, and margarine are usually enriched with vitamin A; and milk

11

Box 4

SOME GOOD SOURCES OF IRON*

- Meats—beef, pork, lamb, and liver and other organ meats†

- Poultry—chicken, duck, and turkey, especially dark meat; liver†

- Fish—shellfish, like clams, mussels, and oysters; sardines; anchovies; and other fish†

- Leafy greens of the cabbage family, such as broccoli, kale, turnip greens, collards

- Legumes, such as lima beans and green peas; dry beans and peas, such as pinto beans, black-eyed peas, and canned baked beans

- Yeast-leavened whole-wheat bread and rolls

- Iron-enriched white bread, pasta, rice, and cereals. Read the labels.

*Does not include complete list of examples. You can obtain additional information from "Good Sources of Nutrients," USDA, January 1990. Also read food labels for brand-specific information.

† Some foods in this group are high in fat, cholesterol, or both. Choose lean, lower fat, lower cholesterol foods most often. Read the labels.

---

is usually enriched with vitamin D. Fortified foods may have one or several nutrients added in extra amounts. The number and quantity of nutrients added vary among products. Fortified foods may be useful for meeting special dietary needs. Read the ingredient list to know which nutrients are added to foods (figure 2). How these foods fit into your total diet will depend on the amounts you eat and the other foods you consume.

Where do vitamin, mineral, and fiber supplements fit in?

Supplements of vitamins, minerals, or fiber also may help to meet special nutritional needs. However, supplements do not supply all of the nutrients and other substances present in foods that are important to health. Supplements of some nutrients taken regularly in large amounts are harmful. Daily vitamin and mineral supplements at or below the Recommended Dietary Allowances are considered safe, but

*Figure 2**

READY-TO-EAT CEREAL

Nutrition Facts

Serving Size 3/4 cup (30g/1.1 oz)
Servings Per Package 11

Amount Per Serving	Cereal	Cereal with 1/2 cup Vitamins A&D skim milk
Calories	120	160
Calories from Fat	15	15

	% Daily Value**	
Total Fat 2g•	3%	3%
Saturated Fat 1g	5%	5%
Cholesterol 0mg	0%	0%
Sodium 210mg	9%	11%
Potassium 45mg	1%	7%
Total Carbohydrate 24g	8%	10%
Dietary Fiber 1g	4%	4%
Sugars 9g		
Protein 2g		

	Cereal	with milk
Vitamin A	15%	20%
Vitamin C	25%	25%
Calcium	0%	15%
Iron	25%	25%
Vitamin D	10%	25%
Thiamin	25%	30%
Riboflavin	25%	35%
Niacin	25%	25%
Vitamin B$_6$	25%	25%
Folate	25%	25%
Phosphorus	2%	15%

*Amount in cereal. One half cup of skim milk contributes an additional 65mg sodium, 6g total carbohydrate (6g sugars), and 4g protein.
** Percent Daily Values are based on a 2,000 calorie diet. Your daily values may be higher or lower depending on your calorie needs:

	Calories	2,000	2,500
Total Fat	Less than	65g	80g
Sat Fat	Less than	20g	25g
Cholesterol	Less than	300mg	300mg
Sodium	Less than	2,400mg	2,400mg
Potassium		3,500mg	3,500mg
Total Carbohydrate		300g	375g
Dietary Fiber		25g	30g

Ingredients: Corn, sugar, whole oats, almonds, partially hydrogenated palm kernel oil, high fructose corn syrup, whole wheat, brown sugar, nonfat dry milk, corn syrup, salt, rice, butter flavor with other natural and artifical flavors, partially hydrogenated cottonseed and soybean oils, modified corn starch, glycerin, butter oil, soy lecithin, polyglycerol esters of fatty acids, malt flavor, guar gum, ascorbic acid (vitamin C), niacinamide, iron, pyridoxine hydrochloride (vitamin B$_6$), riboflavin (vitamin B$_2$), vitamin A palmitate (protected with BHT), thiamin hydrochloride (vitamin B$_1$), folic acid, and vitamin D.

*See page 26 for discussion of Daily Value

13

Figure 2 Continued

LOWFAT MILK

Nutrition Facts

Serving Size 8 fl oz (240 ml)
Servings Per Container 8

Amount Per Serving

Calories 100   Calories from Fat 20

% Daily Value*

Total Fat 2.5g	**4%**
Saturated Fat 1.5g	**8%**
Cholesterol 10mg	**3%**
Sodium 130mg	**5%**
Total Carbohydrate 12g	**4%**
Dietary Fiber 0g	**0%**
Sugars 11g	
Protein 8g	

Vitamin A 10%	•	Vitamin C 4%
Calcium 30%	•	Iron 0%
Vitamin D 25%		

*Percent Daily Values are based on a 2,000 calorie diet. Your daily values may be higher or lower depending on your calorie needs:

	Calories	2,000	2,500
Total Fat	Less than	65g	80g
Sat Fat	Less than	20g	25g
Cholesterol	Less than	300mg	300mg
Sodium	Less than	2,400mg	2,400mg
Total Carbohydrate		300g	375g
Dietary Fiber		25g	30g

Ingredients: Lowfat milk, vitamin A palmitate, vitamin D₃.

14

are usually not needed by people who eat the variety of foods depicted in the Food Guide Pyramid.

Sometimes supplements are needed to meet specific nutrient requirements. For example, older people and others with little exposure to sunlight may need a vitamin D supplement. Women of childbearing age may reduce the risk of certain birth defects by consuming folate-rich foods or folic acid supplements. Iron supplements are recommended for pregnant women. However, because foods contain many nutrients and other substances that promote health, the use of supplements cannot substitute for proper food choices.

Advice for Today

Enjoy eating a variety of foods. Get the many nutrients your body needs by choosing among the varied foods you enjoy from these groups: grain products, vegetables, fruits, milk and milk products, protein-rich plant foods (beans, nuts), and protein-rich animal foods (lean meat, poultry, fish, and eggs). Remember to choose lean and lowfat foods and beverages most often. Many foods you eat contain servings from more than one food group. For example, soups and stews may contain meat, beans, noodles, and vegetables.

Balance the Food You Eat With Physical Activity— Maintain or Improve Your Weight

Many Americans gain weight in adulthood, increasing their risk for high blood pressure, heart disease, stroke, diabetes, certain types of cancer, arthritis, breathing problems, and other illness. Therefore, most adults should not gain weight. If you are overweight and have one of these problems, you should try to lose weight, or at the very least, not gain weight. If you are uncertain about your risk of developing a problem associated with overweight, you should consult a health professional.

How to maintain your weight

In order to stay at the same body weight, people must balance the amount of calories in the foods and drinks they consume with the amount of calories the body uses. Physical activity is an important way to use food energy. Most Americans spend much of their working day in activities that require little energy. In addition, many

15

Box 5

TO INCREASE CALORIE EXPENDITURE BY PHYSICAL ACTIVITY

Remember to accumulate 30 minutes or more of moderate physical activity on most—preferably all—days of the week.

Examples of moderate physical activities for healthy U.S. adults

walking briskly (3-4 miles per hour)

conditioning or general calisthenics

home care, general cleaning

racket sports such as table tennis

mowing lawn, power mower

golf—pulling cart or carrying clubs

home repair, painting

fishing, standing/casting

jogging

swimming (moderate effort)

cycling, moderate speed ($\leq$10 miles per hour)

gardening

canoeing leisurely (2.0-3.9 miles per hour)

dancing

Source: Adapted from Pate, et al., *Journal of the American Medical Association*, 1995, Vol. 273, p. 404.

Americans of all ages now spend a lot of leisure time each day being inactive, for example, watching television or working at a computer. To burn calories, devote less time to sedentary activities like sitting. Spend more time in activities like walking to the store or around the block. Use stairs rather than elevators. Less sedentary activity and more vigorous activity may help you reduce body fat and disease risk. Try to do 30 minutes or more of moderate physical activity on most—preferably all—days of the week (box 5).

The kinds and amounts of food people eat affect their ability to maintain weight. High-fat foods contain more calories per serving than other foods and may increase the likelihood of weight gain. However, even when people eat less high-fat food, they still can gain weight from eating too much of foods high in starch, sugars, or protein. Eat a variety of foods, emphasizing pasta, rice, bread, and other whole-grain foods as well as fruits and vegetables. These foods are filling, but lower in calories than foods rich in fats or oils.

The pattern of eating may also be important. Snacks provide a large percentage of daily calories for many Americans. Unless nutritious snacks are part of the daily meal plan, snacking may lead to weight gain. A pattern of frequent binge-eating, with or without alternating periods of food restriction, may also contribute to weight problems.

Maintaining weight is equally important for older people who begin to lose weight as they age. Some of the weight that is lost is muscle. Maintaining muscle through regular activity helps to keep older people feeling well and helps to reduce the risk of falls and fractures.

How to evaluate your body weight

Healthy weight ranges for adult men and women of all ages are shown in figure 3. See where your weight falls on the chart for people of your height. The health risks due to excess weight appear to be the same for older as for younger adults. Weight ranges are shown in the chart because people of the same height may have equal amounts of body fat but different amounts of muscle and bone. However, the ranges do not mean that it is healthy to gain weight, even within the same weight range. The higher weights in the healthy weight range apply to people with more muscle and bone.

Weights above the healthy weight range are less healthy for most people. The further you are above the healthy weight range for your height, the higher your weight-related risk (figure 3). Weights slightly below the range may be healthy for some people but are sometimes the result of health problems, especially when weight loss is unintentional.

17

Figure 3

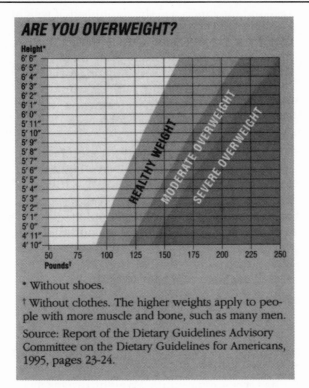

ARE YOU OVERWEIGHT?

* Without shoes.

† Without clothes. The higher weights apply to people with more muscle and bone, such as many men.

Source: Report of the Dietary Guidelines Advisory Committee on the Dietary Guidelines for Americans, 1995, pages 23-24.

Location of body fat

Research suggests that the location of body fat also is an important factor in health risks for adults. Excess fat in the abdomen (stomach area) is a greater health risk than excess fat in the hips and thighs. Extra fat in the abdomen is linked to high blood pressure, diabetes, early heart disease, and certain types of cancer. Smoking and too much alcohol increase abdominal fat and the risk for diseases related to obesity. Vigorous exercise helps to reduce abdominal fat and decrease the risk for these diseases. The easiest way to check your body fat distribution is to measure around your waistline with a tape measure and compare this with the measure around your hips or buttocks to see if your abdomen is larger. If you are in doubt, you may wish to seek advice from a health professional.

Problems with excessive thinness

Being too thin can occur with anorexia nervosa, other eating disorders, or loss of appetite, and is linked to menstrual irregularity and osteoporosis in women, and greater risk of early death in both women and men. Many people—especially women—are concerned about body weight, even when their weight is normal. Excessive concern about weight may cause or lead to such unhealthy behaviors as excessive exercise, self-induced vomiting, and the abuse of laxatives or other medications. These practices may only worsen the concern about weight. If you lose weight suddenly or for unknown reasons, see a physician. Unexplained weight loss may be an early clue to a health problem.

If you need to lose weight

You do not need to lose weight if your weight is already within the healthy range in the figure, if you have gained less than 10 pounds since you reached your adult height, and if you are otherwise healthy. If you are overweight and have excess abdominal fat, a weight-related medical problem, or a family history of such problems, you need to lose weight. Healthy diets and exercise can help people maintain a healthy weight, and may also help them lose weight. It is important to recognize that overweight is a chronic condition which can only be controlled with long-term changes. To reduce caloric intake, eat less fat and control portion sizes (box 6). If you are not physically active, spend less time in sedentary activities such as watching television, and be more active throughout the day. As people lose weight, the body becomes more efficient at using energy and the rate of weight loss may decrease. Increased physical activity will help you to continue losing weight and to avoid gaining it back (box 5).

Many people are not sure how much weight they should lose. Weight loss of only 5-10 percent of body weight may improve many of the problems associated with overweight, such as high blood pressure and diabetes. Even a smaller weight loss can make a difference. If you are trying to lose weight, do so slowly and steadily. A generally safe rate is ½-1 pound a week until you reach your goal. Avoid crash weight-loss diets that severely restrict calories or the variety of foods. Extreme approaches to weight loss, such as self-induced vomiting or the use of laxatives, amphetamines, or diuretics, are not appropriate and can be dangerous to your health.

19

Box 6

TO DECREASE CALORIE INTAKE

- Eat a variety of foods that are low in calories and high in nutrients—check the Nutrition Facts Label.

- Eat less fat and fewer high-fat foods.

- Eat smaller portions and limit second helpings of foods high in fat and calories.

- Eat more vegetables and fruits without fats and sugars added in preparation or at the table.

- Eat pasta, rice, breads, and cereals without fats and sugars added in preparation or at the table.

- Eat less sugars and fewer sweets (like candy, cookies, cakes, soda).

- Drink less or no alcohol.

Weight regulation in children

Children need enough food for proper growth. To promote growth and development and prevent overweight, teach children to eat grain products; vegetables and fruits; lowfat milk products or other calcium-rich foods; beans, lean meat, poultry, fish or other protein-rich foods; and to participate in vigorous activity. Limiting television time and encouraging children to play actively in a safe environment are helpful steps. Although limiting fat intake may help to prevent excess weight gain in children, fat should not be restricted for children younger than 2 years of age. Helping overweight children to achieve a healthy weight along with normal growth requires more caution. Modest reductions in dietary fat, such as the use of lowfat milk rather than whole milk, are not hazardous. However, major efforts to change a child's diet should be accompanied by monitoring of growth by a health professional at regular intervals.

Advice for Today

Try to maintain your body weight by balancing what you eat with physical activity. If you are sedentary, try to become more active. If you are already very active, try to continue the same level of activity as you age. More physical activity is better than less, and any is better than none. If your weight is not in the healthy range, try to reduce health risks through better eating and exercise habits. Take steps to keep your weight within the healthy range (neither too high nor too low). Have children's heights and weights checked regularly by a health professional.

Choose a Diet With Plenty of Grain Products, Vegetables, and Fruits

Grain products, vegetables, and fruits are key parts of a varied diet. They are emphasized in this guideline because they provide vitamins, minerals, complex carbohydrates (starch and dietary fiber), and other substances that are important for good health. They are also generally low in fat, depending on how they are prepared and what is added to them at the table. Most Americans of all ages eat fewer than the recommended number of servings of grain products, vegetables, and fruits, even though consumption of these foods is associated with a substantially lower risk for many chronic diseases, including certain types of cancer.

Most of the calories in your diet should come from grain products, vegetables, and fruits

These include grain products high in complex carbohydrates— breads, cereals, pasta, rice—found at the base of the Food Guide Pyramid, as well as vegetables such as potatoes and corn. Dry beans (like pinto, navy, kidney, and black beans) are included in the meat and beans group of the Pyramid, but they can count as servings of vegetables instead of meat alternatives.

Plant foods provide fiber

Fiber is found only in plant foods like whole-grain breads and cereals, beans and peas, and other vegetables and fruits. Because there are different types of fiber in foods, choose a variety of foods daily. Eating a variety of fiber-containing plant foods is important for proper bowel function, can reduce symptoms of chronic constipation, diverticular disease, and hemorrhoids, and may lower the risk for heart disease and some cancers. However, some of the health benefits associated with a high-fiber diet may come from other components

21

Box 7

SOME GOOD SOURCES OF CAROTENOIDS*

- Dark-green leafy vegetables (such as spinach, collards, kale, mustard greens, turnip greens), broccoli, carrots, pumpkin and calabasa, red pepper, sweet potatoes, and tomatoes

- Fruits like mango, papaya, cantaloupe

*Does not include complete list of examples. You can obtain additional information from "Good Sources of Nutrients," USDA, January 1990. Also read food labels for brand-specific information.

---

present in these foods, not just from fiber itself. For this reason, fiber is best obtained from foods rather than supplements.

Plant foods provide a variety of vitamins and minerals essential for health

Most fruits and vegetables are naturally low in fat and provide many essential nutrients and other food components important for health. These foods are excellent sources of vitamin C, vitamin B_6, carotenoids, including those which form vitamin A (box 7), and folate (box 8). The antioxidant nutrients found in plant foods (e.g., vitamin C, carotenoids, vitamin E, and certain minerals) are presently of great interest to scientists and the public because of their potentially beneficial role in reducing the risk for cancer and certain other chronic diseases. Scientists are also trying to determine if other substances in plant foods protect against cancer.

Folate, also called folic acid, is a B vitamin that, among its many functions, reduces the risk of a serious type of birth defect (box 8). Minerals such as potassium, found in a wide variety of vegetables and fruits, and calcium, found in certain vegetables, may help reduce the risk for high blood pressure (see pages 31 and 9).

The availability of fresh fruits and vegetables varies by season and region of the country, but frozen and canned fruits and vegetables ensure a plentiful supply of these healthful foods throughout the year. Read the Nutrition Facts Label to help choose foods that are rich in carbohydrates, fiber, and nutrients, and low in fat and sodium.

Box 8

SOME GOOD SOURCES OF FOLATE*

• Dry beans (like red beans, navy beans, and soybeans), lentils, chickpeas, cow peas, and peanuts

• Many vegetables, especially leafy greens (spinach, cabbage, brussels sprouts, romaine, looseleaf lettuce), peas, okra, sweet corn, beets, and broccoli

• Fruits such as blackberries, boysenberries, kiwifruit, oranges, plantains, strawberries, orange juice, and pineapple juice

Does not include complete list of examples. You can obtain additional information from "Good Sources of Nutrients," USDA, January 1990.
The Nutrition Facts Label may also provide brand-specific information on this nutrient.

Advice for Today

Eat more grain products (breads, cereals, pasta, and rice), vegetables, and fruits. Eat dry beans, lentils, and peas more often. Increase your fiber intake by eating more of a variety of whole grains, whole-grain products, dry beans, fiber-rich vegetables and fruits such as carrots, corn, peas, pears, and berries (box 9).

Choose a Diet Low in Fat, Saturated Fat, and Cholesterol

Some dietary fat is needed for good health. Fats supply energy and essential fatty acids and promote absorption of the fat-soluble vitamins A, D, E, and K. Most people are aware that high levels of saturated fat and cholesterol in the diet are linked to increased blood cholesterol levels and a greater risk for heart disease. More Americans are now eating less fat, saturated fat, and cholesterol-rich foods than in the recent past, and fewer people are dying from the most common form of heart disease. Still, many people continue to eat high-fat diets, the number of overweight people has increased, and the risk of heart disease and certain cancers (also linked to fat intake) remains high. This guideline emphasizes the continued importance of choosing a diet with less total fat, saturated fat, and cholesterol.

Box 9

FOR A DIET WITH PLENTY OF GRAIN PRODUCTS, VEGETABLES, AND FRUITS, EAT DAILY—

6-11 servings* of grain products (breads, cereals, pasta, and rice)

- Eat products made from a variety of whole grains, such as wheat, rice, oats, corn, and barley.

- Eat several servings of whole-grain breads and cereals daily.

- Prepare and serve grain products with little or no fats and sugars.

3-5 servings* of various vegetables and vegetable juices

- Choose dark-green leafy and deep-yellow vegetables often.

- Eat dry beans, peas, and lentils often.

- Eat starchy vegetables, such as potatoes and corn.

- Prepare and serve vegetables with little or no fats.

2-4 servings* of various fruits and fruit juices

- Choose citrus fruits or juices, melons, or berries regularly.

- Eat fruits as desserts or snacks.

- Drink fruit juices.

- Prepare and serve fruits with little or no added sugars.

*See box 2, page 9, for what counts as a serving.

Foods high in fat should be used sparingly

Some foods and food groups in the Food Guide Pyramid are higher in fat than others. Fats and oils, and some types of desserts and snack foods that contain fat provide calories but few nutrients. Many foods in the milk group and in the meat and beans group (which includes eggs and nuts, as well as meat, poultry, and fish) are also high in fat, as are some processed foods in the grain group. Choosing lower fat options among these foods allows you to eat the recommended servings from these groups and increase the amount and variety of grain

---

Box 10

MAXIMUM TOTAL FAT INTAKE AT DIFFERENT CALORIE LEVELS

Calories	1,600	2,200	2,800
Total fat (grams)	53	73	93

---

products, fruits, and vegetables in your diet without going over your calorie needs.

Choose a diet low in fat

Fat, whether from plant or animal sources, contains more than twice the number of calories of an equal amount of carbohydrate or protein. Choose a diet that provides no more than 30 percent of total calories from fat. The upper limit on the grams of fat in your diet will depend on the calories you need (box 10). Cutting back on fat can help you consume fewer calories. For example, at 2,000 calories per day, the suggested upper limit of calories from fat is about 600 calories. Sixty-five grams of fat contribute about 600 calories (65 grams of fat x 9 calories per gram = about 600 calories). On the Nutrition Facts Label, 65 grams of fat is the Daily Value for a 2,000-calorie intake (figure 4).

Choose a diet low in saturated fat

Fats contain both saturated and unsaturated (monounsaturated and polyunsaturated) fatty acids. Saturated fat raises blood cholesterol more than other forms of fat. Reducing saturated fat to less than 10 percent of calories will help you lower your blood cholesterol level. The fats from meat, milk, and milk products are the main sources of saturated fats in most diets. Many bakery products are also sources of saturated fats. Vegetable oils supply smaller amounts of saturated fat. On the Nutrition Facts Label, 20 grams of saturated fat (9 percent of caloric intake) is the Daily Value for a 2,000-calorie diet (figure 4).

Monounsaturated and polyunsaturated fat. Olive and canola oils are particularly high in monounsaturated fats; most other vegetable oils, nuts, and high-fat fish are good sources of polyunsaturated fats. Both kinds of unsaturated fats reduce blood cholesterol when they

Figure 4

Serving Size reflects the amount typically eaten by many people.

Nutrition Facts
Serving Size 3 cookies (34g/1.2 oz)
Servings Per Container About 5

Amount Per Serving

Calories 180   Calories from Fat 90

	% Daily Value*
Total Fat 10g	**15%**
Saturated Fat 3.5g	**18%**
Polyunsaturated Fat 1g	
Monounsaturated Fat 5g	
Cholesterol 10mg	**3%**
Sodium 80mg	**3%**
Total Carbohydrate 21g	**7%**
Dietary Fiber 1g	**4%**
Sugars 11g	
Protein 2g	

Vitamin A 0%	•		Vitamin C 0%
Calcium 0%	•		Iron 4%
Thiamin 6%	•		Riboflavin 4%
Niacin 4%			

* Percent Daily Values are based on a 2,000 calorie diet. Your daily values may be higher or lower depending on your calorie needs:

		Calories 2,000	2,500
Total Fat	Less than	65g	80g
Sat Fat	Less than	20g	25g
Cholesterol	Less than	300mg	300mg
Sodium	Less than	2,400mg	2,400mg
Total Carbohydrate		300g	375g
Dietary Fiber		25g	30g

Ingredients: Unbleached enriched wheat flour [flour, niacin, reduced iron, thiamin mononitrate (vitamin B₁)], sweet chocolate (sugar, chocolate liquor, cocoa butter, soy lecithin added as an emulsifier, vanilla extract), sugar, partially hydrogenated vegetable shortening (soybean, cottonseed and/or canola oils), nonfat milk, whole eggs, cornstarch, egg whites, salt, vanilla extract, baking soda, and soy lecithin.

The list of nutrients covers those most important to the health of today's consumers.

Calories from Fat are now shown on the label to help consumers meet dietary guidelines that recommend people get no more than 30 percent of the calories in their overall diet from fat.

% Daily Value (DV) shows how a food in the specified serving size fits into the overall daily diet. By using the %DV you can easily determine whether a food contributes a lot or a little of a particular nutrient. And you can compare different foods with no need to do any calculations.

replace saturated fats in the diet. The fats in most fish are low in saturated fatty acids and contain a certain type of polyunsaturated fatty acid (omega-3) that is under study because of a possible association with a decreased risk for heart disease in certain people. Remember that the total fat in the diet should be consumed at a moderate level—that is, no more than 30 percent of calories. Mono-

and polyunsaturated fat sources should replace saturated fats within this limit.

Partially hydrogenated vegetable oils, such as those used in many margarines and shortenings, contain a particular form of unsaturated fat known as trans-fatty acids that may raise blood cholesterol levels, although not as much as saturated fat.

Choose a diet low in cholesterol

The body makes the cholesterol it requires. In addition, cholesterol is obtained from food. Dietary cholesterol comes from animal sources such as egg yolks, meat (especially organ meats such as liver), poultry, fish, and higher fat milk products. Many of these foods are also high in saturated fats. Choosing foods with less cholesterol and saturated fat will help lower your blood cholesterol levels (box 11). The Nutrition Facts Label lists the Daily Value for cholesterol as 300 mg. You can keep your cholesterol intake at this level or lower by eating more grain products, vegetables and fruits, and by limiting intake of high cholesterol foods.

Advice for children

Advice in the previous sections does not apply to infants and toddlers below the age of 2 years. After that age, children should gradually adopt a diet that, by about 5 years of age, contains no more than 30 percent of calories from fat. As they begin to consume fewer calories from fat, children should replace these calories by eating more grain products, fruits, vegetables, and lowfat milk products or other calcium-rich foods, and beans, lean meat, poultry, fish, or other protein-rich foods.

Box 11

FOR A DIET LOW IN FAT, SATURATED FAT, AND CHOLESTEROL

Fats and Oils

• Use fats and oils sparingly in cooking and at the table.

• Use small amounts of salad dressings and spreads such as butter, margarine, and mayonnaise. Consider using lowfat or fat-free dressings for salads.

• Choose vegetable oils and soft margarines most often because they are lower in saturated fat than solid shortenings and animal fats, even though their caloric content is the same.

• Check the Nutrition Facts Label to see how much fat and saturated fat are in a serving; choose foods lower in fat and saturated fat.

Grain Products, Vegetables, and Fruits

• Choose lowfat sauces with pasta, rice, and potatoes.

• Use as little fat as possible to cook vegetables and grain products.

• Season with herbs, spices, lemon juice, and fat-free or lowfat salad dressings.

Meat, Poultry, Fish, Eggs, Beans, and Nuts

• Choose two to three servings of lean fish, poultry, meats, or other protein-rich foods, such as beans, daily. Use meats labeled "lean" or "extra lean." Trim fat from meat; take skin off poultry. (Three ounces of cooked lean beef or chicken without skin—a piece the size of a deck of cards—provides about 6 grams of fat; a piece of chicken with skin or untrimmed meat of that size may have as much as twice this amount of fat.) Most beans and bean products are almost fat-free and are a good source of protein and fiber.

• Limit intake of high-fat processed meats such as sausages, salami, and other cold cuts; choose lower fat varieties by reading the Nutrition Facts Label.

• Limit the intake of organ meats (three ounces of cooked chicken liver have about 540 mg of cholesterol); use egg yolks in moderation (one egg yolk has about 215 mg of cholesterol). Egg whites contain no cholesterol and can be used freely.

Box 11 (Continued)

Milk and Milk Products

- Choose skim or lowfat milk, fat-free or lowfat yogurt, and lowfat cheese.

- Have two to three lowfat servings daily. Add extra calcium to your diet without added fat by choosing fat-free yogurt and lowfat milk more often. [One cup of skim milk has almost no fat, 1 cup of 1 percent milk has 2.5 grams of fat, 1 cup of 2 percent milk has 5 grams (one teaspoon) of fat, and 1 cup of whole milk has 8 grams of fat.] If you do not consume foods from this group, eat other calcium-rich foods (box 3, page 10).

Advice for Today

To reduce your intake of fat, saturated fat, and cholesterol, follow these recommendations, as illustrated in the Food Guide Pyramid, which apply to diets consumed over several days and not to single meals or foods.

- Use fats and oils sparingly.

- Use the Nutrition Facts Label to help you choose foods lower in fat, saturated fat, and cholesterol.

- Eat plenty of grain products, vegetables, and fruits.

- Choose lowfat milk products, lean meats, fish, poultry, beans, and peas to get essential nutrients without substantially increasing calorie and saturated fat intakes.

Choose a Diet Moderate in Sugars

Sugars come in many forms

Sugars are carbohydrates. Dietary carbohydrates also include the complex carbohydrates starch and fiber. During digestion all carbohydrates except fiber break down into sugars. Sugars and starches occur naturally in many foods that also supply other nutrients. Examples of these foods include milk, fruits, some vegetables, breads, cereals, and grains. Americans eat sugars in many forms, and most

Box 12

ON A FOOD LABEL, SUGARS INCLUDE

brown sugar	corn sweetener
corn syrup	fructose
fruit juice concentrate	glucose (dextrose)
high-fructose corn syrup	honey
invert sugar	lactose
maltose	molasses
raw sugar	[table] sugar (sucrose)
syrup	

A food is likely to be high in sugars if one of the above terms appears first or second in the ingredients list, or if several of them are listed.

people like their taste. Some sugars are used as natural preservatives, thickeners, and baking aids in foods; they are often added to foods during processing and preparation or when they are eaten. The body cannot tell the difference between naturally occurring and added sugars because they are identical chemically.

Sugars, health, and weight maintenance

Scientific evidence indicates that diets high in sugars do not cause hyperactivity or diabetes. The most common type of diabetes occurs in overweight adults. Avoiding sugars alone will not correct overweight. To lose weight reduce the total amount of calories from the food you eat and increase your level of physical activity (see pages xx-xx).

If you wish to maintain your weight when you eat less fat, replace the lost calories from fat with equal calories from fruits, vegetables, and grain products, found in the lower half of the Food Guide Pyramid. Some foods that contain a lot of sugars supply calories but few or no nutrients (box 12). These foods are located at the top of the Pyramid. For very active people with high calorie needs, sugars can be an additional source of energy. However, because maintaining a nutritious diet and a healthy weight is very important, sugars should be used in moderation by most healthy people and sparingly by people with low calorie needs. This guideline cautions about eating sugars in large amounts and about frequent snacks of foods and beverages containing sugars that supply unnecessary calories and few nutrients.

Box 13

FOR HEALTHIER TEETH AND GUMS

• Eat fewer foods containing sugars and starches between meals.

• Brush and floss teeth regularly.

• Use a fluoride toothpaste.

• Ask your dentist or doctor about the need for supplemental fluoride, especially for children.

Sugar substitutes

Sugar substitutes such as sorbitol, saccharin, and aspartame are ingredients in many foods. Most sugar substitutes do not provide significant calories and therefore may be useful in the diets of people concerned about calorie intake. Foods containing sugar substitutes, however, may not always be lower in calories than similar products that contain sugars. Unless you reduce the total calories you eat, the use of sugar substitutes will not cause you to lose weight.

Sugars and dental caries

Both sugars and starches can promote tooth decay. The more often you eat foods that contain sugars and starches, and the longer these foods are in your mouth before you brush your teeth, the greater the risk for tooth decay. Thus, frequent eating of foods high in sugars and starches as between-meal snacks may be more harmful to your teeth than eating them at meals and then brushing. Regular daily dental hygiene, including brushing with a fluoride toothpaste and flossing, and an adequate intake of fluoride, preferably from fluoridated water, will help you prevent tooth decay (box 13).

Advice for Today

Use sugars in moderation—sparingly if your calorie needs are low. Avoid excessive snacking, brush with a fluoride toothpaste, and floss your teeth regularly. Read the Nutrition Facts Label on foods you buy. The food label lists the content of total carbohydrate and sugars, as well as calories.

31

Choose a Diet Moderate in Salt and Sodium

Sodium and salt are found mainly in processed and prepared foods

Sodium and sodium chloride—known commonly as salt—occur naturally in foods, usually in small amounts. Salt and other sodium-containing ingredients are often used in food processing. Some people add salt and salty sauces, such as soy sauce, to their food at the table, but most dietary sodium or salt comes from foods to which salt has already been added during processing or preparation. Although many people add salt to enhance the taste of foods, their preference may weaken with eating less salt.

Sodium is associated with high blood pressure

In the body, sodium plays an essential role in regulation of fluids and blood pressure. Many studies in diverse populations have shown that a high sodium intake is associated with higher blood pressure. Most evidence suggests that many people at risk for high blood pressure reduce their chances of developing this condition by consuming less salt or sodium. Some questions remain, partly because other factors may interact with sodium to affect blood pressure.

Other factors affect blood pressure

Following other guidelines in the Dietary Guidelines for Americans may also help prevent high blood pressure. An important example is the guideline on weight and physical activity. The role of body weight in blood pressure control is well documented. Blood pressure increases with weight and decreases when weight is reduced. The guideline to consume a diet with plenty of fruits and vegetables is relevant because fruits and vegetables are naturally lower in sodium and fat and may help with weight reduction and control. Consuming more fruits and vegetables also increases potassium intakes which may help to reduce blood pressure (box 14). Increased physical activity helps lower blood pressure and control weight. Alcohol consumption has also been associated with high blood pressure. Another reason to reduce salt intake is the fact that high salt intakes may increase the amount of calcium excreted in the urine and, therefore, increase the body's need for calcium.

Box 14

SOME GOOD SOURCES OF POTASSIUM*

- Vegetables and fruits in general, especially

  –potatoes and sweet potatoes

  –spinach, swiss chard, broccoli, winter squashes, and parsnips

  –dates, bananas, cantaloupes, mangoes, plantains, dried apricots, raisins, prunes, orange juice, and grapefruit juice

  –dry beans, peas, lentils

- Milk and yogurt are good sources of potassium and have less sodium than cheese; cheese has much less potassium and usually has added salt.

*Does not include complete list of examples. You can obtain additional information from "Good Sources of Nutrients," USDA, January 1990. The Nutrition Facts Label may also provide brand-specific information on this nutrient.

Most Americans consume more salt than is needed

Sodium has an important role in the body. However, most Americans consume more sodium than is needed. The Nutrition Facts Label lists a Daily Value of 2,400 mg per day for sodium [2,400 mg sodium per day is contained in 6 grams of sodium chloride (salt)]. In household measures, one level teaspoon of salt provides about 2,300 milligrams of sodium. Most people consume more than this amount.

There is no way at present to tell who might develop high blood pressure from eating too much sodium. However, consuming less salt or sodium is not harmful and can be recommended for the healthy normal adult (box 15).

Advice for Today

Fresh fruits and vegetables have very little sodium. The food groups in the Food Guide Pyramid include some foods that are high in sodium and other foods that have very little sodium, or can be prepared in ways that add flavor without adding salt. Read the Nutrition Facts Label to compare and help identify foods lower in sodium

Box 15

TO CONSUME LESS SALT AND SODIUM—

- Read the Nutrition Facts Label to determine the amount of sodium in the foods you purchase. The sodium content of processed foods— such as cereals, breads, soups, and salad dressings— often varies widely.

- Choose foods lower in sodium and ask your grocer or supermarket to offer more low-sodium foods. Request less salt in your meals when eating out or traveling.

- If you salt foods in cooking or at the table, add small amounts. Learn to use spices and herbs, rather than salt, to enhance the flavor of food.

- When planning meals, consider that fresh and most plain frozen vegetables are low in sodium.

- When selecting canned foods, select those prepared with reduced or no sodium.

- Remember that fresh fish, poultry, and meat are lower in sodium than most canned and processed ones.

- Choose foods lower in sodium content. Many frozen dinners, packaged mixes, canned soups, and salad dressings contain a considerable amount of sodium. Remember that condiments such as soy and many other sauces, pickles, and olives are high in sodium. Ketchup and mustard, when eaten in large amounts, can also contribute significant amounts of sodium to the diet. Choose lower sodium varieties.

- Choose fresh fruits and vegetables as a lower sodium alternative to salted snack foods.

within each group. Use herbs and spices to flavor food. Try to choose forms of foods that you frequently consume that are lower in sodium and salt.

If You Drink Alcoholic Beverages, Do so in Moderation

Alcoholic beverages supply calories but few or no nutrients. The alcohol in these beverages has effects that are harmful when consumed in excess. These effects of alcohol may alter judgment and can lead to dependency and a great many other serious health problems. Alcoholic beverages have been used to enhance the enjoyment of meals by many societies throughout human history. If adults choose to drink alcoholic beverages, they should consume them only in moderation (box 16).

Current evidence suggests that moderate drinking is associated with a lower risk for coronary heart disease in some individuals. However, higher levels of alcohol intake raise the risk for high blood pressure, stroke, heart disease, certain cancers, accidents, violence, suicides, birth defects, and overall mortality (deaths). Too much alcohol may cause cirrhosis of the liver, inflammation of the pancreas, and damage to the brain and heart. Heavy drinkers also are at risk of malnutrition because alcohol contains calories that may substitute for those in more nutritious foods.

Who should not drink?

Some people should not drink alcoholic beverages at all. These include:

- Children and adolescents.

- Individuals of any age who cannot restrict their drinking to moderate levels. This is a special concern for recovering alcoholics and people whose family members have alcohol problems.

- Women who are trying to conceive or who are pregnant. Major birth defects, including fetal alcohol syndrome, have been attributed to heavy drinking by the mother while pregnant. While there is no conclusive evidence that an occasional drink is harmful to the fetus or to the pregnant woman, a safe level of alcohol intake during pregnancy has not been established.

- Individuals who plan to drive or take part in activities that require attention or skill. Most people retain some alcohol in the blood up to 2-3 hours after a single drink.

- Individuals using prescription and over-the-counter medications. Alcohol may alter the effectiveness or toxicity of medicines. Also, some medications may increase blood alcohol levels or increase the adverse effect of alcohol on the brain.

Box 16

WHAT IS MODERATION?

Moderation is defined as no more than one drink per day for women and no more than two drinks per day for men.

Count as a drink—

* 12 ounces of regular beer (150 calories)

* 5 ounces of wine (100 calories)

* 1.5 ounces of 80-proof distilled spirits (100 calories)

Advice for Today

If you drink alcoholic beverages, do so in moderation, with meals, and when consumption does not put you or others at risk.

Acknowledgments

The U.S. Department of Health and Human Services and the U.S. Department of Agriculture acknowledge the recommendations of the Dietary Guidelines Advisory Committee—the basis for this edition. The Committee consisted of Doris Howes Calloway, Ph.D.(chair), Richard J. Havel, M.D. (vice-chair), Dennis M. Bier, M.D., William H. Dietz, M.D., Ph.D., Cutberto Garza, M.D., Ph.D., Shiriki K. Kumanyika, Ph.D., R.D., Marion Nestle, Ph.D., M.P.H., Irwin H. Rosenberg, M.D., Sachiko T. St. Jeor, Ph.D., R.D., Barbara O. Schneeman, Ph.D., and John W. Suttie, Ph.D. The Departments also acknowledge the staff work of the executive secretaries to the committee: Karil Bialostosky, M.S., and Linda Meyers, Ph.D., from HHS; Eileen Kennedy, D.Sc., R.D., and Debra Reed, M.S., from USDA.

For Additional Information on Nutrition:

* Center for Nutrition Policy and Promotion, USDA, 1120 20th Street, NW, Suite 200 North Lobby, Washington, DC 20036.

- Food and Nutrition Information Center, USDA National Agricultural Library, Room 304, 10301 Baltimore Boulevard, Beltsville, MD 20705-2351. Internet address: fnic@nalusda.gov

- Cancer Information Service, Office of Cancer Communications, National Cancer Institute, Building 31, Room 10A16, 9000 Rockville Pike, Bethesda, MD 20892. Internet address: icic@aspensys.com

- National Heart, Lung, and Blood Institute Information Center, P.O. Box 30105, Bethesda, MD 20824-0105.

- Weight-Control Information Network (WIN) of the National Institute of Diabetes and Digestive and Kidney Diseases, 1 WIN WAY, Bethesda, MD 20892. Internet address: winniddk@aol.com

- National Institute on Alcohol Abuse and Alcoholism, 600 Executive Boulevard, Suite 409, Bethesda, MD 20892-7003.

- National Institute on Aging Information Center, Building 31, Room 5C27, National Institutes of Health, Bethesda, MD 20892.

- Office of Food Labeling, Food and Drug Administration (HFS-150), 200 C Street, SW, Washington, DC 20204.

- Contact your county extension home economist (cooperative extension system) or a nutrition professional in your local public health department, hospital, American Red Cross, dietetic association, diabetes association, heart association, or cancer society.

Chapter 2

The Food Guide Pyramid...Beyond the Basic 4

What's the Best Nutrition Advice?

It's following the **Dietary Guidelines for Americans.** These are seven guidelines for a healthful diet advice for healthy Americans 2 years of age or more. By following the Dietary Guidelines, you can enjoy better health and reduce your chances of getting certain diseases such as heart disease, high blood pressure, stroke, certain cancers, and the most common type of diabetes. These Guidelines are the best, most up-to-date advice from nutrition experts.

- Eat a variety of foods.

- Balance the food you eat with physical activity—maintain or improve your weight.

- Choose a diet low in fat, saturated fat, and cholesterol.

- Choose a diet with plenty of vegetables, fruits, and grain products.

- Choose a diet moderate in sugars.

- Choose a diet moderate in salt and sodium.

- If you drink alcoholic beverages, do so in moderation.

What is the Food Guide Pyramid ?

The Food Guide Pyramid is an outline of what to eat each day based on the Dietary Guidelines. It's not a rigid prescription but a general guide that lets you choose a healthful diet that's right for you.

The Pyramid calls for eating a variety of foods to get the nutrients you need and at the same time the right amount of calories to maintain healthy weight.

Use the Pyramid to help you eat better every day. . . the Dietary Guidelines way. Start with plenty of breads, cereals, rice, pasta, vegetables, and fruits. Add 2-3 servings from the milk group and 2-3 serv-

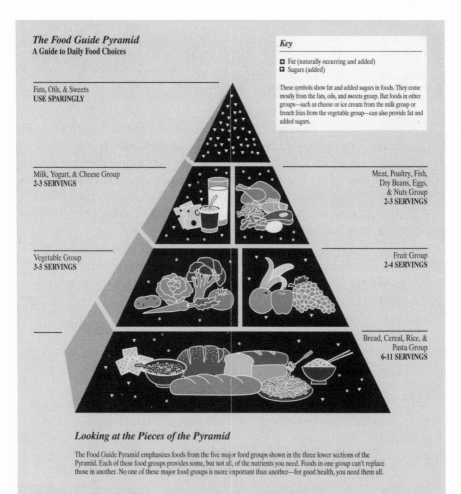

The Food Guide Pyramid
A Guide to Daily Food Choices

Key
□ Fat (naturally occurring and added)
▽ Sugars (added)

These symbols show fat and added sugars in foods. They come mostly from the fats, oils, and sweets group. But foods in other groups—such as cheese or ice cream from the milk group or french fries from the vegetable group—can also provide fat and added sugars.

Fats, Oils, & Sweets
USE SPARINGLY

Milk, Yogurt, & Cheese Group
2-3 SERVINGS

Meat, Poultry, Fish,
Dry Beans, Eggs,
& Nuts Group
2-3 SERVINGS

Vegetable Group
3-5 SERVINGS

Fruit Group
2-4 SERVINGS

Bread, Cereal, Rice, &
Pasta Group
6-11 SERVINGS

Looking at the Pieces of the Pyramid

The Food Guide Pyramid emphasizes foods from the five major food groups shown in the three lower sections of the Pyramid. Each of these food groups provides some, but not all, of the nutrients you need. Foods in one group can't replace those in another. No one of these major food groups is more important than another—for good health, you need them all.

ings from the meat group. Remember to go easy on fats, oils, and sweets, the foods in the small tip of the Pyramid.

What Counts as 1 Serving?

The amount of food that counts as 1 serving is listed below. If you eat a larger portion, count it as more than 1 serving. For example, a dinner portion of spaghetti would count as 2 or 3 servings of pasta.

Be sure to eat at least the lowest number of servings from the five major food groups listed below. You need them for the vitamins, minerals, carbohydrates, and protein they provide. Just try to pick the lowest fat choices from the food groups. No specific serving size is given for the fats, oils, and sweets group because the message is USE SPARINGLY.

Food Groups

Milk, Yogurt, and Cheese

- 1 cup of milk or yogurt

- 1 1/2 ounces of natural cheese

- 2 ounces of processed cheese

Meat, Poultry, Fish, Dry Beans, Eggs, and Nuts

- 2-3 ounces of cooked lean meat, poultry, or fish

- 1/2 cup of cooked dry beans, 1 egg, or 2 tablespoons of peanut butter count as 1 ounce of lean meat

Vegetable

- 1 cup of raw leafy vegetables

- 1/2 cup of other vegetables, cooked or chopped raw

- 3/4 cup of vegetable juice

Fruit

- 1 medium apple, banana, orange

- 1/2 cup of chopped, cooked or canned fruit

- 3/4 cup of fruit juice

Bread, Cereal, Rice, and Pasta

- 1 slice of bread

- 1 ounce of ready-to-eat cereal

- 1/2 cup of cooked cereal, rice, or pasta

How To Make the Pyramid Work for You

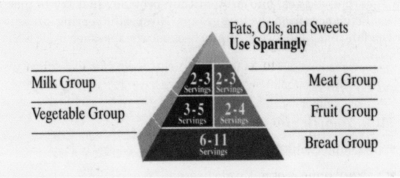

The Food Guide Pyramid shows a range of servings for each major food group. The number of servings that are right for you depends on how many calories you need, which in turn depends on your age, sex, size, and how active you are. Almost everyone should have at least the lowest number of servings in the ranges.

Now take a look at the table below. It tells you how many servings of each major food group you need for your calorie level. It also tells you the total grams of fat recommended for each calorie level; the Dietary Guidelines recommend that Americans limit fat in their diets to 30 percent of calories. This includes the fat in the foods you choose as well as the fat used in cooking or added at the table.

How many servings do you need each day?

	Many women, older adults	Children, teen girls, active women, most men	Teen boys, active men
Calorie level*	about 1,600	about 2,200	about 2,800
Bread Group Servings	6	9	11
Vegetable Group Servings	3	4	5
Fruit Group Servings	2	3	4
Milk Group Servings	2-3**	2-3**	2-3**
Meat Group Servings	2, for a total of 5 ounces	2, for a total of 6 ounces	3, for a total of 7 ounces
Total Fat (grams)	53	73	93

*These are the calorie levels if you choose low fat, lean foods from the 5 major food groups and use foods from the fats, oils, and sweets group sparingly.

**Women who are pregnant or breastfeeding, teenagers, and young adults to age 24 need 3 servings

Pyramid Pointers . . .

Selection Tips for Building a Better Diet

The most effective way to moderate the amount of fat and added sugars in your diet is to cut down on "extras"—foods in the sixth food group (fats, oils, and sweets). Also choose lower fat and lower sugar foods from the other five food groups often. Here are some tips:

Fats Oils and Sweets

Use Sparingly

- Go easy on fats and sugars added to foods in cooking or at the table—butter, margarine, gravy, salad dressing, sugar, and jelly.

- Choose fewer foods that are high in sugars candy—sweet desserts, and soft drinks.

Bread, Cereal, Rice, and Pasta Group

6-11 Servings

- To get the fiber you need, choose several servings a day of foods made from whole grains

- Choose most often foods that are made with little fat or sugars, like bread, english muffins, rice, and pasta.

- Go easy on the fat and sugars you add as spreads, seasonings, or toppings.

- When preparing pasta, stuffing, and sauce from packaged mixes, use only half the butter or margarine suggested; if milk or cream is called for, use lowfat milk.

Vegetable Group

3-5 Servings

- Different types of vegetables provide different nutrients. Eat a variety.

- Include dark-green leafy vegetables and legumes several times a week—they are especially good sources of vitamins and minerals. Legumes also provide protein and can be used in place of meat.

- Go easy on the fat you add to vegetables at the table or during cooking. Added spreads or toppings, such as butter, mayonnaise, and salad dressing, count as fat.

- Use lowfat salad dressings.

Fruit Group

2-4 Servings

- Choose fresh fruits, fruit juices, and frozen, canned, or dried fruit. Go easy on fruits canned or frozen in heavy syrups and sweetened fruit juices.

- Eat whole fruits often—they are higher in fiber than fruit juices.

- Count only 100 percent fruit juice as fruit. Punches, ades, and most fruit "drinks" contain only a little juice and lots of added sugars.

Milk, Yogurt, and Cheese Group

2-3 Servings

- Choose skim milk and nonfat yogurt often. They are lowest in fat.

- 1 1/2 to 2 ounces of cheese and 8 ounces of yogurt count as a serving from this group because they supply the same amount of calcium as 1 cup of milk.

- Choose "part skim" or lowfat cheeses when available and lower fat milk desserts, like ice milk or frozen yogurt. Read labels.

Meat, Poultry, Fish, Dry Beans, Eggs, and Nuts Group

2-3 Servings

- Choose lean meat, poultry without skin, fish, and dry beans and peas often. They are the choices lowest in fat.

- Prepare meats in lowfat ways:

  —Trim away all the fat you can see.

  —Remove skin from poultry.

  —Broil, roast, or boil these foods instead of frying them.

- Nuts and seeds are high in fat, so eat them in moderation.

Chapter 3

Vitamins and Health

This chapter outlines all the major vitamins found on the Food Label. It includes information on recommended daily allowances, function, sources, and information on vitamin deficiency and toxicity for each vitamin.

Vitamin A

U S. Recommended Daily Allowances

Infants (0-12 mo.)	Children (1-3 years)	Adults and Children 4 Years +	Pregnant or Nursing Women
1500 IU*	2500 IU	5000 IU	8000 IU

* International units

(The U.S. RDA amounts are sufficient to meet the needs of practically all healthy people.)

Vitamin A (retinoid) is a fat-soluble vitamin found mainly in animal foods in the vitamin form and in plant foods primarily as carotenes, substances that are formed into vitamin A chiefly in the small intestine.

Function: Essential for growth and for keeping skin and other tissues healthy; helps eyes to adapt to dim light and perceive colors; essential for normal tooth development.

Sources: Beef, chicken and pork livers; whole and vitamin A-fortified milk; cheddar cheese; butter; margarine; egg yolk; deep green, yellow or orange vegetables and fruits (including carrots, spinach, collards, broccoli, kale, nectarines, apricots, mangoes, cantaloupe, pumpkins, winter squash, turnip greens, sweet potatoes, and watermelon).

Deficiency: Vitamin A deficiency is rare in the United States; it mainly occurs among some people in developing countries. Some signs include skin changes, stunted growth, night blindness, and serious eye problems (such as drying, thickening, wrinkling, and muddy pigmentation of the mucous membrane lining the eyelid and eyeball, which eventually can destroy the eye). Inadequate intakes of foods containing vitamin A have been associated with some types of cancer, but the effect, if any, appears related to lack of carotene.

Excess: Because vitamin A is fat soluble, it is stored in the body. As a result, continued high doses (several times the U.S. RDA) have toxic effects. Signs of toxicity include dry and itching skin, headaches, and nausea and diarrhea. High vitamin A intake during pregnancy also may cause birth defects, but it is not known at what level this can occur. Excessive amounts of carotene are not known to be toxic, but will cause the skin to turn deep yellow. The color disappears when the amount of carotene in the diet is decreased.

Vitamin B_1

U.S. Recommended Daily Allowances

Infants (12 mo.)	Children (1-3 years)	Adults and Children 4 Years +	Pregnant or Nursing Women
0.5 mg	0.7 mg	1.5 mg	1.7 mg

Thiamin (vitamin B_1) is a water-soluble vitamin that was the first identified member of the B complex group.

Functions: Helps convert carbohydrates to energy; aids in nerve cell functioning.

Sources: Brewer's yeast: lean cuts of pork; whole-grain or enriched cereal grain products; legumes: liver, heart and kidneys; nuts and seeds.

Deficiency: Thiamin deficiency causes beriberi, a disease whose symptoms include anorexia, weakness, lack of coordination, muscle wasting, paralysis of the eye muscles, mental confusion, rapid heartbeat, edema, and enlarged heart. Deficiency is sometimes seen in this country in people with alcoholism and certain medical conditions.

Excess: High intakes appear nontoxic since excess thiamin is easily excreted by the kidneys.

Vitamin B_2

U.S. Recommended Daily Allowances

Infants (0-12 mo.)	Children (1-3 years)	Adults and Children 4 Years +	Pregnant or Nursing Women
0.6 mg	0.8 mg	1.7 mg	2.0 mg

Riboflavin (vitamin B_2) is a water-soluble vitamin that plays a role in energy production.

Functions: Component of two coenzymes that help convert carbohydrates and protein to energy.

Sources: Meat, poultry and fish; milk and cheese; enriched cereal-grain products; green vegetables, such as broccoli, turnip greens, asparagus, and spinach; eggs.

Deficiency: Signs of deficiency include cracks and sores on the lips and at the corners of the mouth, skin rash, and dimness of vision. Deficiency is rare in the United States because most people have adequate intakes.

Excess: High doses appear nontoxic.

Vitamin B₆

U.S. Recommended Daily Allowances

Infants (0-12 mo.)	Children (1-3 years)	Adults and Children 4 Years +	Pregnant or Nursing Women
0.4 mg	0.7 mg	2.0 mg	2.5 mg

Vitamin B₆ is a water-soluble vitamin that comprises three related forms: pyridoxine, pyridoxal and pyridoxamine.

Functions: Plays many roles in the body, but the most important one is in protein metabolism.

Sources: Fortified instant oatmeal; fortified ready-to-eat cereals; meat, poultry and fish; soybeans; some fruits and vegetables, including bananas, prunes, watermelon, spinach, sweet potatoes, and tomato juice.

Deficiency: Vitamin B6 deficiency can cause anemia, dermatitis and convulsions. In infants, it can lead to a variety of neurological disorders and abdominal distress. Deficiency is rare in the United States; it is mainly seen in people deficient in several B-complex vitamins.

Excess: Long-term megadoses, such as may be taken by women to alleviate premenstrual syndrome, may cause nerve damage and muscular incoordination in the hands and feet.

Vitamin B$_{12}$

U.S. Recommended Daily Allowances

Infants (0-12 mo.)	Children (1-3 years)	Adults and Children 4 Years +	Pregnant or Nursing Women
2 mcg*	3 mcg	6 mcg	8 mcg

* micrograms

Vitamin B$_{12}$ (cobalamin) is a water-soluble vitamin whose primary sources are animal products; plant foods are virtually devoid of it.

Functions: Aids in red blood cell development and the functioning of all cells, particularly those of the bone marrow, nervous system, and intestines. Also helps metabolize protein and fat in the body.

Sources: Animal products, including liver and other organ meats, beef, pork, eggs, milk and milk products, and fish. Bacteria in the intestinal tract produce some vitamin B12 and thus may serve as another source.

Deficiency: Signs include weakness, sore tongue. and anemia. It also is linked to some nerve and psychiatric disorders. However, vitamin B$_{12}$ deficiency is rare, and more than 95 percent of cases seen in the United States are related to the body's inability to absorb the vitamin.

Excess: No toxicity has been reported from high intakes but no benefits have been reported, either.

Vitamin C

U.S. Recommended Daily Allowances

Infants (0-12 mo.)	Children (1-3 years)	Adults and Children 4 years +	Pregnant or Nursing Women
35 mg	40 mg	60 mg	60 mg

Vitamin C (ascorbic acid) is a water-soluble vitamin found in a variety of fruits and vegetables that is easily destroyed when exposed to air, heat and light.

Functions: Essential for growth and maintenance of all cells and tissues; promotes the absorption of iron in the intestines; and acts as a water-soluble antioxidant in the body.

Sources: Many fruits and vegetables, including citrus fruits, cantaloupe, strawberries, tomatoes, green and red peppers, kale, collards, mustard greens, broccoli, cabbage, and potatoes.

Deficiency: Signs of deficiency include delayed wound healing; increased susceptibility to infection; and scurvy, a condition characterized by bleeding under the skin, anemia, joint tenderness and swelling, poor wound healing, weakness, and such oral disorders as bleeding gums, tooth loss, and gingivitis. However, because vitamin C sources are plentiful in the U.S. food supply, deficiency is rarely seen; it mainly occurs in infants fed cow's milk only, or in people whose diets lack adequate sources of vitamin C. In addition, cigarette smokers have lower blood levels of vitamin C than nonsmokers. As a consequence, the National Research Council recommends that smokers consume at least 100 milligrams of vitamin C per day.

Excess: High intakes of 1 gram or more per day may cause nausea, abdominal cramps, and diarrhea in some people.

Vitamin D

U.S. Recommended Daily Allowances

Infants (0-12 mo.)	Children (1-3 years)	Adults and Children 4 years +	Pregnant Nursing Women
400 IU*	400 IU	400 IU	400 IU

* International Unit

Vitamin D is a fat-soluble vitamin available from some foods, as well as from sunlight.

Functions: Forms the hormone 1, 25-dihydrocholecalciferol, which aids in the absorption and metabolism of calcium and phosphorus for bone and tooth formation.

Sources: Sunlight (which stimulates vitamin D production in the skin), fatty fish, fish liver oils, vitamin D-fortified milk, egg yolk. and butter.

Deficiency: In children, vitamin D deficiency causes rickets, a disease in which weak bones lead to bowlegs, knock-knees, and other bone deformities. The disease is rarely seen in the United States because milk and other foods are fortified with vitamin D and because children usually get some sun exposure. In the elderly, especially those in extended-care facilities, vitamin D deficiency has been associated with calcium loss from bones.

Excess: High intakes may cause vomiting, diarrhea, and weight loss and lead to calcium deposits in various organs. Children are especially susceptible, but anyone can have adverse effects from high daily doses.

Vitamin E

U.S. Recommended Daily Allowances

Infants (0-12 mo.)	Children (1-3 years)	Adults and Children 4 Years +	Pregnant or Nursing Women
5 IU*	10 IU	30 IU	30 IU

* International units

Vitamin E is a fat-soluble vitamin not recognized as an essential nutrient until the 1960s, about 40 years after its discovery.

Function: Prevents potentially harmful oxidation of polyunsaturated fatty acids in the body, which would lead to cell damage; important in protecting red blood cell membranes from oxidation.

Sources: Nuts; vegetable oils; fortified ready-to-eat cereals; wheat germ; green leafy vegetables; margarines made from vegetable oils; shrimp and other seafood (including clams, salmon and scallops); some fruits, such as apples, apricots and peaches.

Deficiency: Vitamin E deficiency can cause anemia, as a result of red blood cell destruction, and nerve damage. However, deficiency is rare and mainly occurs in premature, very-low-birth-weight infants and people with fat absorption disorders, such as cystic fibrosis.

Excess: Some evidence suggests that large intakes may cause increased levels of blood cholesterol and lipids.

Vitamin K

U.S. Recommended Daily Allowances

There are no U.S. RDAs for Vitamin K established yet by FDA for food labeling purposes; however, in the 10th edition of *Recommended Dietary Allowances,* the National Research Council of the National Academy of Sciences for the first time recommended allowances for vitamin K—for example, 80 micrograms for males 25 years and older and 65 micrograms for females of same age.

Vitamin K is a fat-soluble vitamin usually formed in the body by intestinal bacteria but also available from some plant and animal sources.

Function: Essential in the formation of prothrombin, a substance necessary for proper clotting of blood, and at least five other blood-clotting factors.

Sources: All green leafy vegetables (including lettuce, spinach, kale, and cabbage), eggs, meats, cereal grain products, fruits, and milk and dairy products.

Deficiency: Vitamin K deficiency may cause bleeding disorders in premature infants with inadequate amounts of stored vitamin K, and in people on blood-thinning medications and those with fat mal-absorption syndromes.

Excess: Natural forms have no known toxic effects; large doses of the synthetic version, menadione, and its derivatives cause anemia and kernicterus, a condition characterized by jaundice, in infants.

Folate

U.S. Recommended Daily Allowances

Infants (0-12 mo.)	Children (1-3 years)	Adults and Children 4 Years +	Pregnant or Nursing Women
100 mcg*	200 mcg	400 mcg	800 mcg

* micrograms

(The U.S. RDA amounts are sufficient to meet the needs of practically all healthy people. FDA set these based on the 1968 Recommended Dietary Allowances by the National Research Council of the National Academy of Sciences. However, in 1989, the council lowered the RDA for folate to 200 micrograms for men and 180 micrograms for women because researchers found that although U.S. diets contain half as much folate as recommended in the 1968 RDAs, such diets do not lead to deficiencies. FDA is in the process of revising its U.S. RDAs.)

Folate (folic acid and related compounds) is a water-soluble vitamin widely distributed in foods.

Functions: Involved in red blood cell production; aids in the formation of genetic material within every body cell.

Sources: Liver; yeast; dried beans, peas and lentils; oranges; fortified ready-to-eat cereals; whole-wheat products; some vegetables (including asparagus, beets, broccoli, brussels sprouts, and spinach).

Deficiency: Signs include cracks on the lips and at the corners of the mouth, anemia, gastrointestinal disorders (such as malabsorption), and infertility. Folate deficiency is believed to be rare, and there is little evidence it constitutes a major problem in the United States. Those who may be most vulnerable are premature infants, women during the last half of pregnancy, women who use oral contraceptives, and people using certain types of anticonvulsants.

[Editor's Note: Recent tests have confirmed that lack of folic acid in early pregnancy can lead to neural tube defects.]

Excess: Very large doses may bring about convulsions in epileptics who are taking the anticonvulsant drug phenytoin. Without evidence of benefit from high doses and with some evidence of potential for toxicity, high intakes of folate supplements are not recommended by the National Research Council of the National Academy of Sciences.

Biotin

U.S. Recommended Daily Allowances

Infants (0-l2 mo.)	Children (1-3 years)	Adults and Children 4 Years +	Pregnant or Nursing Women
50 mcg*	150 mcg	300 mcg	300 mcg

* micrograms

(The U.S. RDA amounts are sufficient to meet the needs of practically all healthy people, FDA set these based on the 1968 Recommended Dietary Allowances by the National Research Council of the National Academy of Sciences. However, in 1989, the Council lowered its ranges of safe and adequate daily dietary intakes for biotin to 10 to 15 micrograms for infants, 20 to 30 mcg for children, and 30 to 100 mcg for adults. FDA is in the process of revising its U.S. RDAs.)

Biotin is a sulfur-containing, B-complex vitamin found in foods and produced by microorganisms in the lower gastrointestinal tract.

Functions: Activates certain enzymes that aid in metabolism of carbon dioxide; involved in metabolism of protein, fats and carbohydrates.

Sources: Widely distributed in foods that are sources of B vitamins, including cereal-grain products, liver, egg yolk, soy flour, and yeast.

Deficiency: Signs include loss of appetite, nausea, vomiting, inflammation of the tongue, pallor, depression, hair loss, and dry, scaly skin, Some rare biotin-related inborn errors of metabolism may cause deficiency; otherwise, deficiency is extremely rare in the United States.

Excess: No effects have been reported.

Niacin

U.S. Recommended Daily Allowances

Infants (0-12 mo.)	Children (1-3 years)	Adults and Children 4 Years +	Pregnant or Nursing Women
8 mg	9 mg	20 mg	20 mg

Niacin (nicotinic acid, nicotinamide) is a water-soluble vitamin whose requirement is partly met by conversion in the body of the essential amino acid tryptophan to niacin.

Functions: Involved in carbohydrate, protein and fat metabolism.

Sources: Enriched cereal-grain products; meat, fish, poultry, cheese, eggs, and milk because they contain tryptophan; peanuts; mushrooms; potatoes.

Deficiency: Severe niacin deficiency causes pellagra, a disease characterized by mouth sores, skin rashes, diarrhea, and dementia. Deficiency is rarely seen in the United States, though, because most people have adequate intakes.

Excess: Large amounts of niacin, when taken in the nicotinic acid form of the vitamin, act as a drug. Nicotinic acid is often prescribed as a cholesterol-lowering drug, and should be taken only under the supervision of a physician. Side effects include vascular dilation of the skin (flushing) and gastrointestinal distress. Prolonged intake may cause liver damage.

Nicotinamide is not known to act as a drug. Effects of high doses are unknown.

Pantothenic Acid

U.S. Recommended Daily Allowances

Infants (0-12 mo.)	Children (1-3 years)	Adults and Children 4 Years +	Pregnant or Nursing Women
3 mg	5 mg	10 mg	10 mg

Pantothenic acid is a B-complex vitamin.

Functions: Involved in release of energy from carbohydrates, metabolism of fats, and synthesis of steroid hormones and other vital substances.

Sources: Milk; beef, pork and poultry; legumes; some fruits and vegetables, including strawberries, dried fruit, avocados, mushrooms, potatoes, and succotash; whole-grain cereal products.

Deficiency: Pantothenic acid deficiency has not been recognized in humans, and it is unlikely to occur in the U.S. population.

Excess: No effects have been reported.

Paula Kurtzweil, Research Director, of FDA's Office of Public Affairs, and Theresa A. Young, of FDA's Philadelphia district office, contributed to this series.

(The above information was derived from a series of articles previously published in *FDA Consumer* from 1990 to 1991.)

Part Two

Applying the Dietary Guidelines

Chapter 4

Good Nutrition for the Highchair Set

"Open the hangar and let the airplane fly in," mother coaxes her reluctant 6-month-old, spoon circling in mid-air. Baby opens her mouth and the "airplane," with its spinach cargo, zooms toward the opening—only to collide with a mouth snapped shut faster than the speed of sound. The green goo dribbles down baby's chin onto her bib. But mother notes with some consolation that baby is tentatively licking some spinach off her lips.

The trials and tribulations of feeding infants are sometimes compounded by uncertainties about when to introduce certain foods and whether homemade varieties offer any benefit over those that are commercially prepared.

About 25 years ago, it was commonly recommended that babies be given "solid" food beginning at 6 weeks of age or sometimes even younger. But a generation of experience has led pediatric experts to conclude that 6 weeks is too early for even cereal mixed with milk, the first traditional solid food. Today the common recommendation is that babies should receive only breast milk or infant formula until they are at least 4 to 6 months old.

Reasons for this are several. Contrary to previous theory, experts now advise that solid food does not make a baby any more likely to sleep through the night than a diet of only formula or breast milk. Such a liquid diet can appease the hunger of an infant under 4 to 6 months of age. The nervous system also needs to mature so the baby

DHHS Publication No. (FDA) 92-2208

can recognize a spoon, coordinate swallowing, and signal if hungry or full. Feeding solids before the baby has these skills is really a kind of force-feeding. Introducing solids too early may contribute to overfeeding and result in food allergies, which can cause gastrointestinal and other problems.

To make baby food more nutritious when babies are ready for it, manufacturers, over the years, have made a number of changes in their products. For example, precooked cereals marketed for infants and usually first offered when the baby is 4 to 6 months old are fortified with iron and B vitamins. Although some forms of iron added to food are not as available to the body as iron naturally present, manufacturers of precooked baby cereals add a form of iron that is absorbed as well as other non-heme (non-meat) iron naturally present in food. Babies need added iron at this age because the iron they had at birth from their mothers is just about used up. Therefore, babies are usually given supplemental iron in the form of drops, or in formula or baby cereal. Most precooked baby cereals contain 45 percent of the U.S. Recommended Daily Allowance (U.S. RDA) of iron per serving.

First Solids: For Ages 4 Months to One Year

When cereal is first fed to babies, to find out if they are allergic to any one type, the single-grain varieties of rice, oatmeal and barley should be given first. Mixed cereals and wheat cereals should be added when the baby is several months older. Cereal made from wheat is a more frequent cause of allergy than the other grains and is slightly rougher on the stomach.

Once they've mastered cereal slurping, babies can be offered a variety of other foods. But these foods must be strained to a very soft, semi-liquid consistency because infants, lacking teeth, cannot yet chew properly and because their swallowing reflex has not yet matured.

For years, commercially prepared baby foods were available only in jars. Then, foil-lined canisters containing dehydrated flakes for mixing with water were introduced. After being opened, baby food in jars lasts about three days in the refrigerator. The flakes do not have to be refrigerated and remain good for about two weeks after opening.

Though it's a time-consuming task, some parents prepare foods at home for their babies in the hope that what they strain and puree (usually with the help of a blender or food processor) may be nutritionally superior to the commercially prepared foods. Often these parents are most concerned about the possible addition of salt, sugar, and other additives to commercial baby foods. A certain amount of sodium is necessary to an infant's health, but an excessive intake is not desirable. Before 1970, baby foods in jars often contained added sodium in the form of salt and monosodium glutamate (MSG). Then the National Academy of Sciences and the American Academy of Pediatrics pointed out that the amount of sodium in baby foods was often far in excess of body needs and that additives (other than vitamins and minerals) were not necessary to the proper nourishment of infants. In response to these points and to the growing concern that high sodium intake early in life might lead to high blood pressure later on, manufacturers of baby food began to limit the amount of added sodium. By 1978, they had entirely stopped adding MSG and salt to products meant for babies under 1 year.

Concerns about sugar and other additives, such as preservatives, have similarly motivated manufacturers to limit the amount of these substances added to their products. Today, commercially prepared baby foods rarely contain preservatives. Sterilization during the manufacturing process contributes to their long shelf life. In most lines of baby food, refined sugar is added only to custards and puddings.

A parent who wants to know what is in baby food need go no further than the label. FDA regulates the labeling of all baby foods with the exception of strained meats, which come under the jurisdiction of the U.S. Department of Agriculture. FDA requires labeling on "infant" food (for babies under a year old) to be more complete than that of other foods so that parents may be well-informed about what they are feeding their youngsters. While the labeling of other foods may list spices and additives simply as such, the labels on infant food must list each ingredient by name, including each spice, flavoring and coloring. In addition, the labeling must specify the plant or animal source of an ingredient. For example, rather than vegetable oil, the label must say "coconut oil" or "palm oil." As with other foods, ingredients are listed in descending order of predominance. Most manufacturers also include on the label the amounts (or percentages of U.S. RDAs) of calories, protein, carbohydrate, fat, sodium, vitamins, and minerals.

Along with solid foods, parents usually start to feed babies fruit juices at about 6 to 7 months of age. Initially, fruit juices for babies were marketed in cans. However, concern about lead from the cans getting into the juice after the can was opened and left partly filled caused manufacturers to switch to small glass bottles. (Unopened cans do not pose this problem.) The juices are fortified with vitamin C (as are many strained fruits) and most brands do not contain added refined sugar. Juice should be served to the baby in a cup. It is especially important not to put a baby to bed with a bottle of fruit juice because if, as the baby dozes, its mouth remains in contact with the fruit juice, the acid and natural sugars have more of a chance to promote tooth decay.

Toddler Foods: For Ages One Year and Above

A separate line of products is marketed for babies over a year old. These are commonly referred to as "toddler" foods. Chunkier than infant foods, these foods help in the transition to regular table food. Unlike infant foods, the sodium content of some toddler foods has not been significantly reduced. The National Academy of Sciences has set 325 to 975 milligrams of sodium as the safe and adequate daily dietary intake for children 1 to 3 years old. Yet some products marketed for this age group have 500 to 700 milligrams of sodium per serving, so that a child eating more than one serving a day might get an excessive amount of sodium. FDA has been encouraging manufacturers to reduce the amount of sodium in these products. The U.S. Department of Agriculture, which regulates the meat products that compose the majority of "toddler" food lines, is also working with manufacturers on this problem.

Because children under 4 years do not have a full set of teeth and therefore cannot chew as well as older children, extra care is needed when giving them toddler foods such as meat sticks and biscuits. The same precautions should be taken when feeding them "finger" foods, such as hot dogs, nuts, and hard candies. (See "Parents: Guard Against Food-Related Chokings" in the November 1984 *FDA Consumer* and "Determining When a Food Poses a Hazard" in the June 1983 *FDA Consumer*.)

In response to these concerns, the following was added to the labeling of toddler biscuits:

> "For Your Information: Biscuits, cookies, toast and crackers should be eaten in an upright position—never while lying down—to reduce the possibility of choking on crumbs."

The following has been added to the labeling of toddler meat sticks:

"This product is intended for children with teeth. To reduce the possibility of choking, serve these sticks only to toddlers who have learned to chew solid foods properly. It is important that mealtime and snack time of small children be supervised. They should be fed in an upright position and never during vigorous activities."

Despite these few problems, commercially prepared baby and toddler foods offer an adequate and safe alternative that most parents prefer to home-prepared foods for babies. FDA continues to monitor these foods and shares parents' concern that what zooms into their babies' mouths be as safe and nutritious as possible.

Introducing Baby To Solid Foods

Foods are usually (but not necessarily) introduced in the order shown below, with several weeks between different types of foods. Ages of introduction are approximate and may vary with individual babies. The baby's doctor is the best source for advice on when and how often any particular food is appropriate for that baby. Cereals should be mixed with formula or breast milk.

Age	Food	Frequency
4-6 months	precooked baby cereal	twice a day
	baby juices	between meals
5-6 months	strained single fruits	twice a day
6-7 months	strained vegetables	once a day
7-8 months	strained meats	once a day
	plain yogurt	once a day
	baby juices	between meals
8-9 months	egg yolk, strained	once a day

Nutritional Needs Of Infants

Recommended Dietary Allowances*

Nutrient	Birth to 6 months	6 to 12 months
Protein (grams/kilogram of baby's weight)	13 g	14 g
Vitamins		
A (micrograms [µg])	375	375
D (µg)	7.5	10
E (milligrams [mg])	3	4
Vitamin K (µg)	5	10
C (mg)	30	35
Thiamine (mg)	0.3	0.4
Riboflavin (mg)	0.4	0.5
Niacin (mg)	5	6
B_6(mg)	0.3	0.6
Folacin (µg)	25	35
B_{12} (µg)	0.3	0.5
Minerals		
Calcium (mg)	400	600
Phosphorus (mg)	300	500
Magnesium (mg)	40	60
Iron (mg)	6	10
Zinc (mg)	5	5
Iodine (µg)	40	50
Selenium (µg)	10	15

Babies under 1 year get most of their vitamins and minerals from formula or milk. When solid foods are introduced, they are to supplement, not replace, milk or formula. Only gradually should solid foods become major sources of nutrients.

* Source: Food and Nutrition Board, National Academy of Sciences-National Research Council, Revised 1989.

by Judith Willis

Judith Willis is editor of *FDA Consumer*

Chapter 5

Healthy Eating is a Family Affair

All healthy Americans, 2 years of age or older, should eat in a way that is low in saturated fat and cholesterol. We now know that eating this way lowers blood cholesterol levels and reduces the risk of heart disease.

Heart disease is still the number one killer of both men and women in the United States. More than 6 million Americans have symptoms of heart disease. High blood pressure, smoking, and obesity, as well as high blood cholesterol increase your risk of getting heart disease. The good news is that you can change these risk factors and reduce your family's risk of heart disease.

How Does Blood Cholesterol Affect Heart Disease?

Heart Disease Has Its Start Early in Life

Atherosclerosis may start very early in life, yet not produce symptoms for many years. Over the years, cholesterol and fat build up in the arteries. This narrows the arteries and can slow or block the flow of blood to the heart. This process is known as "atherosclerosis." Most heart attacks are caused by a clot forming at a narrow part of an artery which cuts off the blood and oxygen supply to the heart muscle. Most coronary heart disease is due to blockages in these same arteries.

NIH Publicaton No.92-3099

We know that lowering blood cholesterol in adults slows the fatty buildup in the walls of the arteries and reduces the risk of heart disease and heart attack. Lowering blood cholesterol levels in children is likely also to help reduce their risk of heart disease when they become adults.

Cholesterol: Your Body Needs It And Makes Its Own

Cholesterol is a soft, waxy substance. Your body needs cholesterol to function normally. Cholesterol is present in all parts of the body, including the brain, nerves, muscle, skin, liver, intestines, and heart. It is a part of cell membranes. And it is important for the production of hormones, vitamin D, and bile acids—which help to absorb fat.

Your blood cholesterol level is affected not only by the saturated fat and cholesterol in your diet, but also by the cholesterol made in your liver. In fact, your body makes all the cholesterol it needs. The saturated fat and cholesterol in your diet only help to increase your blood cholesterol level.

Lipoproteins Carry Cholesterol in Your Blood

Cholesterol travels in your blood in packages called lipoproteins. They are often referred to as LDLs and HDLs.

- LDLs—Low density lipoproteins (LDLs) carry most of the cholesterol. If your LDL level is high, cholesterol and fat can build up in your arteries and cause atherosclerosis. This is why LDL cholesterol is often called "bad cholesterol."

- HDLs—Cholesterol is also packaged in high density lipoproteins (HDLs). HDLs carry cholesterol back to your liver. Here it is processed or removed from your body. Removal helps prevent cholesterol from building up in your arteries. So, HDLs are often referred to as "good cholesterol."

What Affects Blood Cholesterol Levels?

Many Factors Influence Blood Cholesterol Levels

Diet. Among the factors you and your family can do something about, diet has the greatest effect on blood cholesterol levels.

- Saturated fat raises blood cholesterol levels more than anything else you eat.

- Dietary cholesterol also increases blood cholesterol levels.

Changing your family's way of eating will be a very important step to control or lower blood cholesterol.

Weight. In children, as in adults, obesity is related to increased total blood cholesterol levels. Losing weight has been shown to lower these levels. Children who are obese are more likely than other children to become obese adults. Obesity, by itself, also increases the risk of heart disease.

Physical activity. Regular exercise throughout life is associated with a lower risk of heart disease. We also know that regular exercise may help control weight and increase HDL-cholesterol. Aerobic exercise helps strengthen the heart and improve the circulatory system as well.

Smoking. Cigarette smoking is related to lower HDL-cholesterol levels, and also increases the risk of heart disease.

Genetic factors. Genes, i.e., heredity, play a major role in determining blood cholesterol levels and how well your child will be able to lower the level by diet. Because of their genes, a very small number of people have a high blood cholesterol level even if they eat a cholesterol-lowering diet.

Sex and age. In the United States, the average total cholesterol level in children is about 160 mg/dL. At birth, total cholesterol levels are about 70 mg/dL and rise to between 100 to 150 mg/dL during the first few weeks of life. At 2 years of age, these levels increase to about 160 mg/dL in boys and to 165 mg/dL in girls. They stay at about these levels until puberty. Between 12 and 18 years, total cholesterol in boys declines slightly to about 150 mg/dL. Levels in girls also decline slightly. At age 20, blood cholesterol levels in both men and women start to rise.

Alcohol. You may have heard that modest amounts of alcohol can improve HDL-cholesterol levels. However, it is not known whether this protects against heart disease. Because drinking alcohol can have serious harmful effects, it is not recommended as a way to prevent heart disease.

Shared Habits and Genes

Families share similar habits including eating, exercise, smoking, and drinking. Families also share similar genes. The shared habits and genes influence cholesterol levels in families. Clearly, as a family you can do something about your shared habits.

- Eat foods lower in saturated fat and cholesterol. This will help to lower blood cholesterol levels and maintain a healthy weight. In fact, most people are able to control their blood cholesterol levels by eating this way.

- Exercise regularly.

- If you smoke, STOP. As your child's role model, help him or her avoid taking up the habit.

- Be aware that friends, fads, and advertising also influence eating, exercise, smoking, and other habits.

Does Your Child Need A Cholesterol Test?

As a Parent, You Need To Know Your Cholesterol Level

If your blood cholesterol was ever "high" (240 mg/dL or greater), your child's blood cholesterol level will need to be checked. Any cholesterol level above 200 mg/dL, even in the "borderline-high" group, increases your risk for heart disease. Levels less than 200 mg/dL put you at lower risk.

Most Children Do Not Need To Have Their Cholesterol Levels Checked

Most children do not need to have their blood cholesterol tested. The National Cholesterol Education Program and the American Academy of Pediatrics agree that children, 2 years of age or older, and teenagers should have their blood cholesterol levels measured if they have one of the following:

- At least one parent who has ever had high blood cholesterol (240 mg/dL or greater).

- A parent or grandparent who got heart disease before 55 years of age.

- Parents whose medical history is not known, especially in children with other risk factors for heart disease.

Getting your child's total cholesterol level measured is easy and can be part of a regular visit. The doctor will take a small sample of blood from the finger or arm. Your child can usually eat and drink before this test.

Even if you do not know your blood cholesterol level or your family history for heart disease your doctor may measure your child's cholesterol level. If your child's cholesterol is high, heart disease may run in your family. So, be sure to ask your doctor to measure your cholesterol level too. Your spouse and any other children in the family should also have their levels checked. All family members who have an elevated cholesterol level need to take steps to lower it—it is a family affair.

What Is a Cholesterol Profile?

The "cholesterol profile" is a detailed set of blood measurements. It includes measurements of LDL-cholesterol, HDL-cholesterol, and triglyceride levels. This is done because LDL and HDL provide more accurate information on the risk of getting heart disease.

Your doctor should check your child's cholesterol profile if:

- Your child's total cholesterol is "high" (200 mg/dL or greater).

- Your child's total cholesterol level is "borderline" (170 mg/dL or greater) after two measurements are averaged, or

- A parent or grandparent had heart disease before age 55.

In order to do a cholesterol profile, your doctor will take a blood sample from your child's arm. Your child must not eat or drink anything, except water, for 12 hours before the test.

Next Steps Based on Your Child's Cholesterol Level

Acceptable. Children with an acceptable total or LDL-cholesterol level should adopt the same eating pattern as all healthy Americans, namely one lower in saturated fat and cholesterol. This will help keep their cholesterol level low.

Borderline and High. If your child's total cholesterol level is either high or borderline, your doctor will likely do a cholesterol profile. This will show your child's LDL-cholesterol level. If the LDL level is high or borderline, your child will require a Step-One Diet. This diet is basically the same eating pattern suggested for all healthy children. However, children given the Step-One Diet will have to follow the eating pattern more closely. The doctor will check their cholesterol levels more often to see how they are responding to the diet.

A few children who are not able to lower their cholesterol level enough may need the Step-Two Diet. This diet is lower in saturated fat and cholesterol to help produce the biggest change. Information about the Step-One and Step-Two Diets is given below.

Aim for Acceptable Blood Cholesterol Levels

Your child's blood cholesterol level should begin to fall within a few weeks after starting the Step-One Diet. Ideally the goal should be:

- Acceptable total cholesterol— less than 170 mg/dL, or

- Acceptable LDL-cholesterol— less than 110 mg/dL.

After starting the Step-One Diet, your doctor will most likely check your child's cholesterol level on a regular basis. If the goal is not met after a certain period of time on the Step-One Diet, your doctor will likely have your child try the Step-Two Diet. If the goal is still not met after 6 months to 1 year on the diet, some children with extremely high levels may need to be given drugs along with the diet.

Make Heart-Healthy Eating A Family Routine

What your family eats has a large impact, not only on their blood cholesterol levels, but on their general health as well. All children and teenagers need to eat a nutritious diet. They need to eat a variety of foods that provide enough calories and nutrients—carbohydrates, protein, fat, vitamins, and minerals. This helps them grow and develop properly. It is also important as they become more physically active. A nutritious and "heart-healthy" diet is also low in saturated fat, total fat, and dietary cholesterol. As you know, this type of diet is important to lower blood cholesterol and maintain it at acceptable levels.

Did you know that what parents eat influences what their children eat? Do you make a habit of eating fatty fried foods or rich, high-fat desserts? Children learn these eating patterns early in life. They learn to enjoy the taste of high-fat foods. They can also learn to enjoy the taste of fruits, vegetables, and grains if you show them how. Changing established eating habits can often be difficult for you and your children, especially teenagers. It is much easier to start by making changes at home that everyone in your family over 2 years old can follow. Buy and prepare foods low in saturated fat, total fat, and dietary cholesterol for the whole family.

Help Your Child Eat Right And Exercise

Telling children and teenagers to eat right and exercise is good; showing them is better. Here are some tips to help your children develop healthful habits.

Be a model. Set a good example. Adults, particularly parents, are a major influence on children's behavior. Children are also influenced by television, radio, magazines, newspapers, ads, friends, brothers and sisters, and others who may not conform to your ways. So, eat a heart-healthy diet and your children will be more likely to do the same. Exercising with your child also sets a good example.

Know the dietary guidelines to lower blood cholesterol. Knowing how diet, blood cholesterol and heart disease are related will help you guide your family to lower their blood cholesterol levels. Knowing the basics on choosing foods low in saturated fat, total fat, and cholesterol is important to your success.

Know the food groups. Know the food groups and the low-saturated fat, low-cholesterol choices within each group. This will help you buy and provide such foods and snacks at home.

Stock the kitchen. Stock the kitchen with low-saturated fat, low-cholesterol foods from each of the food groups. Prepare these foods in large quantities to be frozen for quick use later. Foods such as casseroles, soups, and breads can be frozen in individual servings for a quick meal. The whole family will then have low-saturated fat, low-cholesterol meals on hand. Teach children how to choose healthy snacks.

Teach basic food preparation skills. Teach children how to clean vegetables, make salads, and safely use the stove, oven, microwave, and toaster. Children who have basic cooking skills appreciate food more and are more inclined to try new foods.

Let children help. Let children help with or even do the grocery shopping. The supermarket is an ideal place to teach children about foods. Teach them how to read food labels. Involve children in meal planning and preparation. Encourage them to prepare snacks, bag lunches, and breakfast. This will help them become responsible and fulfill a need for independence.

Plan family meals. Eating meals together as a family can really help foster heart-healthy eating habits in children. The more you create a "family setting" where everyone shares the same nutritious meals, the more children will accept healthful eating as a way of life. Try to maintain regular family meals every day—breakfast, lunch or dinner, or all three. This way, the whole family can learn about healthful eating and build good eating habits.

Encourage physical activity. Make time for physical activity. Encourage children to get some exercise throughout the day and especially on the weekends. Take trips that involve activities like hiking, swimming, and skiing. Join in the fun. Ride bikes, run, skate, or walk to places close by. Give your child a splash or dance party. Use your backyard or park for basketball, baseball, football, badminton, or volleyball.

Know the Dietary Guidelines for Lowering Blood Cholesterol Levels

In order to help your family eat in a way that is lower in saturated fat and cholesterol, you need to know some dietary guidelines. They are consistent with the "Dietary Guidelines for Americans" and include choosing a variety of foods that provide the following nutrients:

- Less than 10 percent of calories from saturated fat,

- An average of no more than 30 percent of calories from fat,

- Less than 300 milligrams of dietary cholesterol a day,

- Enough calories to support growth, and to reach or maintain a healthy weight.

The whole family (except infants under 2 years who need more calories from fat) should follow these guidelines. This may look complicated, but you will soon see that it is really easy if you take some general steps shown on this and the next page.

These guidelines are basically the same as the Step-One Diet. The Step-Two Diet, however, is different because it is lower in saturated fat and cholesterol as shown below:

- Less than 7 percent of calories from saturated fat,

- Less than 200 milligrams of dietary cholesterol a day.

Briefly, each gram of fat (of any type) provides 9 calories per gram. So, if your child eats 1,800 calories per day, 10 percent of those calories from saturated fat is equal to 20 grams of saturated fat allowed per day. This information is provided because food labels list fat information in grams, not percent of calories.

Remember, the Step-One and Step-Two Diets are recommended for children with elevated blood cholesterol levels. If your doctor prescribes one of these diets, help your child to follow it closely. Registered dietitians or qualified nutritionists can provide additional information to help children and their families adjust to this way of eating and still include some favorite foods.

Eating Patterns Help Your Child Follow the Guidelines

Following the dietary guidelines to lowering blood cholesterol levels can be easy if you think of them in terms of food. Foods make up your eating patterns. So, knowing the foods to choose is the first step. The appendix, at the end of this chapter, "Foods to Choose and Decrease," lists those foods lower in saturated fat, total fat, and cholesterol as the foods to "choose." Choosing these foods from each of the food groups every day will help assure that your family is following the guidelines recommended for all healthy Americans. And, eating a variety of foods will help assure your child is getting all of the nutrients needed for growth. Don't worry about whether your child eats specific numbers of servings from each group every day as long as your child's cholesterol level is in the acceptable range.

The appendix also lists specific eating patterns to help meet the Step-One and Step-Two Diets recommended for children with elevated levels. The eating patterns for these two diets are provided by food group with serving sizes (ounces, cups, teaspoons) and listings of the number of servings. Note that the patterns depend on the child's age and sex.

These patterns are only examples and should be adjusted according to your child's weight, level of activity, and food preferences. This is especially important to younger children. Children ages 2 to 3 are gradually starting to eat like the rest of the family. Once your child is put on the Step-One or Step-Two Diet, allow him or her time to grow into the pattern. Be flexible, yet encourage your child to eat enough of the right kinds of foods. Remember, these diets can also be enjoyed by the whole family.

Calories. Children and teenagers need calories to grow and develop. The suggested eating patterns are not low in calories, they are low in saturated fat, total fat, and cholesterol. Some calories from fat are replaced by calories from carbohydrates to maintain normal growth. Do not restrict your child's calorie level while on a low-fat diet. This can cause growth problems. Children with high blood cholesterol who follow the Step-One or Step-Two Diet should be followed closely by their doctor.

Obesity. Most children who are obese and still growing taller should not lose weight. Instead, they should eat in a way that keeps their weight the same while they continue to grow taller. Obese teenagers who are at their adult height should be encouraged to follow a weight-loss diet under a doctor's care to achieve desirable weight. It's also good to develop lifelong habits of regular exercise to help in weight control.

Saturated Fat. Saturated fat raises your blood cholesterol level more than anything else in your diet. The best way to lower your blood cholesterol level is to reduce the amount of saturated fat that you eat. Animal products are a major source of saturated fat in the average American diet. Butter, cheese, whole milk, ice cream, and cream all contain high amounts of saturated fat. It is also concentrated in the fat that surrounds meat and in the white streaks of fat in the muscle of meat. Poultry, fish, and shellfish also contain saturated fat, although generally less than meat. Some vegetable oils such as coconut, palm, and palm kernel are rich in saturated fat. They are often found in commercially baked goods such as cookies and crackers, cake mixes, and some snack foods like chips, buttered popcorn and candy bars.

Protein and Vegetarianism. Protein is vital to growth and development. An eating pattern low in saturated fat, total fat, and dietary cholesterol does not mean cutting out all animal products or becoming a vegetarian. It means you replace fatty cuts of meat with lean meat, fish, and poultry, and whole-milk dairy products with low-fat or nonfat dairy products.

Vegetarian diets, if well planned, are not low-protein diets and may offer nutrition and health benefits which include lower blood cholesterol levels. But, not enough calories and other nutrients from strict vegetarian diets have caused poor growth and vitamin and mineral deficiencies. Vegetarian diets for children and teenagers require careful thought. Meeting with a registered dietitian can be helpful.

Protein and Building Muscle. Some teenagers, especially boys, believe that protein builds muscle. Most Americans eat more protein than they need. So, eating even more won't necessarily build muscle. Some foods high in protein, such as fatty cuts of meat and whole milk products, are also high in fat and saturated fats. If your teenager insists on eating more protein, choose those high-protein foods that are lower in total fat and saturated fat. Skim milk, for example, has as much protein as whole milk. Carbohydrate foods from the breads, cereals, pasta, rice, dry peas and beans group are important for athletes of all ages and also provide protein.

Total Fat. The two types of dietary fat are saturated and unsaturated. Unsaturated fats are more likely to be solid, while unsaturated fats are more likely to be liquid. Unsaturated fats are further grouped as either polyunsaturated or monounsaturated fats. In a food, saturated and unsaturated fats together equal total fat. All foods containing fat contain a mixture of fats. All fats regardless of their type provide 9 calories per gram. Carbohydrate and protein provide 4 calories per gram. Because fat is the richest source of calories, eating less fat will help reduce your calorie intake.

Dietary Cholesterol. Dietary cholesterol is found only in foods that come from animals (eggs, dairy products, meat, poultry, fish, and shellfish). Egg yolks and organ meats (liver, kidney, sweetbread, brain) are particularly rich sources of cholesterol. It is not found in any food coming from plants; which means it is never found in peanut butter, bran products, or vegetable oils. Although, different from saturated fat, dietary cholesterol also can raise your blood cholesterol level. So, it is important to eat fewer foods high in cholesterol.

Unsaturated Fats. Unsaturated fat actually helps to lower cholesterol levels when it replaces saturated fat. So, when you can, replace part of the saturated fat with unsaturated fats (polyunsaturated and monounsaturated fats). Unsaturated fats are found mostly in vegetable oils.

Complex Carbohydrates. Foods high in complex carbohydrates (starch and fiber) are excellent substitutes for foods high in saturated fat and cholesterol. As fat is reduced in the diet, carbohydrates will likely increase to maintain an appropriate calorie level.

Read Food Labels. Many foods have labels that tell you how much saturated fat and cholesterol they have. Did you know that even low-fat foods can be high in cholesterol? And some products may not contain cholesterol but are still high in fat and saturated fat. Make a habit of reading food labels to help you select foods low in both saturated fat and cholesterol as shown below.

Shop For Foods That Are Low In Saturated Fat And Cholesterol

Stocking your kitchen with a variety of foods that are low in saturated fat, total fat, and cholesterol will help you and your family eat in a heart-healthy way. These heart-healthy choices are described by food group beginning on this page and summarized in the appendix. You will find this information very helpful when making out your shopping list. Reading labels is an important step in heart-healthy grocery shopping. See below for more help with label reading.

Food Groups

Meat, Poultry, Fish and Shellfish

Meat, poultry, fish, and shellfish are important sources of protein and other nutrients in your child's diet. They also provide saturated fat and cholesterol. Examples of lean and fatty choices are shown below. Lean cuts of beef, such as top round, are lower in saturated fat and cholesterol than fattier cuts such as regular ground beef. Chicken without skin has less saturated fat and less total fat than chicken with skin. And even though two chicken hot dogs have a lot less saturated fat than beef hot dogs they have more saturated fat than even chicken with the skin. Fish such as haddock has less saturated fat and cholesterol than either chicken or beef. And, foods with less fat contain fewer calories as well.

To help lower your child's blood cholesterol level, choose leaner meats as well as chicken, turkey, fish, and shellfish more often. Remember, all of these foods contain some saturated fat and cholesterol. So, the number of servings and serving size your child eats are also important. For variety, consider dry beans or legumes as a main dish instead of meat. They are high in protein and very low in fat. Or, stretch small amounts of meat with pasta, rice, or vegetables for hearty dishes.

Meat. Lean cuts of beef, veal, pork, and lamb are available (see the table below). These cuts of meat can be tender and tasty if prepared the right way. Some people think that only the well-marbled cuts of meat (meat with white fat running through it) taste good. However, tasty cuts do not have to be high in fat.

Beef, veal, and lamb cuts are "graded" based on the amount of marbling in the meat. "Prime" is the top grade and has the most fat. "Choice" has less fat and "select" least of all. "Select" grades of meat can also be tender if braised or stewed. Before preparing any meat, be sure to trim the fat off.

Remember, your child's diet can include meat, especially the lean cuts. For teenage girls, who are more likely to get iron deficiency anemia, lean meat is an especially important source of iron.

High-fat processed meats (like bologna, salami, beef or pork hot dogs, and sausage) should be eaten less often. Sixty to eighty percent of their calories come from fat—much of which is saturated. The good news is that a few lower-fat beef hot dogs have recently been developed. Organ

81

meats (like liver, sweetbreads, and kidneys) are relatively low in fat, but are high in cholesterol. They too should be eaten less often—once a month is okay on the Step-One Diet—and even less often on the Step-Two Diet.

Lean Cuts of Meat

Beef	Veal	Pork	Lamb
Round	All trimmed cuts	Tenderloin	Leg
Sirloin		Leg (fresh)	Arm
Chuck		Shoulder (arm	Loin
Loin		or picnic)	

Poultry. In general, poultry has less saturated fat than meat, especially when the skin is removed. Chicken and turkey are excellent choices for your family's new eating pattern. When choosing poultry, keep these tips in mind:

- Eat chicken and turkey without skin to reduce the saturated fat.

- Bake, roast, or broil—do not fry.

- In choosing processed poultry products like chicken hot dogs, bear in mind that they contain more fat and cholesterol than fresh chicken. However, some are lower in fat than similar beef or pork products.

Fish and Shellfish. Most fish, such as haddock or halibut, is lower in saturated fat and cholesterol than meat and poultry. Fish also provides protein and other nutrients, so it is a good choice.

Shellfish varies in cholesterol content. Some, like shrimp and crayfish, are relatively high, and some, like clams and lobster, are low. All shellfish has less fat than meat, poultry, and most fish. So, shellfish can certainly be eaten occasionally.

Some fish, like tuna, salmon, and mackerel—the high-fat fish—are rich in "omega-3" fatty acids, a polyunsaturated fatty acid. Some people believe that these omega-3 fatty acids, commonly called "fish oils," lower blood cholesterol levels. This does not appear to be the case. However, eating fish is a good choice since it is low in saturated fat. Taking fish oil supplements for treating high blood cholesterol is not recommended. It may lead to undesirable side effects over time.

Meat, Poultry, and Fish: A Comparison

Product (3 oz. cooked— the size of a deck of cards)	Saturated Fat (grams)	Dietary Cholesterol (milligrams)	Total Fat (grams)	Total Calories
Beef, top round, braised	2	76	4	169
Regular ground beef, baked, well done	7	92	18	269
Beef hot dogs (2)	11	54	26	284
Chicken, broiler/fryer breast, without skin, roasted	1	73	3	141
Chicken, broiler/fryer, breast, with skin roasted	2	71*	7	168
Chicken hot dogs (2)	5	90	18	232
Haddock, baked	0.1	63	<1	95
Shrimp	0.3	166	1	84

*On an equal weight basis, chicken without skin has slightly more cholesterol than chicken with skin. That's because cholesterol is found mostly in chicken meat, not the fatty skin. Skinless chicken is still the better choice since it is lower in saturated fat.

To figure calories from fat or saturated fat, multiply grams of fat or saturated fat by 9.

Dairy Products

Whole milk dairy products are major sources of saturated fat and cholesterol. However, dairy products are also a great source of calcium. Children and adolescents need calcium for the proper growth and development of strong bones. Girls, especially, need to eat foods high in calcium. By choosing low-fat, skim, and nonfat dairy products more often than high-fat dairy products you not only cut back on saturated fat and cholesterol but in most cases you get more calcium per serving. Dairy products are often added to foods, like casseroles, pizza, cookies, and sauces. So, even if your children do not eat much cheese or drink much milk, they may be getting quite a lot of high-fat dairy products without knowing it.

Milk. Milk provides many nutrients, especially calcium, that are essential for growth and development. Choose more often either 1 percent or skim milk instead of whole milk (3.3 percent) or 2 percent milk. The lower fat types provide as much or more calcium and other nutrients as whole milk. Yet they have much less saturated fat and cholesterol and fewer calories. Children over age 2 can drink 1 percent or skim milk and still get the nutrients they need.

Cheese. When people cut back on meat, they often eat more cheese. Most cheeses, particularly those prepared with whole milk or cream, are actually higher in saturated fat than meat or poultry. Cholesterol, however, is about the same in the high-fat cheeses, meat, and poultry. The table below compares the saturated fat and cholesterol content in chicken, fatty and relatively lean cuts of meat, and some cheeses.

Determining which cheeses are high or low in saturated fat and cholesterol can be confusing. Cheeses are often labeled as part-skim milk, low-fat, imitation, processed, natural, hard, or soft. As a rule, imitation cheeses (made with vegetable oil), part-skim milk cheese, and cheeses advertised as "low-fat" are usually lower in saturated fat and cholesterol than are natural and processed cheeses (which are made with whole milk). However, even part-skim milk cheese and low-fat cheeses are not necessarily lower in fat than many meats.

Remember it this way:

- Natural, processed, and hard cheeses, like cheddar, Swiss or American, are highest in saturated fat.

- Low-fat and imitation cheeses may have less saturated fat.

- Many meats have less saturated fat than many of these cheeses.

Therefore, when you can, replace natural, processed and hard cheeses with low-fat and imitation cheeses. Read the label.

When your child has the urge for cheese, try the following:

- String cheese.

- Part-skim mozzarella.

- Low-fat cottage cheese.

- Farmer cheese.

If your child is on the Step-One Diet, choose low-fat cheeses that have no more than 6 grams of fat in 1 ounce. If your child is on the Step-Two Diet, choose low-fat cheeses that have no more than 2 grams of fat in 1 ounce.

Choosing Cheese

Step-One Diet	Step-Two Diet
6 grams of fat/ounce	2 grams of fat/ounce

Ice Cream. Children love ice cream. But, ice cream is made from whole milk and cream. It contains a large amount of saturated fat and cholesterol. Try frozen desserts, like ice milk and low-fat frozen yogurt, which are lower in saturated fat. Also try sorbet and popsicles, which contain no fat.

Make your own ice cream substitutes:

- Tangy yogurt cubes. Combine 6 ounces of undiluted frozen fruit juice concentrate with 8 ounces plain low-fat yogurt and freeze in ice cube trays or paper cups.

- Homemade popsicles. Freeze orange and other juices on a stick.

- Floats. Combine ice milk with carbonated fruit juice.

85

Meat, Poultry, and Cheese: A Comparison

Product (3 oz. serving)	Saturated Fat (grams)	Dietary Cholesterol (milligrams)	Total Fat (grams)	Total Calories
Chicken, broiler/fryer, breast, without skin, roasted	1	73	3	141
Beef bottom round, roasted	2	66	6	160
Beef, porterhouse steak, broiled	8	70	19	260
Low-fat cottage cheese	<1	4	<1	62
Part-skim mozzarella	9	48	14	216
Mozzarella	11	66	18	240
American cheese food	13	54	21	279
Cream cheese	19	93	30	297

To figure calories from fat or saturated fat, multiply grams of fat or saturated fat by 9.

Eggs

Egg yolks are high in cholesterol: each contains about 213 mg. So, they should be eaten in moderation. On the Step-One Diet your child can eat 3 to 4 yolks a week. This includes those in processed foods and many baked goods. On the Step-Two Diet your child should eat even less. Egg whites which contain no cholesterol can be eaten freely.

In recipes, whole eggs can be replaced with egg whites. For most cake or cookie recipes, you can substitute egg whites for one to two eggs; in some, up to three to four. Since egg substitutes are made mainly of egg white, they also may be used to replace eggs (all or some) in dishes such as scrambled eggs, omelets and some baked items.

How Eggs Add Up

Approximate Portion of Whole Egg

Eggnog (about 1/2 cup)	1/4
Cornbread (1/9 of 9"x9" pan)	1/4
Muffin (1)	1/10
Pancakes, 4" (2)	1/4
Baked custard (6 oz. custard cup)	1/2
Chocolate, lemon meringue	
or pumpkin pie (1/8 of 9" pie)	1/3
Pound cake (1/12 of loaf)	1/2
Sponge cake (1/12 of 9"x9" cake)	1/3
Tapioca pudding (1/2 cup)	1/3
Yellow or chocolate	
two-layer cake (1/16 of 9" cake)	1/8
Cheese soufflé (1 cup)	1/2
Chicken salad (1/2 cup)	1/3
Corn pudding (1/2 cup)	1/2
Omelet (depends on size)	1 to 3
Mayonnaise (1/4 cup)	1/4
Thousand Island dressing (1/4 cup)	1/3

Source: Adapted from *Dietary Treatment of Hypercholesterolemia, A Manual for Patients,* American Heart Association and National Heart, Lung, and Blood Institute, 1988.

Fats and Oils

Foods included in this group will be high in either saturated, polyunsaturated, or monounsaturated fatty acids. Lard, fatback, and butter are high in saturated fat. Solid shortenings and some commercial salad dressings contain moderate amounts of saturated fats. So, limit how much you use of these foods, especially in your cooking.

Instead of butter, use margarine since it is higher in polyunsaturated fatty acids. Choose those liquid vegetable oils that are highest in unsaturated fats, like canola (rapeseed oil), safflower, sunflower, corn, olive, sesame, and soybean oils in cooking and salad dressings. When you shop, read food labels. Choose margarines and oils that have more polyunsaturated fat than saturated fat.

Some vegetable oils, like coconut, palm, and palm kernel oil, are saturated. These vegetable fats, often called "tropical oils," can be found in commercially baked goods such as cookies and crackers, non-dairy substitutes such as whipped toppings and coffee creamers, cake mixes, and even frozen dinners. They also can be found in some snack foods, like chips, candy bars, and buttered popcorn. Many companies have removed tropical oils from their products in order to help reduce their saturated fat content.

Also, vegetable oils can become saturated by hydrogenation—a process that makes them solid. They are called hydrogenated vegetable oils.

When choosing foods that contain tropical oils or hydrogenated vegetable oils, read the label before you buy. Choose those products lowest in saturated fat.

Since avocados, olives, nuts, and seeds are high in fat, they are often grouped with fats and oils. Although the fat in nuts and seeds is mostly unsaturated fat, they are very high in calories. They can fit into the eating plan if used in small amounts and not too often. Peanut butter can be a good choice for children's sandwiches, and nuts and seeds can be an after school treat.

Fruits and Vegetables

Fruits and vegetables contain no cholesterol, are very low in saturated fat, and are low in calories, except for avocados and olives (see Fats and Oils). Cutting back on high-fat foods cuts out some calories. Eating more fruits and vegetables is a good way for the whole family to replace those calories. Fruits can be a tasty snack or dessert. Even vegetables can be disguised as snacks and interesting side dishes. When chopped into small pieces, vegetables can be added to most favorite recipes without the child even noticing. By eating more of these foods your child can get more vitamins, minerals, and fiber and less saturated fat and cholesterol.

Breads, Cereals, Pasta, Rice, and Dry Peas and Beans

Breads, cereals, pasta, rice, and dry peas and beans are all high in complex carbohydrates and low in saturated fat. Replace foods high in saturated fat with those high in complex carbohydrates.

Your child might like some of the following suggestions:

- Try pasta with tomato sauce, or spaghetti with oil and herbs for supper as the main dish. Add low-fat cheese or small amounts of meat or fish and vegetables for extra punch.

- Combine rice with vegetables or smaller portions of meat, chicken, or fish

- Use dry peas and beans (like split peas, lentils, kidney beans, and navy beans) as main dishes, casseroles, soups, or other one-dish meals without high-fat sauces. Chili without lots of meat is a good low-fat, one-dish meal.

Cereals, both cooked and dry, are usually low in saturated fat. Some that contain coconut or coconut oil, like many types of granola, are not. In fact, most granolas are high in fat. Compare the cereal labels. Choose those lower in fat, particularly saturated fat.

Most breads and rolls also are low in fat. Choose the whole-grain types for more fiber. Some commercially baked goods, like those listed below, are often made with large amounts of saturated fats.

- Croissants

- Muffins

- Biscuits

- Butter rolls

- Doughnuts

Read the labels on baked goods to figure out their fat content. Instead of buying the high-fat types, you can make your own muffins and quick breads using unsaturated vegetable oils and egg whites or substitutes. In most recipes, you can replace one whole egg with two egg whites.

Foods from this group can be great snacks for children at any age. Instead of snacks high in saturated fat, encourage your child to try lowfat crackers (like graham crackers); ready-to-eat cereal; and whole-grain bread with low-fat cheese, peanut butter, or lean meat. Even pizza can be lower in fat and saturated fat when made with low-fat cheese on an English muffin or low-fat crackers. Remember to leave off the pepperoni, sausage, and extra cheese toppings.

Sweets and Snacks

Sweets and snacks often are high in saturated fat, cholesterol, and calories. Commercial cakes, pies, cookies, cheese crackers, and some types of chips are examples of such foods. Once again, the key is to read labels carefully. Choose those that contain primarily unsaturated fats and are low in total fat and calories.

Candy made mostly of sugar (for example, hard candy, gum drops, candy corn) has very little or no fat. It can be a snack now and then. Other candies, especially chocolate, should be limited because they are high in saturated fat.

If your child likes to eat pies, cakes, or cookies, try some tasty alternatives to the high-saturated fat and high-cholesterol types. Fig bars, ginger snaps, graham crackers, homemade cake and cookies made with vegetable oils and egg whites or substitutes, or angel food cake are all options. New baked goods have been developed which contain no cholesterol and very little fat. Some items, like frozen dairy desserts and puddings, are even made with fat substitutes. Even though these new products may be low in saturated fat and cholesterol, they are not always low in calories. Pay attention to serving sizes, especially for children who are overweight.

Remember, most desserts can be made at home. Substitute unsaturated oil or margarine for butter and lard, skim milk for whole milk, and egg whites or substitutes for egg yolks. This reduces their saturated fat and cholesterol, although total fat remains high. If your child has a weight problem, they should be eaten only once in a while. For snacks, try instead a piece of fruit, some vegetable sticks, unbuttered popcorn, or breadsticks.

Changing Eating Patterns Takes Time

All of the changes suggested above don't have to happen at once. Take it day by day. Aim for the target of change: less saturated fat, total fat, and cholesterol in your child's diet each day. This is especially important if your child has a high blood cholesterol level.

The first step is to look at your child's current eating pattern and begin to plan alternatives. (See "Take a Look" at the end of this chapter.) Write down a typical day's menu for your child. Is your child eating too many high-fat foods? Is your child eating from all the food groups?

Don't try to cut out all the high saturated fat and high-cholesterol foods at one time. Instead, try to substitute one or two more appropriate foods each day. If your child rarely eats foods high in saturated fat, these foods once in a while won't raise your child's blood cholesterol level. If you expect a high-saturated fat, high-cholesterol day, have your child eat a low-saturated fat, low-cholesterol diet the day before and the day after.

Changing eating patterns takes time. Start with easy-to-do changes followed by harder ones. For example, instead of limiting pizza, try pizza with vegetables and low-fat cheese. Make "lasting" changes rather than rapid changes that will last only a short time. Soon enough your child will be eating in a way that is lower in saturated fat and cholesterol.

Heart-Healthy Meals And Snacks

Heart-Healthy Meals Can Be Fun and Taste Good

Breakfast

Children as they get older, especially girls, may often skip breakfast. It is important to begin the day with a good breakfast. Breakfast is an easy meal to introduce good-tasting heart-healthy foods.

- Serve toast (whole-grain types), English muffins, bagels, and hot or cold cereal with skim milk. These are quick and easy to prepare.

- Serve unsweetened or barely sweetened cereals as often as you can. Adding fruit to unsweetened cereal makes it special, and at the same time, increases nutrients and fiber without adding fat.

- For special events or weekend treats, try pancakes, muffins, or French toast made with egg whites or egg substitutes and skim milk. Add some sweet syrup or fruit sauce, neither of which contains fat, to make it more appealing to children.

- For a more hearty breakfast, add some low-fat meat such as sliced poultry or lean ham to a bagel or an English muffin.

Lunch

Choosing lunch at school gives children the chance to make the right food choices for themselves. Packing a lunch offers them the chance to plan their own heart-healthy meals. Whether your child buys a school lunch or takes a packed lunch, discuss some tips for eating right. Try some of these:

91

- Sliced turkey, lean roast beef, chicken, or tuna fish are good choices for lower-fat sandwiches. Even add a bit of sliced processed low-fat cheese.

- Peanut butter and jelly is also okay, especially on whole grain bread. For more nutritional punch, create peanut butter and mashed bananas with raisins or carrots.

- Whole-wheat, rye, pumpernickel, or bran breads add more fiber to a sandwich and taste good too.

- Try some of last night's pasta salad or cold baked chicken with herbs for a switch from sandwiches for lunch.

- Pack some snacks such as apples, bananas, grapes, raisins, nuts, or seeds. Also, put in prepackaged juices or other types of unsweetened beverages.

Some lunches provided at school may be high in saturated fat and cholesterol. Check the menu in advance. If low-fat choices are not available on a certain day, you and your child can pack a lunch. However, if your child's school never offers heart-healthy choices, try to arrange that it does so. Work with your PTA or school system to promote a school lunch program which offers heart-healthy choices.

Dinner

Dinner may pose a problem for busy parents who have little time to shop and cook. Many rely on high-fat convenience foods like creamy, canned soups and boxed macaroni and cheese dinners. Replace these with foods lower in saturated fat and cholesterol that are quick and easy to prepare:

- Chicken breasts, fish fillets, and lean hamburgers take little time to prepare. Broil, bake, or microwave rather than fry.

- Vegetables can be steamed or microwaved in minutes.

- Vegetable stew can be made with rice or pasta and shavings of lean meat instead of a lot of chunks. Meat contributes protein, vitamins, and minerals like iron. Children should not avoid eating meat. It is a good idea to "stretch" meat by using it in a combination dish, like stew.

- Many ethnic dishes can also be low in fat and quick and easy to prepare. Try Chinese stir fries of rice, peppers, mushrooms, and water chestnuts with thin strips of beef or chicken. Pizza can be made with low-fat cheese and vegetable toppings rather than sausage or pepperoni.

- Some TV dinners and other convenience meals can be low in saturated fat and cholesterol. Look for dinners that provide foods from different food groups including vegetables, fruits, and breads. Choose less often those that contain battered, fried, or deep fried items. Read the labels and compare. Choose the one lowest in total fat and saturated fat.

Snacking Is Okay

Snacking is not a bad word. What your child eats matters more than when it is eaten. Children are growing quickly and need calories. Young children's appetites and stomachs may be small, so they may tend to eat smaller amounts at one time. They may not be able to eat enough calories at a meal to meet their energy needs. So, snacks may need to be part of their eating pattern. See the sample menus below.

Preteens and teenagers also may need extra nutrition and calories to get them through their growth spurts or athletic programs. Snacks can help meet their energy needs without being high in saturated fat and cholesterol. Instead, they can be rich in carbohydrates and fiber.

Plan for snacks. We all tend to eat what's handy. So, stock your kitchen with nutritious, low-saturated fat, low-cholesterol snack foods from all of the food groups. See below for some suggestions.

Let the snack foods you serve at home be the "good eating guide" when your child is away from home. Some of these snacks are now also found in vending machines. Your child just needs to choose them.

Like anything else, snacking can be overdone. If snacking leads to eating too much, it can lead to weight gain. Or, if snacks come mainly from the "Sweets and Snacks" group, your child may not get enough of the nutrients provided by other foods.

Low-Saturated Fat, Low-Cholesterol Snacks

- Snack mix of cereal, dried fruit, and small amounts of nuts and seeds

- Cold cereal, dry or with low-fat milk

- Peanut butter and jelly sandwich

- Fruit juice and vegetable juice

- Peanuts in a shell or other dry roasted nuts

- Toast with jam or jelly

- Fruit Leather

- Lowfat cheese pizza on English muffin

- Celery stalk filled with peanut butter

- Vegetable soup and low-fat crackers

- Candy (non-chocolate fat-free types)

- Skim milk with graham crackers

- Raisins and other dried fruit

- Frozen grapes or bananas

- Flavored low-fat yogurt

- Low-fat cookies

Recipes And Healthy Fast Foods

Most Families Have Favorite Recipes

There is no reason to stop using your favorite recipes and cookbook. You can change tried and true recipes to low-saturated fat, low-cholesterol recipes. The tips for substitutes in the table below will help you get started.

Experiment! Find the recipes that work best with these changes.

Substitutes

In place of	Use
1 tablespoon butter	1 tablespoon margarine or 3/4 tablespoon oil
1 cup shortening	2/3 cup vegetable oil
1 whole egg	2 egg whites
1 cup sour cream	1 cup yogurt (plus 1 tablespoon cornstarch for some recipes)
1 cup whole milk	1 cup skim milk

Convenience Foods and Fast Foods Can Be Heart Healthy

Stopping now and then at a fast food restaurant with friends or family does no harm. However, these days children may be eating fast and convenience foods three or more times week. By serving heart-healthy meals and snacks at home, you can plan for fast-food meals once in a while. Also some fast and convenience foods are now lower in saturated fat and cholesterol than they used to be. See the table below for a comparison of some of children's fast food favorites.

Here are some ways to avoid eating too much saturated fat and cholesterol while enjoying convenience. Try some of these tips:

- Order a small plain hamburger. It is lower in fat than fried or battered fish and chicken or anything with cheese.

- Try lean roast beef and grilled or broiled chicken sandwich or pita pockets filled with small pieces of meat and vegetables.

- Select the small serving; order the regular hamburger instead of the jumbo.

- Order a plain baked potato instead of French fries.

- Create a salad at the salad bar. Limit toppings of cheese, fried noodles, bacon bits, and salads made with mayonnaise. Also, limit salad dressings that add saturated fat and cholesterol.

- Try ethnic cuisine—many such as Chinese and Mid-Eastern are becoming fast food.

- Choose pizza with vegetable toppings such as mushrooms, onions, or peppers. Avoid extra cheese, pepperoni, or sausage.

- Create convenience foods at home by freezing low-fat casseroles, soups, and leftovers in single serving sizes.

The table of fast food meals below shows how some of these small changes can add up to big savings in saturated fat, total fat, cholesterol, and calories.

Sample Menus: Step-One And Step-Two Diets

Putting It All Together—Sample Menus

The differences between the eating pattern suggested for all healthy Americans, the Step-One Diet, and Step-Two Diet appear to be small. BUT they are very important for lowering your child's blood cholesterol level. All of the small changes add up to improve your child's blood cholesterol level.

Take a look at the sample menus. There are three sets of menus, each set for a different age range. The samples of the suggested eating pattern, Step-One, and Step-Two Diets have the same number of calories as the sample menu of the current eating pattern. However, they have much less saturated fat, total fat, and cholesterol. And, the sample menus show that because the fat in the current eating pattern was so calorie rich, the new eating patterns actually allow your child to eat more food!

The menus show how you can change a child's current eating pattern to one that is lower in saturated fat, total fat, and cholesterol, and be consistent with the Step-One and Step-Two Diets. (The nutrient analysis for each sample menu is provided below.)

Look across the menus and compare the highlighted items.

- Some items show simple changes in the type of food offered which lowers the saturated fat and cholesterol content of the menu. For example, across the sample menus for breakfast, you will see a change from whole milk to 1% milk to skim milk. Likewise, the dinners in sample menu 2 show a

96

Fast Food Favorites: A Comparison

Product	Saturated Fat (grams)	Dietary Cholesterol (milligrams)	Total Fat (grams)	Total Calories
Cheese pizza, 1 slice	2	9	3	140
Pepperoni pizza, 1 slice	2	14	7	181
Bean burrito	3	3	7	224
Beef and cheese burrito	5	85	12	317
Hamburger	4	36	12	275
Cheeseburger	6	50	15	320
French fries, regular	4	0	12	310
French fries, large	6	0	19	355
Grilled chicken breast sandwich	1	60	9	310
Chicken nuggets, 6 pieces	6	62	17	290
Beef hot dog, on bun	6	27	15	265
Vanilla low-fat frozen yogurt cone	0	2	1	105
Vanilla soft serve ice milk cone	4	28	6	164
Vanilla shake	5	32	8	314
Vanilla ice cream, 1 cup (10% fat)	9	59	14	269
Cola, 12 oz.	0	0	0	151

Source: USDA handbook 8-21; individual manufacturers for items not available from USDA.

Sample Fast Food Meals: How Small Changes Add Up

Meal	Saturated Fat (grams)	Dietary Cholesterol (milligrams)	Total Fat (grams)	Total Calories
Typical meal #1 Chicken nuggets Large French fries Vanilla Shake	17	94	45	959
Lower-fat choice #1 Grilled chicken breast sandwich 1/2 small French fries 12 Oz. cola Low-fat frozen yogurt cone	3	62	16	684
Typical meal #2 Cheeseburger Large French fries 12 oz. cola Vanilla ice milk cone	16	78	40	990
Lower-fat choice #2 Hamburger 1/2 small French fries 12.oz cola low-fat frozen yogurt	6	38	19	649

change from fried chicken to skinless broiled chicken, and change the butter on the vegetables to regular or tub margarine.

• Other changes in the actual foods offered can also help to reduce saturated fat and cholesterol. For example, the lunches in sample menu 2 show replacing a cheeseburger with a hamburger for Step-One, and with a tuna sandwich made with water-pack tuna for Step-Two. Sample menu 3 suggests choosing a roast beef sandwich instead of a beef hot dog with chili for lunch, and chicken cacciatore (made with skinless chicken and pasta) instead of lasagna (made with regular ground beef and whole milk mozzarella) for dinner.

You may notice that the Step-Two Diet calls for adding more margarine as tub margarine, which is highly unsaturated. By using only skim milk, low-fat cheese, and the leanest meat on the Step-Two Diet, you have removed many hidden sources of saturated fat. Since the Step-Two Diet has the same amount of total fat and calories as the other eating patterns it's okay to replace these saturated fats with more tub margarine.

As you can see, learning to eat the heart-healthy way means choosing more foods low in saturated fat and cholesterol. The appendix gives you more ideas of foods to choose. It's important to remember that you can have variety within any given day.

You Can Lead Your Child To Food, But You Can't Make Him Eat

The most carefully planned heart-healthy meal is no good if your child does not eat it. Younger children may just be picky eaters going through a stage. Older children may have "reasons" for being picky. Children can be encouraged to eat foods lower in saturated fat and cholesterol but should not be made to eat them. You need to be creative and give them choices:

- Let your child help fix the meal. Helping makes eating more fun.

- Make the meal attractive. For younger children, make a face on top of casserole or cut foods with a cookie cutter to make fun shapes.

- If your child doesn't like a certain lower fat food, serve it with something your child does like. Disguise an unliked food in other foods. For example, add the food to casseroles or soups, or bake it into muffins or quick breads.

- Above all, be a good role model yourself—let your eating patterns be the example for others.

Choosing to eat in a heart-healthy way is a family affair. It becomes even more important if someone in the family has high blood cholesterol. If your child has high blood cholesterol, talk to them about it. They may not understand why they need to eat this way and may be afraid of sudden changes. Encourage children to eat for the health of their heart, yet don't make too big a deal about it. If your child is growing well, he or she is probably getting enough to eat. So don't worry about it. If your child gets stuck on one food or refuses to make any changes, discuss the problem with your doctor or a dietitian.

HELP!

If you want more help in planning low-saturated fat, low-cholesterol eating patterns, visit a registered dietitian or other qualified nutritionist. They can help you design an eating pattern suited to your own child's needs and likes. Dietitians may be found at local hospitals, and state and district chapters of the American Dietetic Association (ADA). The ADA keeps a list of registered dietitians. By calling the Division of Practice, you can request names of dietitians in your area. Others can be found in public health departments, health maintenance organizations, cooperative extension services, and colleges.

Dietitians can help you by giving further advice on shopping and preparing foods, eating away from home, and changing your child's eating habits to help maintain the new eating pattern. Their skill will help you and your child set short-term targets for change. This will help your child reach the blood cholesterol goal without greatly changing your family's eating patterns and lifestyle.

The National Cholesterol Education Program has produced booklets for children of different age groups: ages 7 to 10, 11 to 14, and 15 to 18. These booklets are designed to help children understand blood cholesterol levels and the need to eat in a way that is low in saturated fat, total fat, and cholesterol. To order these booklets and others for adults with high blood cholesterol, contact:

National Cholesterol Education Program
NHLBI Information Center
P.O. Box 30105
Bethesda, Maryland 20824-0105

Appendices

Foods To Choose and Decrease

Eating in a way that is lower in saturated fat, total fat, and cholesterol is a balancing act: eating the variety of foods to supply the nutrients your child needs without too much saturated fat and cholesterol or extra calories.

One way to assure variety and a balanced diet is to choose foods every day from each of the food groups. You may question why children would need to choose foods from the fats and oils group and the sweets and snacks group. They don't have to since the nutrients provided by the foods in these groups are easily provided by other foods. But, it is likely that they will choose foods from these groups. This chart is meant to be a guide in making those choices.

Choose different foods from within groups, too, especially foods low in saturated fat and cholesterol (the choose column). Foods in the decrease column are higher in saturated fat and cholesterol.

The number of servings should be adjusted to promote your child's growth and development and to maintain or achieve your child's healthy weight. As a guide, examples of the number of servings needed from each food group to achieve the eating patterns for the Step-One and Step-Two Diets are listed. Common serving sizes are listed next to the different food types in the choose column.

Meat, Poultry, Fish, and Shellfish

Recommended Ounces Per Day

Age	Step-1	Step-2*
2-3	2	2
4-6	5	5
7-18	6	6

*Note: Step-2 Diet allows only the leanest cuts of meat, fish, and poultry.

Choose	**Decrease**
Lean cuts of meat with fat trimmed, like:	Fatty cuts of meat, like:

Choose	Decrease
Beef—round, sirloin, chuck, loin	Beef—regular ground, short ribs, corned beef brisket
Lamb—leg, arm, loin, rib	Pork—spareribs, blade roll
Pork—tenderloin, leg, shoulder (arm or picnic)	Bacon, sausage
Veal—all trimmed cuts except ground	Organ meats, like liver, kidney, sweetbreads, brain
Poultry—without skin	Poultry with skin, fried chicken
Fish	Fried fish and shellfish
Shellfish	Regular luncheon meat, like bologna, salami, sausage, and beef or pork hot dogs
Luncheon meat like turkey ham, turkey, lean ham, lean roast beef, or chicken hot dogs	

Eggs

Recommended Servings Per Week

Age	Step-I	Step-2
2-3	3	2
4-6	3	2
7-18	3	1

Choose	Decrease
Egg whites (2 whites equal 1 whole egg in recipes)	Egg yolks beyond suggested number of servings per week (includes egg used in cooking)
Cholesterol-free egg substitutes	

Dairy Products

Recommended Servings Per Day

Age	Step-I	Step-2*
2-3	3	3
4-6	3	3
7-18	4	4

*Note: Step-2 Diet allows only milk and yogurt with 1% fat or less, and cheeses with not more than 2 grams of fat per ounce.

Choose

Milk (1 cup)—skim milk, 1% milk (fluid, powdered evaporated); buttermilk

Yogurt (1 cup)—nonfat or low-fat yogurt; yogurt beverages

Cottage cheese (½ cup)—low-fat, nonfat, or dry curd (0 to 2% fat)

Cheese (1 oz.)—low-fat cheeses labeled no more than 6 grams of fat per ounce on Step-I (no more than 2 grams of fat per ounce on Step-2)

Frozen dairy dessert ½ cup)— ice milk, frozen yogurt (low-fat and nonfat)

Decrease

Whole milk (fluid, evaporated, condensed); 2% low-fat milk; imitation milk

Whole-milk yogurt; custard-style yogurt; whole-milk yogurt beverages

Cottage cheese (4% fat)

High-fat cheese, like American, blue, brie, cheddar, colby, edam, monterey jack, parmesan, Swiss, Neufshatel

Cream cheese

Ice cream

Cream, half-&-half, whipping cream, nondairy creamer, whipped topping, sour cream

Fats and Oils

Recommended Servings Per Day

Age	Step-1	Step-2*
2-3	4	5
4-6	5	6
7-10	5	7
11-14		
males	7	9
females	5	8
15-18		
males	10	12
females	5	8

*Note: Step-2 Diet allows tub margarines and oils very low in saturated fats. In order to keep total calories from fat at about 30%, while reducing saturated fats, Step-2 Diet allows more servings of unsaturated fats.

Choose

Unsaturated oils (1 tsp.)—corn, olive, peanut, rapeseed (canola oil), safflower, sesame, soybean

Margarine (1 tsp.)—made from unsaturated oils listed above; light or diet margarine (2 tsp.)

Salad dressings (1 tbsp.)—dressings made with unsaturated oils listed above: low-fat or oil-free dressings (serving size depends on amount of oil)

Seeds and nuts (1 tbsp.)—peanut butter, other nut butters

Decrease

Coconut oil, palm kernel oil, palm oil

Butter, lard, bacon fat, shortening

Dressings made with egg yolk, cheese, sour cream, whole milk

Coconut

Chocolate

Choose	Decrease
Cocoa powder (as desired)	
Olives (5 small)	
Avocado (1/8 of whole)	

Breads, Cereals, Pasta, Rice, Dry Peas and Beans

Recommended Servings Per Day

Age	Step-l	Step-2
2-3	5	5
4-6	6	6
7-10	7	7
11-14		
males	9	9
females	8	8
15-18		
males	12	12
females	8	8

Choose	Decrease
Bread (1 slice)—whole grain bread; hamburger and hot dog bun (½); corn tortilla (1)	Bread in which eggs are a major ingredient; croissants
	Granola-type cereals
Cereal (1 cup ready-to-eat, 1/3 cup bran or 1/2 cup cooked)—oat, wheat, corn, multigrain	Egg noodles and pasta containing egg yolk
Pasta (1/2 cup cooked), like plain noodles, spaghetti, macaroni	Pasta and rice prepared with cream, butter, or cheese sauces

Choose	Decrease
Rice (1/2 cup cooked)	High-fat crackers, like cheese crackers, butter crackers, those made with saturated fats
Low-fat crackers— animal crackers (8); graham (3); saltine-type (6)	Commercial baked pastries, muf fins,biscuits, doughnuts, sweet rolls,
Homemade baked goods using unsaturated oil, skim or 1% milk, and egg substitutes— quick bread (1 slice); 2" biscuit (1); cornbread muffin (1); bran muffin (1); 4" pancake (1); 9" diameter waffle (1/4)	Danish pastry using saturated fats Dry peas and beans prepared with butter, cheese, or cream
Dry peas and beans (1/2 cup cooked),like split peas, black-eyed peas, chick peas, kidney beans, navy beans, lentils, soybeans, soybean curd (tofu)	

Vegetables

Recommended Servings Per Day

Age	Step-l	Step-2
2-3	3	3
4-6	3	3
7-10	3	3
11-18		
males	4	4
females	3	3

Choose	Decrease
Vegetables (1/2 cup) fresh, frozen, or canned	Vegetables prepared with butter, cheese, or cream sauce

Fruits

Recommended Servings Per Day

Age	Step-I	Step-2
2-3	2	2
4-6	3	3
7-10	3	4
11-14	3	3
15-18		
males	5	5
females	3	3

Choose

Fruit (1/2 cup or medium-size piece) fresh, frozen, canned, or dried

Fruit juice (1/2 cup) fresh, frozen. or canned

Decrease

Fried fruit or fruit served with butter or cream sauce

Sweets and Snacks

Recommended Servings Per Day

Age	Step-I	Step-2
2-3	1	1
4-6	2	2
7-10	2	2
11-18		
males	4	4
females	3	3

Choose

Beverages (6 fluid oz.)—fruit-flavored drinks; lemonade, fruit punch

Decrease

Candy made with chocolate, butter, cream, coconut oil, palm oil, palm kernel oil, coconut oil

Choose	Decrease

Sweets (1-l/2 tbsp.)—sugar, syrup, honey, jam, preserves; candy(3/4 oz.) made primarily with sugar (candy corn, gumdrops, hard candy); fruit-flavored gelatin (1/2 cup)

Ice cream and frozen treats made with cream and whole milk

Commercial baked high-fat cookies, cakes, cream pies, doughnuts

Low-fat frozen desserts (1/3 cup)— sherbet, sorbet, fruit ice, popsicles, low-fat frozen yogurt

Cookies (2), cake (1 slice), pie (1 slice), pudding (1/2 cup)— (all prepared with egg whites, egg substitute, skim milk or 1% milk, and unsaturated oil or margarine) gingersnaps (2); fig barcookies (I); angel food cake

Take A Look

What is your child's current eating pattern? Is it low in saturated fat and cholesterol? Does your child get brisk, sustained exercise at least 3 times a week?

To answer these questions, take a look at your child's eating and exercise habits. Use a chart to have your child keep a record of everything he or she eats and drinks (except water) for 3 days. This includes the dressing on the salad, the butter on toast—all the "little" extras. Also, record any exercise.

Keep an accurate record. To do this, you may want your child to record foods right after a meal or snack. This might mean carrying paper and pen in a pocket or pocketbook for 3 days. You could also sit down together after school or work to recall all the foods eaten during the day. Find a method that works best for you and your child.

When the 3 days are over, take a look. Together you and your child can compare what your child ate to the foods to choose and decrease in the appendix. Next to the foods your child wrote down, check off whether they are foods to choose or decrease.

- Are there many foods higher in saturated fat and cholesterol?

- Are there low-fat foods your child would eat instead?

Remind your child of the need to eat in a way that is lower in saturated fat and cholesterol. Discuss options with your child. Let your child join you in planning a grocery list based on what changes may have to be made in the eating pattern. You may want to do this exercise again in several months to see if there appear to be lasting changes.

Exercise, especially aerobic exercise, is important in helping your child lower cholesterol and achieve a healthy weight. Has your child had some aerobic exercise in these 3 days? If your child was getting exercise 3 times a week, it would be likely that on at least 1 day he got some. If not, be sure next week is different.

Keep in mind that your child's eating and exercise habits may reflect yours. Eating right and exercising is a family affair.

Chapter 6

On the Teen Scene: Good News About Good Nutrition

You've heard it all before. For as long as you can remember, your parents, your teachers, perhaps even your doctor, have been telling you to eat your vegetables, limit sweets, drink your milk.

Now, in your teen years, this advice takes on new meaning for a lot of very different reasons: How can you gain weight to put on muscle instead of fat? What's a healthy weight for you? How can you squeeze in a good, quick meal after school and before you have to be at your part-time job? All good questions, and because of the enormous changes that are going on in your body, the way you decide to deal with your nutrition needs now can make a big difference not only in how you feel today, but also in your well-being in years to come.

If you are between 15 and 18, you're completing your final major growth spurt, and are in the process of putting on nature's finishing touches for adulthood. For girls, the finishing touch means adding some fat padding. For boys, it means adding muscle and increasing the volume of blood. These changes often encourage girls to diet unnecessarily to stay slim, while boys may overeat to satisfy their appetites. Both can lead to health problems down the road, and, incidentally, probably will not do the job you want right now.

So what is the right approach to healthy eating?

A good start is to eat a variety of foods, as suggested in the Dietary Guidelines for Americans, published by the U.S. Departments of Agriculture and Health and Human Services. Get the many nutri-

FDA Consumer/April 1992

ents your body needs by choosing a variety of foods from each of these groups:

- vegetables

- fruits

- breads, cereals, rice, and pasta

- milk, yogurt and cheese

- meat, poultry, fish. dried beans and peas, eggs. and nuts.

What's So Junky About "Junk" Food?

The pace for teens is fast and getting faster. Added to pressures from school to prepare for college or a job, many teens take part in sports and work part-time. This often means eating on the run. Stack that on top of the snack foods you eat on dates or when you and your friends just get together, and the balance of your nutrients can get way out of kilter.

Many snacks, such as potato chips, fast-food cheeseburgers, and fries, have high levels of fat, sugar or salt—ingredients that are usually best limited to a small portion of your diet. Healthy eating doesn't mean that you can't have your favorite foods, but the Dietary Guidelines advise you to be selective and limit the total fat, saturated fat, cholesterol, and sodium you eat. Our main source of saturated fat comes from animal products and hydrogenated vegetable oils, with tropical oils—coconut and palm—providing smaller amounts. Only animal fat provides cholesterol. Sodium mostly comes from salt added to foods during processing, home preparation, or at the table.

Fats are our most concentrated source of energy and supply about 40 percent of the total calories in typical American diets. Scientists know that eating too much fat, especially saturated fat and cholesterol, increases blood cholesterol levels, and therefore increases your risk of heart disease. Too much fat also may lead to overweight and increase your risk of some cancers.

Dietitians recommend that no more than 30 percent of your calories come from fats, and not more than 10 percent of these calories should be from saturated fat. Choose lean meats, fish, poultry without skin, and low-fat dairy products whenever you can. When you eat out, particularly at fast-food restaurants, look for broiled or baked rather than fried foods. Try the salad bars more often, but pass up creamy items and limit the amount of salad dressing you use to keep down the fat and calories. Look for milk-based high-calcium foods with reduced fat.

Spare the Sugar and Salt

Most people like the taste of table sugar. But did you know that other sweeteners are sometimes "hidden" in foods? There are sugars in honey, dried fruits, concentrated fruit juices, and ingredients such as corn syrup that are added to soft drinks, cookies, and many other processed foods. You can see what sugars are in packaged foods by looking at the ingredient list.

If you are a very active teen with high energy needs, sweets can be an additional source of calories. But keep in mind that they contain only limited nutrients and that both sugars and starches can contribute to tooth decay.

A moderate amount of sodium in your diet is necessary, because sodium, along with potassium, maintains the water balance in your body. But for some people, too much sodium can be a factor in high blood pressure. Since processed foods often contain large amounts of sodium, it's wise to use salt sparingly when cooking or at the table— and to avoid overeating salty snacks like pretzels and chips.

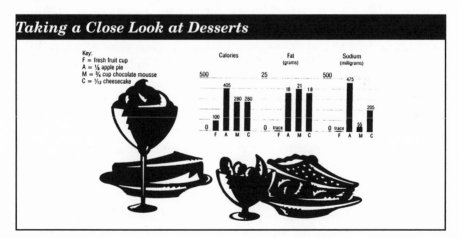

Taking a Close Look at Desserts

Key:
F = fresh fruit cup
A = ⅛ apple pie
M = ¾ cup chocolate mousse
C = 1/12 cheesecake

Here's how much fat, sodium and calories you get from a few popular desserts. The estimates are based on usual portion sizes, which take into account that cheesecake is often served in portions half the size of a slice of apple pie.

(Source: U.S. Department of Agriculture)

When you exercise heavily and sweat profusely, you can deplete your sodium reserve, unbalance your body chemistry, and possibly become dehydrated. In extreme cases of profuse sweating, such as during training or competition, a dilute glucose-electrolyte drink may become necessary, but always with an abundance of water to make up for sweat losses.

What's All This About Fiber?

Whole-grain breads and cereals, dried beans and peas, vegetables, and fruits contain various types of dietary fiber essential for proper bowel function. Eating plenty of these fiber-rich foods may reduce you risk of cancer and heart disease.

The benefits from a high-fiber diet may be related to the foods themselves and not to fiber alone. For this reason, it's best to get fiber from foods rather than from the fiber supplements you can purchase in a store.

Be Aware of Alcohol

Alcoholic beverages deserve special mention. Drinking them risks good health and can cause other serious problems for teens. And although it is illegal for teens to buy alcoholic beverages, a 1991 survey conducted by the Department of Health and Human Services shows that over half of 10.7 million junior and senior high school students have had at least one drink within the past year. Eight million students drink weekly, and almost half a million binge (five or more drinks at one time) weekly.

Teens who drink risk impaired judgment in their social relationships and endanger their own and others' lives if they drive after drinking. The U.S. Department of Transportation reports that in 1989, 2,800 students between 15 and 19 years of age died in alcohol-related traffic accidents. Almost half of all traffic accidents involving this age group, whether or not someone died, were alcohol-related.

Alcoholic beverages contain calories, but few if any nutrients. Drinking heavily can lead to poor nutrition if alcoholic beverages replace foods with needed nutrients, and alcoholism is not unknown among teenagers.

What About Vegetarians?

There are many types of vegetarian diets, but the two most common are the lacto-ovo, which includes eggs and milk products but not meat, and vegan, which eliminates all forms of animal products. Teens who are lacto-ovo vegetarians can usually get enough nutrients in their diets, with the possible exception of iron, says Marilyn Stephenson, a dietitian with the Food and Drug Administration's Office of Nutrition and Food Sciences.

Getting enough iron is especially important to teens. The need for iron for both boys and girls increases between the ages of 11 and 18. The National Academy of Sciences recommends teenage boys get 12 milligrams of iron a day, mostly to sustain their rapidly enlarging body mass. For girls, the recommended daily requirement is 15 milligrams to offset menstrual losses that begin during this time.

It's important to plan how to get adequate iron in your diet. Iron from meat, poultry and fish is better absorbed by your body than the iron from plant sources. However, the absorption of iron from plants is improved by eating fruit or drinking juice that contains vitamin C with the iron-rich food.

Vegan vegetarians are vulnerable to deficiencies of several nutrients, particularly vitamins D and B_{12}, calcium, iron, zinc, and perhaps other trace elements. Like all essential nutrients, these vitamins and minerals are required to maintain proper growth.

Teens need extra calcium to store up an optimal amount of bone (called "peak" bone mass). The richest sources of calcium are milk and other dairy products. Building optimal bone mass through a balanced diet, including adequate calcium, may help delay the onset or limit your chances of developing osteoporosis later in life. Osteoporosis is a disease in which reduced bone mass causes bones to break easily. It occurs in both men and women, but is more common among older women.

If it is important to you to be a vegetarian, it is easier to achieve good nutrition with the lacto-ovo form. A dietitian (or your school nurse) can help you plan a vegetarian diet that provides you with the nutrients you need for growth and development during the teen years.

What's a Healthy Weight?

Some teens have a difficult time projecting a healthy weight for themselves. Girls especially may think they need to be thinner than they are, or should be. Extraordinary concern or obsession for thinness leads some teens to the eating disorders of anorexia nervosa (dieting to starvation) or bulimia (overeating and then vomiting).

If you're concerned about your weight, it's important to talk to a health professional such as your family doctor or the school nurse. That person can help you decide whether you do need to lose weight and, if so, the best way to achieve and maintain a weight that is healthy for you.

If health professionals recommend that you need to lose weight, most experts say it's best to increase your exercise as the first step. Often that's all teens need to do for weight control because they're rapidly growing. If eating less is also necessary, it is best to continue eating a variety of foods while cutting down on fats and sugars.

Losing weight quickly on a very low-calorie diet is never a good idea for anyone. And if you're into sports, you should be aware that it could affect your athletic performance. Under no circumstances should you drink less fluid to lose weight. A steady loss of a pound or so a week until you reach your goal is generally safe, and you're more likely to be able to maintain your weight loss. [See Chapter 7 for more information on teens and dieting.]

Skipping meals to lose weight is another poor idea. You're likely to overeat at the next meal just because you're so hungry. And surveys show that people who skip breakfast or other meals tend to have poorer nutrition than those who don't.

Help for Healthy Eating Is on the Way

Food processors and many grocery stores are preparing now to help nutrition-conscious people make wise food choices. This can be important to teens who sometimes shop not only for themselves, but also for the whole family. While many food labels already voluntarily show nutrition information, new legislation, the Nutrition Labeling and Education Act, enforced by FDA, requires food products to be labeled with the nutritive values they contain per serving size (which will be standardized and realistic). There will be no implied or misleading claims. And all this must be in easy-to-read and easy-to understand terms.

All food labels must have this information in place by 1993. Look for more information about the new labeling from FDA and USDA.

Thanks to growing scientific knowledge about several diet and health relationships, healthy eating is more socially "in" than ever before. Eating a healthy diet is not difficult with knowledge of a few of the basics, and can help you excel on the playing field, in school, and in your social life.

Dietary Guidelines for All Americans

What should Americans eat to stay healthy? These guidelines, published by the U.S. Departments of Agriculture and Health and Human Services, reflect recommendations of nutrition authorities who agree that enough is known about the effect of diet on health to encourage certain dietary practices. The guidelines are:

- Eat a variety of foods.

- Balance the food you eat with physical activity—maintain or improve your weight.

- Choose a diet low in fat, saturated fat, and cholesterol.

- Choose a diet with plenty of vegetables, fruits, and grain products.

- Choose a diet moderate in sugars.

- Choose a diet moderate in salt and sodium.

- Children and adolescents should not drink alcoholic beverages.

The Dietary Guidelines suggest at least the following number of servings from each of these food groups:

Vegetables	3-5 servings
Fruits	2-4 servings
Breads, cereals, rice, and pasta	6-11 servings
Milk, yogurt and cheese	2-3 servings*
Meats, poultry, fish, dried beans and peas, eggs, and nuts	2-3 servings

* People aged 12 through 24 years should have three or more servings daily of foods rich in calcium.

by Judith E. Foulke

Judith Foulke is a staff writer for FDA Consumer.

Chapter 7

On the Teen Scene: Should You Go On A Diet?

What do the hula hoop, "grapefruit diet," and wearing your clothes backwards have in common? They are all fads. Fads come and go, but when it comes to fad diets, the health effects can be permanent—especially for teenagers. Not all teens who go on diets need to lose weight. Pressure from friends—and sometimes parents—to be very slim may create a distorted body image. Having a distorted body image is like looking into a funhouse mirror: You see yourself as fatter than you are.

A national survey of 11,631 high school students conducted by the National Centers for Disease Control and Prevention found that more than a third of the girls considered themselves overweight, compared with fewer than 15 percent of the boys. More than 43 percent of the girls reported that they were on a diet—and a quarter of these dieters didn't think they were overweight. The survey found that the most common dieting methods used were skipping meals, taking diet pills, and inducing vomiting after eating.

"The teenage years are a period of rapid growth and development," points out Ronald Kleinman, M.D., chief of the Pediatric Gastrointestinal and Nutrition Unit of Massachusetts General Hospital in Boston, and chairman of the Committee on Nutrition of the American Academy of Pediatrics. He explains that fad dieting can keep teenagers from getting the calories and nutrients they need to grow properly and that dieting can retard growth. Stringent dieting may cause

(FDA) 94-1214

girls to stop menstruating, and will prevent boys from developing muscles, he says. If the diet doesn't provide enough calcium, phosphorus and vitamin D, bones may not lay down enough calcium to help reduce the risk of osteoporosis later in life.

Instead of dieting because "everyone" is doing it or because you are not as thin as you want to be, first find out from a doctor or nutritionist whether you are carrying too much weight or too much body fat for your age and height.

What if You Need to Lose Weight?

The flip side to feeling pressured to be thin is having legitimate concerns about overweight that adults dismiss by saying, "It's just baby fat" or "You'll grow into your weight." Most girls reach almost their full height once they start to menstruate, notes Kleinman. Although boys usually don't stop growing until age 18, data from a study suggest that adolescent obesity can carry serious lifelong health consequences for them.

The study, which followed the medical histories of 508 people from childhood to age 70, found that men who had been overweight teenagers were more likely to develop colon cancer and to suffer fatal heart attacks and strokes than their thinner classmates. Women who had been overweight teens had an increased tendency to develop clogged arteries (atherosclerosis) and arthritis. By age 70, these problems made it difficult for them to walk more than a quarter mile, lift heavy objects, or climb stairs.

While this study linked adolescent obesity to health problems decades down the road, some adverse effects show up much earlier. Sometimes teens develop high blood pressure, elevated cholesterol, and conditions that often precede diabetes. Also, as Kleinman points out, "The longer you remain overweight, the greater the likelihood that the problem will persist into adulthood."

As with most everything else, there's a right way and a wrong way to lose weight. The wrong way is to skip meals, resolve to eat nothing but diet bread and water, take diet pills, or make yourself vomit. You may make it through the end of the week and maybe even lose a pound or two, but you're unlikely to keep the weight off for more than a few, months—if that. And inducing vomiting can lead to an eating disorder called bulimia, which can result in serious health problems.

(See "On the Teen Scene: Eating Disorders Require Medical Attention" in the March 1992 FDA Consumer.)

"The more you deprive yourself of the foods you love, the more you will crave those foods. Inevitably, you'll break down and binge," says Jo Ann Hattner, a clinical dietitian at Packard Children's Hospital in Palo Alto, Calif. Then you'll not only gain those pounds back, you'll likely add a couple more.

Experts call this cycle of weight loss and weight gain "yo-yo" dieting, and believe that the repeated stress on your body of losing and gaining weight may be at least as bad for long-term health as being overweight.

Additionally, low-calorie diets that allow only a few types of foods can be bad for your health because they don't allow you to get enough vitamins and minerals. Kleinman warns that rapid weight loss from very low-calorie "starvation diets" can cause serious effects in teenagers, such as gallstones, hair loss, weakness, and diarrhea.

Diet Pills

Last year, FDA banned 111 ingredients in over-the-counter (OTC) diet products—including amino acids, cellulose, and grapefruit extract—after manufacturers were unable to prove that they worked.

A number of products (Cal-Ban 3000, Cal-Lite 1000, Cal-Trim 5000, Perma Slim, Bodi Trim, Dictol 7 Plus, Medi Thin, Nature's Way, and East Indian Guar Gum) were also recalled because they posed serious health risks. The products contained guar gum, which supposedly swelled in the stomach to provide a feeling of fullness. However, the swelling from the guar gum caused blockages in the throat and stomach.

In May 1991, FDA also began a formal inquiry into the safety of phenylpropanolamine hydrochloride (abbreviated PPA), an ingredient in many OTC diet pills, because of concern that the drug may increase the risk of stroke when taken at or over recommended doses. FDA has determined that additional studies need to be done to resolve this safety concern.

Previously, an advisory review panel of outside experts in 1982 advised FDA that PPA was an effective appetite suppressant. But questions remain about PPA use by teenagers and those with eating disorders.

Recently, manufacturers of OTC diet pills proposed a voluntary program in which they would include on the product labels a statement cautioning: "Persons between 12 and 18 are advised to consult their physician before using this product."

Michael Weintraub, M.D, a consultant to FDA's Office of OTC Drug Evaluation, says, "PPA is not recommended for use by teenagers because they are still growing and if they suppress their appetite, they may not get proper nutrition." The author of studies on PPA published in scientific journals, Weintraub adds, "This is especially true of teens who don't need to lose weight but think that they do."

The Real Skinny on Weight Loss

If going to extremes won't do the trick, what will? Believe it or not, it's as simple as making a few changes in your eating habits to emphasize healthy foods and exercise—good advice even if you don't need to lose weight.

Hattner describes a good diet as one that has balance, variety and moderation in food choices. "Balance your favorite foods [which are usually high in fat] with fruits and vegetables [which are almost always very low in fat]; eat a wide variety of foods to keep from getting bored and to make sure your diet is nutritionally sound; and keep portion sizes reasonable so that you can have your [thin] slice of cake and lose weight, too."

In devising a healthy diet, Hattner suggests using the U.S. Department of Agriculture's "Food Pyramid." These guidelines call for six to 11 servings a day of grains (bread, cereal, rice and pasta), three to five servings of vegetables, two to four servings of fruit, and two to three servings each of dairy (milk, cheese and yogurt) and protein-rich foods (meat, eggs, poultry, fish, dry beans, and nuts). (See "The Food Pyramid-Food Label Connection" in the June 1993 FDA Consumer.)

"Teens who need to lose weight should limit the number of recommended servings to the lower end of the scale for each category except dairy," Hattner advises. "The most important dietary change you can make is to limit the amount of high-fat foods that you eat," she adds.

To keep fat intake down, Hattner recommends making simple lower fat substitutions for the foods that you eat: Switch to 1 percent or skim milk instead of whole milk, nonfat frozen yogurt sweetened with a low-calorie sugar substitute instead of ice cream, pretzels instead of corn chips. High-fat foods such as french fries, candy bars, and milkshakes that have no low-fat substitutes should only be eaten once in a while or in very small amounts.

Move It and Lose It

Whether you are overweight or not, regular exercise (at least three times a week) is important to look and feel your best. If you do need to lose weight, stepping up your activity level will cause you to burn calories more quickly and help make weight loss easier.

"Exercise increases lean body weight. Also, you will appear slimmer as you develop your muscles because muscles give shape and form to your body," notes Hattner.

Fad or starvation diets and diet pills offer temporary solutions, at best. At worst, they may jeopardize your health. To lose weight and keep it off, your best bet is to reduce fat intake and to exercise.

by Ruth Papazian

Ruth Papazian is a writer in Bronx, N.Y.

Chapter 8

All About Eating for Two: Diet and Pregnancy

The nutritional needs of women differ not only from those of men, but they also vary at different times during a women's life. This article discusses how pregnancy and lactation affect a woman's nutritional needs.

"Pickles and ice cream" conjures up a picture of a woman whose pregnancy has caused her food preferences to become a bit offbeat.

Although the tastes of mothers-to-be usually run along far more normal lines, the "pickles and ice cream" image is accurate in portraying the food cravings—and aversions—that sometimes accompany pregnancy. These tastebud changes often reflect changes in nutritional needs.

Such changes are partly due to the nourishment demands of the fetus and partly to other physiological variations that affect absorption and metabolism of nutrients. These changes help insure normal development of the baby and fill the subsequent demands of lactation, or nursing.

Exactly how nutrients are exchanged between mother and fetus is not understood. In the past it was viewed as a host-parasite relationship, with the fetus in the role of the parasite, taking whatever nourishment it required from the host mother. But recent research has shown that the fetus is not a perfect parasite. The fetus is sometimes more affected than the mother by lack of nourishment, and there is a relationship between maternal weight gain and growth and development of the fetus.

DHHS Publication No. (FDA) 90-2183

Pedro Rosso, M.D., of Columbia University's Institute of Human Nutrition, wrote in *Nutritional Disorders of American Women* that "contrary to the idea of fetal parasitism, there seem to be feedback mechanisms operating in the mother that would reduce the maternal supply line to the fetus when nutrients are in short supply."

Writing in *Nutritional Impacts on Women*, two English researchers, Frank E. Hytten, M.D., and Angus Thomson, said that changes in nutritional needs in pregnancy appear to be related to the body's adaptation to pregnancy because the changes occur too early to be responding solely to fetal needs. Such changes include a reduction of electrolytes, proteins, glucose, vitamin B_{12}, folate, vitamin B_6, and a rise in lipids, triglycerides, and cholesterol in blood.

The consequences of maternal malnourishment may include health problems for the mother and an infant of low birth weight who may have nutritional and other deficiencies.

Nutrients for the fetus come from the mother's diet, stored nutrients in the mother's bones and tissues, and synthesis of certain nutrients in the placenta. The placenta facilitates the transfer of nutrients, hormones, and other substances from mother to fetus.

According to a booklet by Roslyn B. Alfin-Slater, Ph.D., titled *Nutrition and Motherhood*, if the mother is poorly nourished, the placenta does not perform its functions as well.

Recommendations for Vitamins and Minerals

The Food and Nutrition Board of the National Academy of Sciences specifies certain increases in the Recommended Daily Dietary Allowances (RDAs) for pregnant and lactating women (see chart). More iron is needed not only because of fetal demands, but also because the mother's blood volume may be increased as much as 30 percent. Because the additional requirement for iron cannot be met by the usual American diet nor by existing stores in many women, iron supplements of 30 to 60 milligrams under supervision of a health-care professional are recommended.

The main effect of inadequate iron during pregnancy is iron deficiency anemia, which makes the mother less able to fight off an infection and less able to tolerate hemorrhaging during childbirth. It has been suggested that pica, the craving for substances with little or no nutritional value, may be associated with iron deficiency. Although pica occurs during pregnancy in a number of ethnic groups and geographic areas, in this country it is most prevalent among southern blacks. The most common substances eaten are dirt, clay, starch, and ice. The National Research Council has noted that as many as 75 percent of the pregnant women attending southern health department clinics consumed starch and 50 percent ate clay. Concerns about the practice are several. First, eating these substances may take the place of eating nutritionally adequate food. Second, some pica substances, such as starch, are high in calories and may contribute to obesity. Third, some pica substances (such as charcoal, air fresheners, and mothballs) contain toxic substances. Fourth, the chemical makeup of some of these substances interferes with the absorption of minerals. Although it is not known whether anemia is the cause of or the effect of pica, the craving abates when the anemia is corrected.

To a certain extent, Mother Nature lends a hand in pregnancy by improving iron absorption. A woman who is not pregnant absorbs about 10 percent of the iron present in food consumed. A pregnant woman, however, can absorb up to twice as much. In addition, the fetus stores iron during the last month or two of gestation. Some good sources of iron are meat (especially liver and other organs), egg yolks, and legumes.

Pregnancy doubles a woman's need for folate (folic acid or folacin). Women can get additional folate by eating more green leafy vegetables, certain fruits, and liver and other organ meats. Severe folate deficiency can result in a condition called megaloblastic anemia, which occurs most often in the last trimester of pregnancy. In this condition the mother's heart, liver and spleen may become enlarged, and the life of the fetus may be threatened.

Because folic acid is crucial to cell multiplication, the fetus's needs are met before those of the mother. Therefore, the mother's health is more adversely affected at first. In contrast to the increased absorption of iron in pregnancy, folic acid absorption may be impaired by hormonal changes in pregnancy.

Pregnant women also have an increased need for vitamin B_6 and B_{12}. B_6 requirements usually can be met by eating more whole grains, milk, egg yolks, and organ meats. Vitamin B_{12} is found in foods of animal origin, including eggs and milk products. Because B_{12} occurs only in such foods, vegetarians who eat no eggs or cheese (vegans) should ask their health-care professionals about the necessity of B_{12} supplements. Severe vitamin B_{12} deficiency in pregnancy is rare.

A word about using vitamin and mineral supplements in pregnancy: If taken, they should be at about RDA levels. Large doses of vitamins and minerals should be avoided. In animal studies, megadoses of vitamins A and D have resulted in fetal defects. The same is likely to be true in humans.

Pregnant adult women need an extra 400 milligrams of calcium daily. That's about 50 percent more than recommended for women 25 and older. Nearly all of the extra calcium goes into the baby's bones. This need can usually be met by consuming more dairy products. If there is not enough calcium in the mother's diet, the fetus may draw calcium from the mother's bones. Calcium deficiency in pregnancy may result in osteopenia (decreased bone density) in the mother.

Nature also helps supply the extra calcium needed in pregnancy by improving calcium absorption. Less is lost in urine and feces, and passage of calcium through the placenta to the fetus is facilitated.

A pregnant woman needs three or more servings of milk or other dairy products a day to get 1,200 milligrams of calcium. For women who are lactose intolerant, there are a variety of low-lactose and re-duced-lactose food products available. Sometimes calcium supplements are recommended by a woman's doctor. But pregnant women should not take calcium supplements such as bone meal and dolomite. FDA surveys have shown that some bone meal and dolomite products contain substantial amounts of lead. Lead can be harmful to both mother and fetus.

Weight Gain

Attitudes have changed about weight gain in pregnancy. In the past, pregnant women were told to limit gain to about 15 pounds. Higher weight gain was thought to be related to a number of prob-lems. The most worrisome of these problems was toxemia (also called Pregnancy Induced Hypertension—PIH), a condition of unknown ori-gin occurring after the twentieth week of pregnancy and involving high blood pressure and protein in the urine or water retention or both. Although sudden large weight gain, water retention, and blood pressure elevation continue to be recognized danger signs of toxemia, most physicians have come to agree that weight gain does not cause toxemia. The consequences of restricting weight gain, in fact, appear to be potentially more harmful, particularly to the fetus, than unre-stricted weight gain, even in women who are overweight before be-coming pregnant.

If a woman's calorie intake is restricted in pregnancy, she may not get enough protein, vitamins and minerals to adequately nourish her unborn child. Low-calorie intake can result in a breakdown of stored fat in the mother, leading to the production of substances called ketones in her blood and urine. The production of ketones is a sign of starvation or a starvation-like state. Chronic production of ketones can result in a mentally retarded child.

For these reasons, the National Academy of Sciences recommends that pregnant women eat an average of 150 calories more per day in the first trimester and 350 calories more per day in the two subsequent trimesters than they did before becoming pregnant. A total weight gain of about 25 to 30 pounds is usually recommended, with the actual pattern of gain considered more important than the number of pounds. Weight gain should be at its lowest during the first trimester, and should steadily increase, with the mother-to-be gaining the most weight in her third trimester, when the fetus and placenta are growing the most.

The effects of undernutrition on infant size is greatest when nutritional deprivation occurs during the final three months. Weight gain in the second trimester is due mostly to increases in tissue, blood volume, and fat stores, and enlargement of the uterus (womb) and breasts.

Arthur Alfin-Slater estimates that a 25-pound weight gain breaks down as follows: baby, 8 pounds; placenta, 1 pound; amniotic fluid, 1.5 pounds; breasts, 3 pounds; uterus, 2.5 pounds; and stored fat and protein, water retention, and blood volume, 8 pounds.

Along with increased total calories, pregnant women need high-quality protein daily, the approximate amount contained in two large eggs and 2 ounces of cheese or a 4-ounce serving of meat.

During pregnancy, fat deposits may increase by more than a third the total amount a women had before she became pregnant. Most women lose this extra weight in the birth process or within several weeks thereafter. Breast-feeding helps to deplete the fat deposited during pregnancy. A woman who breast-feeds expends 600 to 800 more calories than one who doesn't. The woman who nurses her baby also has increased needs for specific nutrients (see chart).

The extra 600 to 800 calories a day includes both the nutritive value of the milk produced as well as the energy needed to synthesize the milk from lactose, protein and fat. Severely undernourished women produce less milk. However, obese women produce the same amount of milk as those of average weight. The amount of vitamins in human milk, particularly water-soluble vitamins such as C and the B complex, is closely related to that in the mother's diet. The concentrations of trace elements such as copper and fluoride, and of fat-soluble vitamins, seem to be less dependent on the fluctuations in maternal eating habits.

Restricting Sodium and Sugar

Pregnancy is a natural, healthy state, and most changes in pregnant women occur without harmful effects. But some physiological changes have been topics of particular medical concern. In past years, the tendency of pregnant women to retain water has led to restriction of sodium intake. When water retention was severe, diuretics were frequently prescribed to avoid toxemia. However, views on sodium restriction have changed. Today, there is considerable medical opinion that pregnancy is a "salt-wasting" condition—that is, one in which the body can use more salt than usual. Further, sodium deprivation may be harmful to the fetus. The sodium intake usually recommended in pregnancy is 2,000 to 8,000 milligrams a day, compared to the normally recommended 1,100 to 3,300 milligrams per day. However, pregnant women should be careful that their sodium intake does not greatly exceed this allowance.

Sugar is also an occasional concern in pregnancy. Virtually all women excrete more glucose (a form of sugar) in their urine when they are pregnant. This is one of the normal physiological adjustments to pregnancy and is not a cause for concern in the majority of women. It is significant only in the few women who have a tendency towards diabetes and who may thus become diabetic during pregnancy.

Diabetic women should be closely monitored to make sure their blood sugar values are at or near normal. If maternal blood sugar rises too high, the increased sugar crossing the placenta can result in a large, overdeveloped fetus and an infant with blood sugar level abnormalities. Diabetic women may also suffer from a greater loss of some nutrients.

Nausea in early pregnancy is another condition that often can be managed nutritionally. Dr. Alfin-Slater's booklet suggests the following:

* Keep meals small, and avoid long periods without food.

* Drink fluids between, but not with, meals.

* Avoid foods that are greasy, fried or highly spiced.

Current Research into Diet and Fetal Development

Improvements in the technological ability to diagnose birth defects early in pregnancy have focused attention on ways to correct certain fetal defects by manipulating the mother's diet. For example, researchers are investigating the use of vitamin-mineral supplements to prevent neural tube defects—that is, failure of the fetus's neural tube to close because of spinal cord abnormalities. Other investigators are researching ways maternal nutrition can help fetuses with inherited birth defects, usually inborn errors of metabolism, in which certain nutrients are not processed normally.

The effects of a woman's diet on her children start long before she becomes pregnant. Stores of fat, protein, and other nutrients built up over the years are called upon during pregnancy for fetal nourishment.

According to Roy M. Pitkin, M.D., of the University of Iowa College of Medicine, in *Nutritional Impacts on Women*, pre-pregnant weight and pregnancy weight exert independent and added influences on the infant's birth weight.

To what extent pregnancy affects a woman long after she has given birth is another subject under investigation. FDA's Jean Pennington, Ph.D., says it is known that a woman who has a large number of children may deplete calcium stores. Walter H. Glinsmann, M.D., chief of FDA's clinical nutrition branch, counsels that having babies should be considered a major life effort that begins long before conception.

"Getting pregnant is like running a race," Dr. Glinsmann says. "You have to get yourself in condition."

Recommended Daily Dietary Allowances for Women (Revised 1989)

From the Food and Nutrition Board of the national Academy of Sciences / Nutritional Research Council

Fat-Soluble Vitamins

Age (years)	Weight (lbs.)	Height (inches)	Protein (g)	Vit. A (mcg)	Vit. D (mcg)	Vit. E (mg)	Vit. K (mcg)
11-14	101	62	46	800	10	8	45
15-18	120	64	44	800	10	8	55
19-24	120	65	44	800	10	8	60
25-50	120	64	44	800	5	8	65
Pregnant			60	800	10	10	65
Lactating							
1st 6 months			65	1300	10	12	65
2nd 6 months			62	1200	10	11	65

Water-Soluble Vitamins

Age (years)	Weight (lbs.)	Height (inches)	Vit.C (mg)	Thiamine (mg)	Riboflavin (mg)	Niacin (mg)	Vit.B$_6$ (mg)	Folate (mcg)	Vit.B$_{12}$ (mcg)
11-14	101	62	50	1.1	1.3	15	1.4	150	2.0
15-18	120	64	60	1.1	1.3	15	1.5	180	2.0
19-24	120	65	60	1.1	1.3	15	1.6	180	2.0
25-50	120	64	60	1.1	1.3	15	1.6	180	2.0
Pregnant			70	1.5	1.6	17	2.2	400	2.2
Lactating									
1st 6 months			95	1.6	1.8	20	2.1	280	2.6
2nd 6 months			90	1.6	1.7	20	2.1	260	2.6

Minerals

Age (years)	Weight (lbs.)	Height (inches)	Cal- cium (mg)	Phos- phorus (mg)	Mag- nesium (mg)	Iron* (mg)	Zinc (mg)	Iodine (mcg)	Sele- nium (mcg)
11-14	101	62	1200	1200	280	15	12	150	45
15-18	120	64	1200	1200	300	15	12	150	50
19-24	120	65	1200	1200	280	15	12	150	55
25-50	120	64	800	800	280	15	12	150	55
Pregnant			1200	1200	320	30	15	175	65
Lactating									
1st 6 months			1200	1200	355	15	19	200	75
2nd 6 months			1200	1200	340	15	16	200	75

* The increased requirement during pregnancy cannot be met by the iron content of typical American diets nor by the existing iron stores of many women; therefore, the use of 30 to 60 mg of supplemental iron is recommended. Iron needs during lactation are not substantially different from those of non-pregnant women, but continued supplementation for mothers of two to three months after parturition is advisable to replenish stores depleted by pregnancy.

Key:
g = grams
mcg = micrograms
mg = milligrams

by Judith Levine Willis

Judith Levine Willis is editor of *FDA Consumer*.

Chapter 9

Food Facts for Older Adults

Introduction

What should you eat to stay healthy? New information about nutrition seems to come out each day. Often, the information does not address the concerns of older adults. Sometimes the advice is confusing. This bulletin focuses on nutrition topics of particular interest to older adults and gives suggestions on how you can improve your diet by following the Dietary Guidelines for Americans.

The Dietary Guidelines for Americans

- Eat a variety of foods

- Balance the food you eat with physical activity—maintain or improve your weight

- Choose a diet low in fat, saturated fat, and cholesterol

- Choose a diet with plenty of vegetables, fruits, and grain products

- Choose a diet moderate in sugars

- Choose a diet moderate in salt and sodium

- If you drink alcoholic beverages, do so in moderation

U.S. Department of Agriculture, Human Nutrition Service Home and Garden Bulletin No. 251 (April, 1993)

135

Sorting out information on nutrition, figuring out what it means for you personally, and making changes in how you eat are well worth the effort. What you eat may affect your risk for several of the leading causes of death in the United States, such as coronary heart disease, stroke, diabetes, and some types of cancer. More importantly, healthy eating and regular exercise can give you the energy and strength to enjoy an active, independent lifestyle as long as possible.

Americans of all ages need to eat healthier. Making changes doesn't have to be difficult. You don't have to give up your favorite foods or stop eating out. With some basic information and a look at your current eating habits, you can begin to make gradual changes that can help you improve or maintain your health.

This chapter provides information and suggestions that can help you follow the guidelines, including—

1. Facts about fat, cholesterol, and sodium;

2. A discussion of the special needs of older adults, including getting enough nutrients, fluids, and fiber, and precautions when taking medications;

3. Tips on making healthy food choices when you shop and cook;

4. How to maintain a healthy weight

5. Questions older people ask about nutrition

6. A roundup of tips and recipes for preparing foods Dietary Guidelines style; and

7. A list of resources for more information.

Please note that this information is for people who are generally in good health. If your doctor has prescribed a special diet for you because of a health condition, follow that advice. However, this chapter will help you better understand current nutrition information and may raise questions for you to discuss with your doctor or dietitian about your special nutrition needs.

What You Should Know About Fat, Cholesterol and Sodium

Every day you hear some news items about fat, cholesterol or sodium. What should you know about them, and what should you do about them when making food choices?

Some Facts About Fat and Cholesterol

Fats are the most concentrated source of food energy (calories). Fats are mixtures of three kinds of fatty acids—saturated, monounsaturated and polyunsaturated. A fat that contains a lot of saturated fatty acids is usually firm, like butter or lard. Some vegetable fats like coconut oil, palm kernel oil and palm oil are also high in saturated fatty acids. Vegetable oils such as olive oil, canola oil, corn oil or soybean oil contain a lot of monounsaturated and polyunsaturated fatty acids. When vegetable oils are hydrogenated to form solid shortenings or margarine, some of the unsaturated fatty acids become saturated, and the fat becomes firm.

Did You Know?

Some fat is necessary in the diet. It provides energy, helps your body absorb vitamins such as A, D and E, and provides essential fatty acids needed by everyone in small amounts. Fat also helps make food taste good, providing flavor, aroma and texture.

Cholesterol is a fatlike substance found in almost all your body cells. Your body can make it, but it also comes from the food you eat. Cholesterol is present in all animal foods—meat, poultry, fish, dairy products, and egg yolks. Both the cholesterol that comes from your food (dietary cholesterol) and the cholesterol made by your body circulate in your blood (blood cholesterol). Cholesterol is used by your body to make hormones, substances needed for digestion, and new cells.

Why Be Concerned About Fat and Cholesterol?

If you have a high blood cholesterol level, you have a greater chance of having a heart attack or a stroke. Eating too much saturated fat, cholesterol, and too many calories can increase your blood cholesterol. A diet containing too much total fat and too many calories may increase your risk for certain cancers.

The way diet affects blood cholesterol varies among individuals. However, blood cholesterol does increase in most people when they eat a diet high in saturated fat and cholesterol and excessive in calories. Of these, dietary saturated fat has the greatest effect; dietary cholesterol has less.

Should You Be Concerned?

A blood cholesterol level of 200 mg/dl or less is considered desirable for adults. The relation of blood cholesterol to the risk for heart disease is less clear in older adults than in middle-aged people. However, heart disease is still the number one cause of death in older Americans, both men and women. Smoking, high blood pressure, diabetes, lack of exercise, heredity, and being overweight are other risk factors. If you don't know what your blood cholesterol level is, ask your doctor to check it the next time you go for a visit. Your doctor can help you evaluate your risk and determine whether your cholesterol level is too high. Your doctor can also explain the different kinds of blood cholesterol (HDL and LDL), triglycerides, and other blood lipids and explain how they affect your risk for heart disease.

Most of us eat too much fat. Even if your blood cholesterol level is not high, you may want to make some changes in your food choices to reduce the amount of fat and saturated fat you eat. If you're like most Americans, 36 percent of your calories come from fat. A diet with 30 percent or less of calories from total fat (**and** less than 10 percent of calories from saturated fat) would be healthier. Reducing fat may help you control your weight if necessary. This is important because obesity increases your risk for high blood pressure, stroke, high blood cholesterol, and diabetes and also aggravates arthritis by putting added stress on your joints.

Did You Know?

Fat is not the same as cholesterol. Some foods contain a lot of cholesterol, but are low in fat, like liver; and some foods have no cholesterol, but are high in fat, like nondairy creamers, vegetable oil or margarine. A food that says "no cholesterol" can still be high in fat. Read the label to see how much and which kinds of fats are included in the product before you buy it.

All types of fat have the same number of calories—both butter and margarine have about 36 calories per teaspoon. So, go easy on all fats and foods made with a lot of fat.

Easy Ways To Cut Fat, Saturated Fat, and Cholesterol in Your Diet

At the Store:

- Choose lean cuts of meat, such as beef round, loin, sirloin, pork loin chops, and roasts

- Consider fish and poultry as alternatives; they are somewhat lower in saturated fat.

- Buy lowfat versions of dairy products.

- Read the food label and choose those foods that are lower in fat, saturated fat, and cholesterol.

At the Table:

- Use less of all fats and oils, especially saturated fats such as butter, cream, sour cream, and cream cheese.

- Try reduced-calorie salad dressings—they are usually low in fat.

- As a beverage, gradually replace whole milk with 2 percent fat milk, then 1 percent fat or skim milk.

In the Kitchen:

- When cooking, replace saturated fats such as butter and lard with small amounts of polyunsaturated and monounsaturated fats in vegetable oils such as corn oil, soybean oil, olive oil, peanut oil, or canola oil.

- Broil, roast, bake, steam, or boil foods instead of frying them, or try stirfrying with just a little fat.

- Trim all visible fat from meats before cooking and remove the skin from poultry.

- Spoon off fat from meat dishes after they are cooked.

- Use skim milk or lowfat milk when making "cream" sauces, soups, or puddings.

- Substitute lowfat yogurt or whipped lowfat cottage cheese for sour cream and mayonnaise in dips and dressings.

- Substitute two egg whites for each whole egg in recipes for most quick breads, cookies, and cakes. (The cholesterol and fat are in the yolk, not in the white.)

- Try lemon juice, herbs, or spices to season foods instead of butter or margarine.

Some Facts About Sodium

Sodium occurs naturally in most foods. It is also added to many foods and beverages, usually as salt. One teaspoon of salt contains about 2,000 milligrams of sodium. The body needs sodium to maintain normal blood volume and for the nerves and muscles. But, populations with diets high in salt have more high blood pressure, a condition that increases your risk for heart attack, stroke, and kidney disease. People with high blood pressure are usually advised to restrict their salt and sodium. It is also important to maintain a healthy weight, exercise regularly, and stay on your medication.

No one can predict who will develop high blood pressure, but many Americans eat more sodium than they actually need. Some health authorities suggest that healthy adults try to limit their sodium intake to 2,400 milligrams (mg) a day.

Much of the sodium in the American diet comes from salt added in cooking or at the table. The taste for salt is learned—you can "unlearn" it by gradually cutting down on your salt intake. Start by thinking about how much sodium you add every time you use that salt shaker.

Sodium is an ingredient in many foods— even ones that might not taste salty, such as luncheon meats, ready-to-eat cereals, and many mixes and prepared foods at the supermarket. Sodium is found in soy sauce and other prepared sauces and dressings, cured meats, canned soups and vegetables, most cheeses, and many convenience foods such as frozen dinners and casserole mixes.

Did You Know?

Salt substitutes are not for everyone. People who are under medical supervision, particularly for kidney problems, should check with their doctor before using salt substitutes.

Try commercial seasoning blends that are mixtures of spices and herbs without added salt. These, as well as homemade seasoning blends, can be used to flavor foods without adding sodium.

Some Tips on Reducing Sodium in Your Diet:

At the Store:

- Read labels for information on the sodium content.

- Try fresh or plain frozen vegetables and meats instead of those canned or prepared with salt.

- Look for low or reduced sodium or "no-salt added" versions of foods.

In the Kitchen:

- Cook plain rice, pasta, and hot cereals using less salt than the package calls for (try 1/8 teaspoon of salt for two servings). "Instant" rice, pasta, and cereals may contain salt added by the processor.

- Adjust your recipes, gradually cutting down on the amount of salt. If some of the ingredients already contain salt, such as canned soup or vegetables, you may not need to add any more salt at all.

- Use herbs and spices as seasonings for vegetables and meats instead of salt.

At the Table:

- Taste your food before you salt it. Does it really need more salt? Try one shake instead of two. Gradually cut down on the amount of salt you use. Your taste will adjust to less salt.

Where's the Salt?

The following table will give you an idea of the amount of sodium in different types of food. Individual products vary. Information on food labels can also help you make choices to moderate your sodium intake.

FOOD GROUP	SODIUM, milligrams
Breads, Cereals	
Cooked cereal, rice, pasta, unsalted	trace per ½ cup
Ready-to-eat cereal	100-350 per oz.
Bread	110- 175 per slice
Fruits	
Fruit, fresh, frozen, canned	trace per ½ cup
Vegetables	
Vegetables, fresh or frozen cooked without salt	less than 70 per ½ cup
Vegetables, canned, or frozen with sauce	140-460 per ½ cup
Tomato juice, canned	660 per ¾ cup
Vegetable soup, canned	810 per cup

FOOD GROUP	SODIUM, milligrams
Meat, Poultry, Fish	
Fresh meat, poultry, fish	less than 90 per 3 oz.
Tuna, canned, water pack	300 per 3 oz.
Bologna	580 per 2 oz.
Ham, lean roasted	1,025 per 3 oz.
Milk, Yogurt, Cheese	
Milk	120 per cup
Yogurt	170 per 8 oz.
Natural cheeses, such as Cheddar or swiss	110-275 per 1-1/2 oz.
Process cheeses, such as American or swiss	790 per 2 oz.
Other	
Salad dressing	80-220 per tbsp.
Catsup, steak sauce	180-230 per tbsp.
Soy sauce	1020 per tbsp.
Salt	2,000 per tsp.
Dill pickle	930 per 1 medium
Potato chips, salted	135 per oz.
Corn chips, salted	235 per oz.
Peanuts, roasted in oil, salted	120 per oz.

Summing Up:

It's natural to think about fat, saturated fat, cholesterol, or sodium as separate parts of your diet, but the best idea is to look at your diet as a whole. You can have small amounts of any food as part of a balanced diet. For example, if one of your food choices is relatively high in fat and sodium, such as baked ham, choose low fat and low sodium foods to eat with it, such as fresh or plain frozen vegetables cooked with little salt and seasoned with herbs instead of butter or margarine.

A Food Choice Checkup

Think about your own food choices. Use these quizzes to check your diet for fat and sodium and see where you might begin to make some small changes as suggested in this section.

How do you score on FAT?

How often do you eat—

	Seldom or never	1 to 2 times a week	3 to 5 times a week	Almost daily
1. Fried, deep-fat fried, or breaded foods?	☐	☐	☐	☐
2. Fatty meats, such as sausage, luncheon meats, fatty steaks and roasts?	☐	☐	☐	☐
3. Whole milk, high-fat cheeses, ice cream?	☐	☐	☐	☐
4. Pies, pastries, rich cakes?	☐	☐	☐	☐
5. Rich cream sauces and gravies?	☐	☐	☐	☐
6. Oily salad dressings, mayonnaise?	☐	☐	☐	☐
7. Butter or margarine on vegetables, dinner rolls, toast?	☐	☐	☐	☐

How do you score on SODIUM?

	Seldom or never	1 to 2 times a week	3 to 5 times a week	Almost daily

How often do you—

1. Eat cured or processed meats, such as ham, sausage, frankfurters, and other luncheon meats? ☐ ☐ ☐ ☐

2. Choose canned vegetables or frozen vegetables with sauce? ☐ ☐ ☐ ☐

3. Use frozen TV dinners, entrees, or canned or dehydrated soups? ☐ ☐ ☐ ☐

4. Eat cheese? ☐ ☐ ☐ ☐

5. Eat salted nuts, popcorn, pretzels, corn chips, or potato chips? ☐ ☐ ☐ ☐

6. Add salt to cooking water for vegetables, rice, pasta, or cereals, or add seasoning mixes or sauces containing salt when preparing foods? ☐ ☐ ☐ ☐

7. Salt your food before tasting it? ☐ ☐ ☐ ☐

Take a look at your answers.

Several checks in the last two columns mean you may have a high fat or sodium intake. Perhaps you could use those types of foods less often, or in smaller quantities. Watching your fat and sodium can be a real challenge at certain meals or snacks. See below for ideas on healthful snacks, desserts, and tips for eating out.

145

Special Advice for Older Adults

As you age, health conditions may limit what you can eat. This can make eating a balanced diet more difficult. You may need to pay more attention to getting adequate nutrients and fluids and to achieving and maintaining a healthy weight. You may also need to consider possible interactions between foods and medications.

Meeting Your Nutrient Needs

Until recently, research on nutritional requirements has focused on younger people. No one really knows enough about how nutritional needs change as people age. Researchers believe you need the same variety of foods as younger people, but different quantities of some nutrients. Furthermore, individual health and level of activity differ widely among the older population. The best strategy is to figure out a balanced approach to eating that fits your general health and preferences. Use the food guide on the next page to help you make food choices for a healthy diet.

Use the guide below to help you remember what foods and how much to eat each day. Each of the food groups in the three lower levels of the Pyramid supplies specific vitamins and minerals, so it's important to include them all to get the nutrients you need for good health. Try to have at least the lowest number of suggested servings from each of these food groups every day. The lowest number of servings, with modest amounts of fat and sweets, provides about 1,600 calories—right for many older women. Older men need somewhat more (see chart below). But remember, individual needs vary, depending on your body size, health, and how active you are. If you need more food, eat more from each of these food groups, and go easy on foods from the fats, oils, and sweets group.

A Guide to Daily Food Choices

Fats, Oils, & Sweets
USE SPARINGLY

KEY
☐Fat (naturally occurring   ▧ Sugars
and added)   (added)
These symbols show that fat and added sugars come mostly from fats, oils, and sweets, but can be part of or added to foods from the other food groups as well.

Milk, Yogurt,
& Cheese
Group
2-3 SERVINGS

Meat, Poultry, Fish,
Dry Beans, Eggs,
& Nuts Group
2-3 SERVINGS

Vegetable
Group
3-5 SERVINGS

Fruit
Group
2-4 SERVINGS

Bread, Cereal,
Rice, & Pasta
Group
**6-11
SERVINGS**

What counts as 1 serving?

Breads, Cereals, Rice, and Pasta
1 slice of bread
½ cup of cooked rice or pasta
½ cup of cooked cereal
1 ounce of ready-to-eat cereal

Fruits
1 piece of fruit or melon wedge
¾ cup of juice
½ cup of canned fruit
¼ cup of dried fruit

Vegetables
½ cup of chopped raw or cooked vegetables
1 cup of leafy raw vegetables

Milk, Yogurt, and Cheese
1 cup of milk or yogurt
1-1/2 to 2 ounces of cheese

Meat, Poultry, Fish, Dry Beans, Eggs, and Nuts
2-1/2 to 3 ounces of cooked lean meat, poultry, or fish
Count ½ cup of cooked beans or 1 egg or 2 tablespoons of peanut butter
as 1 ounce of lean meat (about 1/3 serving)

Fats, Oils, and Sweets
LIMIT CALORIES FROM THESE
especially if you need to lose weight

The amount you eat might be more than one serving. For example, a
dinner portion of spaghetti would count as two or three servings of pasta.

Suggested numbers of servings for older adults

Bread group	*6-9
Vegetable group	*3-4
Fruit group	*2-3
Milk group	2
Meat group	2

*Lower numbers of servings are suggested for older women. The higher numbers are suggested for older men.

A Closer Look at Fat and Added Sugars

The small tip of the Pyramid shows fats, oils, and sweets. These
are foods such as salad dressings, cream, butter, margarine, sugars,
soft drinks, candies, and sweet desserts. Alcoholic beverages are also
part of this group. These foods provide calories but few vitamins and
minerals. Most people should go easy on foods from this group.

Some fat or sugar symbols are shown in the other food groups.
That's to remind you that some foods in these groups can also be high
in fat and added sugars, such as cheese or ice cream from the milk
group, or french fries from the vegetable group. When choosing foods
for a healthful diet, consider the fat and added sugars in your choices
from all the food groups, not just fats, oils, and sweets from the Pyramid tip.

Did You Know?

Learning to estimate serving sizes can be helpful in following the guide to food choices on the previous pages. Here are some typical portion sizes:

- a 1/4-inch-thick slice of cooked lean meat or poultry measuring about 3 x 4 inches weighs about 2 ounces.

- a 3-ounce, cooked, lean hamburger patty starts out as 4 ounces or 1/4 pound of raw meat. The cooked patty will measure about 3 inches across and about 1/2 inch thick, about the size of the palm of a woman's hand, or the size of a large mayonnaise far lid.

- a 1-inch cube of hard cheese, like Cheddar or swiss, weighs about 1/3 ounce.

- a cooked chicken breast half, without skin, weighs about 3 ounces.

Of Special Interest for Older Adults—Calcium and Vitamin D

All nutrients are important for good health at any age, but some that have been mentioned in the news lately have special importance for older adults. For example, inadequate calcium has been linked to osteoporosis, a condition in which bones become weak and brittle. The exact cause of osteoporosis is not known. Several nutrients in addition to calcium are involved.

However, many scientists believe that women particularly need to get adequate amounts of calcium throughout life. Milk, yogurt, cheese, and other dairy products are the best sources of calcium. Some dark-green leafy vegetables, canned fish eaten with the bones (canned sardines and salmon), and tofu also provide calcium.

To absorb calcium, your body needs vitamin D. Vitamin D is added to most fluid milk; it can also be made by your skin when exposed to sunlight. Dietary supplements of vitamin D are usually not necessary. Your doctor or dietitian should advise you on your need for additional vitamin D. If they recommend supplements, they should tell you how much you should take. Generally, vitamin D supplements should not exceed the U.S. Recommended Daily Allowance (U.S. RDA) of 400 International Units (IU) per day, because continued use of high doses is harmful. (U.S. RDA's are nutrient standards developed for food product labels by the U.S. Government.)

In addition to getting adequate calcium and vitamin D, it's important to note that moderate exercise that places weight on your bones, such as walking, helps maintain and may even increase bone density and strength in older adults.

Who's at Risk for Osteoporosis?

Anyone can get osteoporosis, but women are at greatest risk, especially white women who are thin, fair-skinned, and small in build. Aging itself, extreme immobility, and genetics, as well as smoking and drinking alcoholic beverages, are believed to contribute to risk for osteoporosis. Loss of calcium from the bones increases in women after menopause, when levels of the hormone estrogen decrease. Estrogen replacement therapy can be prescribed by a doctor to help decrease bone loss after menopause. Because estrogens may have negative side effects in some women, the decision to take estrogen should be made by each woman with the help of her doctor.

How To Get Enough Calcium If You Don't Drink Milk

Milk is the most obvious and popular source of both calcium and vitamin D, but some people don't drink it and need to consider other ways to get calcium. Some people have trouble digesting lactoses, the sugar occurring naturally in milk.

If you have trouble digesting milk—

•   Drink milk that has had lactase added or add it yourself. Lactase is an enzyme that breaks down milk sugar. It can be purchased at many drug stores.

•   Drink only a small amount of milk at a time.

•   Eat yogurt or cheese. Lactose has been partially broken down in these foods.

•   Try cooked foods made with milk such as soups, puddings, or custards.

If you don't like milk, eat more of other foods with calcium, such as—

• foods made with milk or cheese.

• tofu, a soy product that is sometimes made with calcium sulfate (check the label); ½ cup (4 ounces) of tofu made with calcium sulfate has about the same amount of calcium, protein, and fat as 1 cup of whole milk.

• dark-green leafy vegetables, such as kale, collards, and broccoli.

• tortillas made with cornmeal that is fortified with calcium; label may state that the cornmeal is processed with lime, or may list the cornmeal as 'masa harina."

• canned or dried fish with edible bones, such as salmon and sardines.

Should You Take a Vitamin Supplement?

Thirty-seven percent of American adults take a daily multivitamin pill. Some even take extra vitamins and minerals as well, especially vitamin C. Yet most of these supplements are unnecessary for people of any age. A well-balanced diet should provide all of your nutritional needs. High doses of some vitamins, such as A and D, can be harmful. Large amounts of some supplements can upset the natural balance of nutrients normally maintained by the body. Large doses, called megavitamins, containing 10 to 100 times the RDA for a vitamin or mineral, can act like drugs, with potentially serious results.

While researchers continue to learn more about how nutrient requirements change during aging, eating a balanced diet containing foods from each food group (listed on the table above) is the best approach to getting the nutrients you need. Supplements may be beneficial for people who cannot eat a balanced diet or who do not eat enough food, or people who take medicines that interact with nutrients. Before you decide to take a nutritional supplement, discuss it with your doctor or dietitian. If you have specific health problems, or likes and dislikes that greatly limit your food choices, consult a registered dietitian (R.D.) for help in planning the best diet for you.

Drink Enough Fluids

The sense of thirst declines with age, so older people may not drink enough water and other fluids. Sometimes people intentionally drink less to avoid going to the bathroom often. But if you aren't getting enough fluids you can become dehydrated, especially during hot weather.

Drinking plenty of fluids is important to help your body flush out wastes—it's worth a few more trips to the bathroom. Most adults should drink at least eight glasses of water a day. This water can come from any beverage—juice, coffee, tea, milk, or soft drinks—as well as from soup. However, the caffeine in coffee and other drinks may increase your urge to urinate. The sugar in regular soft drinks is an added source of calories you may not need. Plain water, unsweetened fruit juices, and lowfat milk are better choices. Or, for a refreshing carbonated drink, mix fruit juice with club soda or seltzer water. To make plain water more appealing, try it chilled with a twist of lemon or lime.

What About Constipation?

Constipation bothers many older adults. The frequency of bowel movements among healthy people varies from three a day to three a week. Know what is normal for you and avoid relying on laxatives. Drinking enough fluids; eating plenty of fruits, vegetables, and whole grain products for fiber; and exercising regularly can help with this condition.

Prevention of constipation is the best approach:

- Eat foods with dietary fiber, such as whole-wheat breads and cereals, fruits, and vegetables every day.

- Drink plenty of liquids.

- Exercise regularly.

- Go to the bathroom when you feel the need. Don't delay.

Facts About Fiber

Dietary fiber (sometimes called "roughage") is the part of plant foods that humans can't digest. The fiber passes through the intestines, forming bulk for the stool. There are two major types of fiber—insoluble and soluble. Each has different health benefits, so both are needed in the diet. Insoluble fiber is most often found in whole-grain products, such as whole-wheat bread and cereals, fruits and vegetables with their peels, and dry beans and peas. Insoluble fiber helps prevent constipation. Diets high in insoluble fiber and low in fat may also reduce your risk of colon cancer.

Soluble fiber is found in fruits, vegetables, dry beans and peas, and some cereal products such as oatmeal, oat bran, and rice bran. Some research indicates that diets that are low in fat and saturated fat and rich in soluble fiber may help reduce blood cholesterol levels.

How Much Fiber Should You Eat?

It isn't clear yet exactly how much fiber you should eat each day. Some health experts have suggested that an increase to a range of 20 to 30 grams is a good idea. That's about twice what the average adult eats now. Because plant foods differ in the types and amounts of fiber they contain, it's a good idea to eat different kinds of foods rich in fiber. You can get about 20 grams of fiber if you eat three servings of whole-grain foods, two to three servings of fruit, and three to four servings of vegetables daily. You don't need to take fiber supplements or sprinkle bran on all your foods.

Five Quick Tips To Increase Fiber in Your Diet:

- Try a whole-grain breakfast cereal, hot or cold. It doesn't have to be 100-percent bran—look for a cereal with at least 2 grams of dietary fiber per serving.

- Choose baked goods made with whole grains, such as corn muffins; cracked wheat bread; graham crackers; oatmeal bread or muffins; and whole-wheat, pumpernickel or rye breads, rolls, and bagels.

- Eat fresh fruit or stewed fruit—an orange, half a grapefruit, prunes, or apricots—instead of drinking fruit juice.

- Eat fruits and vegetables with their peels— apples, pears, peaches, potatoes, or summer squash.

- Add cooked or canned dry beans, split peas, and lentils to your favorite soups, stews, and salads.

If you're not used to eating foods with fiber, increase fiber gradually to avoid gas or cramping. Be sure to drink enough water or other fluids when you eat more high-fiber foods.

Are You Getting Enough Fiber in Your Diet?

	Seldom or never	1 to 2 times a week	3 to 5 times a week	Almost daily
How often do you eat—				
1. Three or more servings of breads and cereals made with whole grains?	☐	☐	☐	☐
2. Starchy vegetables such as potatoes, corn, peas, or dishes made with dry beans or peas?	☐	☐	☐	☐
3. Several servings of other vegetables?	☐	☐	☐	☐
4. Whole fruit with skins and/or seeds (berries, apples, pears, etc.)?	☐	☐	☐	☐

The best answer is ALMOST DAILY. Whole-grain products, fruits, and vegetables provide fiber. Eating a variety of these foods daily will provide you with adequate fiber, both soluble and insoluble types.

Avoiding Problems When Medications and Foods Don't Mix

Many older adults take several medications, both prescription and over-the-counter types. It's important to find out from your doctor or pharmacist if these medicines are affected by food or beverages. Some medicines must be taken with meals, while others work better on an empty stomach. Some medicines may have serious or unpleasant side effects or may not work as well if taken in combination with certain foods or alcoholic beverages. Writing out a schedule for your meals and medicines can help you take your medicines properly and get adequate nutrition—both are important to your health.

Ask your doctor or pharmacist if there are special instructions about diet and if there are foods you should avoid when taking your medicine. You may need special advice about diet and—

- diuretics and other high blood pressure medicines,

- some antibiotics,

- some pain relievers,

- some antidepressants,

- anticoagulants (drugs for blood thinning),

antacids.

Do You Take Medicines Properly?

When you get a new prescription medicine, be sure you understand **when** to take it, **how much** to take, **how long** to take it, and **what to do** if you miss a dose.

Tell your doctor about any other medicines you may be taking, including those prescribed by other doctors, over-the-counter medicines, and any vitamins or other supplements.

Ask whether there are foods or over-the counter medicines you should not take with your new prescription.

Contact your doctor or pharmacist right away if you experience any side effects. If you are taking several medicines for long periods, ask your doctor every once in a while if you should still be taking all of them. Don't stop taking any prescribed medicines without consulting your doctor.

Make sure you understand the name of the drug and directions printed on the container. Ask your pharmacist to use large type if necessary. If child-proof containers are hard to handle, ask for easy-to-open containers.

Discard old prescription medicines and expired over-the-counter drugs. Never take drugs that were prescribed for a friend or relative, even though your symptoms may be the same.

Planning a Menu Using the Food Guide

The sample menu on the next page shows how you might use the Food Guide Pyramid above. The 1,600-calorie menu includes the lower numbers of servings from the food groups, and the 2,400-calorie menu includes the higher numbers of servings shown in the table above. Jelly, margarine, sherbet, and lemonade are extras, from the Fats, Oils, and Sweets group. Listed below are nutrient values for the two menus:

	1,600 Calorie Menu	2,400 Calorie Menu
Total fat, grams	46	75
% of calories	26	28
Saturated fat. grams	18	24
% of calories	10	9
Cholesterol, mg	185	235
Sodium, mg	2,190	3,010
Dietary fiber, grams	18	30

Ask Yourself...

- Do I eat foods from all the food groups each day?

- Am I getting enough calcium-rich foods?

- Do I need to take a vitamin supplement, or can I add foods to my diet that will provide me with the nutrients I need?

- Have I discussed the vitamins I take with my doctor or a dietitian?

- How much fluid do I drink each day?

- Are these fluids high in calories?

- Do I know how all of the medications I am taking interact with foods or drinks?

Menu

1,600 calories   **2,400 calories**

Breakfast

1,600	Food	2,400
½ medium	Grapefruit	½ medium
2 slices	Whole-wheat toast	2 slices
1 tsp.	Margarine, soft	2 tsp.
None	Jelly	1tbsp.
1 cup	Milk, skim	1 cup

Lunch

1,600	Food	2,400
6 fl. oz.	Vegetable juice, no salt added	6 fl. oz
	Luncheon salad:	
1 oz.	Turkey	2 oz.
1 oz.	Ham	1 oz.
1-1/2 oz.	Swiss cheese	1-1/2 oz.
1-1/2 cups	Mixed greens	1-1/2 cups
1 tbsp.	French dressing, low calorie	1-1/2 tbsp.
2 small	Corn muffins	3 small
1 medium	Peach, fresh	2 medium

Dinner

1,600	Food	2,400
3 oz.	Sirloin steak, broiled (lean only)	3 oz.
½ cup	Yellow corn, fresh or frozen	1 cup
½ cup	Stewed tomatoes, no salt added	½ cup
1 small	Whole-grain roll	2 small
1 tsp.	Margarine, soft	1 tsp.
½ cup	Lime sherbet	½ cup
As desired	Coffee, tea, or water	As desired

1,600 calories		2,400 calories
	Snacks	
None	Peanut butter sandwich 2 slices of whole-wheat bread 2 tbsp. of peanut butter 2 tsp. of jelly	1 sandwich
3 squares	Graham crackers	None
8 fl. oz.	Lemonade	8 fl. oz.

Making Healthy Food Choices When You Shop and Cook

Many older adults who once cooked and shopped for families now find they must adjust their shopping and preparation to fit the appetite of one or two people. Others find themselves on their own in the kitchen or supermarket for the first time. Most are becoming more concerned about calories, fat, and sodium in their diets. Here are some tips on how to manage in an increasingly complex marketplace.

Use Food Labels

Food labels are the best source of specific information about the foods you buy and eat. They can help you choose between similar products. Here is what you need to know:

Ingredients are listed in order by weight, from the largest amount to the least amount.

Check the ingredient list for ingredients you may want to limit, such as salt, saturated fats, or sugars, or those you want to increase, such as whole grains in baked products.

Nutrition information lists calories, protein, carbohydrates, fat, sodium, and various vitamins and minerals contained in a serving of the food. Saturated fat, cholesterol, and dietary fiber may also be listed. Amounts of vitamins and minerals are listed as percentages of the U.S. Recommended Daily Allowances (U.S. RDAs), nutrient standards developed for food product labels by the U.S. Government.

Did You Know?

Food ingredient statements on labels may list different forms of the same ingredient separately. For example, a product may list several forms of sugar, such as sugar, corn syrup, honey or molasses. If several forms are listed, the product probably is high in sugar.

Some Hints on Using the Nutrition Label:

Check the nutrition information for:

- **Serving size**—Is it the amount you usually eat?

- **Amounts of fat and sodium per serving**—Is the fat or sodium high? For a point of reference, compare the amount per serving of the product to the total amounts suggested per day:

  –Fat: Suggested amount is 30 percent of daily calories—53 grams per day for 1,600-calorie diets 80 grams per day for 2,400-calorie diets. For example, a food that provides 20 grams of fat would provide over one third of the day's fat in a 1,600-calorie diet.

  –Sodium: 2,400 mg or less per day is suggested by some health authorities.

- **Amounts of vitamins or minerals** of special interest to you, such as calcium. Look for foods that have a significant amount of the vitamin or mineral (10 percent or more of the U.S. RDA), but not too many calories.

Is It Fresh?

Many products now have **open dating**, which provides information on freshness in several ways:

- the **pull-by** or **sell-by** date tells you when the product should be sold or taken off the shelves by the grocery store.

- **best used by** date is typically found on bakery goods and packaged cereals—it's the last day the product can be expected to be at its peak quality.

- **expiration** or **use by** date, usually on refrigerated products, is the last date the food should be used.

- **pack date** is the date the food was processed or packaged and is usually found on foods like canned goods that have a long shelf life. Be sure not to buy any bulging or leaking cans. The food is unsafe.

These dates tell you how long you can store and use the product. This will be helpful if you can't shop often.

Food Shopping, Dietary Guidelines Style

Whether you are age 7 or 70, you need a variety of foods from each of the food groups. There are many choices available in today's typical supermarket. Here are some food choices that will help you get the variety you need while watching your fat, cholesterol, and sodium intake. Try a few the next time you shop.

Breads, cereals, rice, and pasta:

- whole-wheat, rye, pumpernickel, mixed grain, and enriched breads and rolls, bagels, and english muffins

- whole grain crackers, such as graham crackers, wheat crackers, and rice cakes

- whole-grain breakfast cereals

- plain rice, pasta (cook with less salt)

Fruits:

- fresh fruit

- canned fruit, in juice rather than heavy syrup

- canned or frozen fruit juice, unsweetened

Vegetables:

- fresh leafy vegetables and other vegetables (use within a few days)

- carrots, potatoes, onions (will keep longer)

- frozen vegetables without sauce

- canned vegetables, tomato sauces, and soups; try those with reduced sodium, or no salt added, if available

- dry beans or split peas; canned beans; bean and pea soups.

Meat, poultry, fish:

- fresh, well-trimmed, lean meats—beef round, loin, sirloin, chuck arm; pork loin, roasts, and chops; leg of lamb—(½ pound trimmed boneless raw meat will make about two 3-ounce cooked servings)

- for leaner ground beef, ask the butcher to trim fat off and grind a piece of beef round steak

- fresh chicken, turkey parts; boneless, skinless breasts or thighs

- fresh or plain frozen fish; tuna fish canned in water

- eggs (you may want to buy only a half-dozen)

- peanut butter

Milk, yogurt, cheese:

- lowfat (2 percent or 1 percent) or skim milk

- lowfat or nonfat yogurt, plain or flavored

- part-skim and lowfat cheeses such as mozzarella, ricotta, cottage cheese

- frozen yogurt or ice milk

Spreads and seasonings:

- margarine, with liquid vegetable oil listed as the first ingredient

- vegetable oils, such as canola, olive, corn, and soybean oils, for cooking and salad dressings

- low-calorie mayonnaise and salad dressings

- salt-free herb blends for seasoning

Did You Know?

You can ask the grocer to divide packages of fresh vegetables or eggs and cut smaller portions of meat for you. You don't have to buy more than you can use.

New on the Market—Lower Fat, Lower Sodium, Lower Sugar Products

Many new foods are available to help you choose a diet that is low in fat, sugars, and sodium. One no longer has to go to the dietetic section of the supermarket to find fruits canned in juice instead of heavy syrup, canned vegetables with no salt added, and soups with reduced sodium content. Even frozen dinners come in varieties that are low in fat and sodium. Some manufacturers also have reformulated their baked products and frozen dairy desserts to produce "ice creams", cookies, cakes, and pastries that are nearly fat and cholesterol free.

Low-calorie sweeteners are widely used to sweeten soft drinks, fruit punches, puddings, gelatin desserts, yogurts, frozen dairy desserts, and many other foods. Low-calorie, low-cholesterol fat substitutes processed from egg white and skim milk proteins are used in gourmet-style frozen dairy desserts and may be used in other cold products, such as salad dressings, sour cream, and cheese spreads. Food scientists are developing other heat-stable substances that may partially substitute for fat in frying.

Are fat and sugar substitutes safe? The Food and Drug Administration (FDA) must approve food additives and novel ingredients such as fat and sugar substitutes before they can be used in foods. If you have questions about the safety of a food additive or ingredient, contact the FDA Consumer Affairs Office on the resource list included in this chapter. As always, moderation in use of these products is the best advice. It is not necessary to use products containing fat or sugar substitutes to have a healthy diet.

What's To Eat?—Quick and Easy Meals for One or Two People

Here are some ideas to get you started on making easy and nutritious meals for one or two people:

- Cook once and eat twice, or even three times. Cook a small roast; eat one portion now and freeze additional portions to mix with vegetables for quick soups, stews, or chili.

- Buy frozen vegetables in 1-pound bags. Cook what you need for single or double servings or mix several kinds for an interesting vegetable medley.

- Keep several kinds of pasta on hand. Many cook quickly. Pasta makes an attractive side dish, or it can be used as a base for stews or topped with a lowfat sauce. Make single servings or cook extra to add to soups or casseroles. Mix with vegetables and a lowfat dressing for pasta salad.

- Try a baked fruit for dessert—one or two servings cook quickly in a microwave oven, or bake the fruit along with another food prepared in the oven. Serve warm, with a dash of cinnamon or nutmeg.

Dinner's in the Freezer!

Frozen dinners and entrees are becoming staples in many one and two-person households. They offer convenient, quick-cooking, tasty meals with little waste and clean up. Even if you don't use them regularly, it's nice to have one or two on hand for those times when you just don't feel like cooking. Here are some hints for choosing frozen dinners and entrees and using these foods as part of a healthy diet:

1. **Read the label.** Use the nutrition label, the ingredient label, and even the name and the picture of the product to see what you are getting.

- Read the ingredient label to see what ingredients are present and in what amounts. Products containing cream sauces, cheese, and ground meat are likely to be higher in fat than products made with lean cuts of meat, vegetables, and broth. Oriental-style products containing soy sauce or teriyaki sauce are likely to be higher in sodium.

- Read the nutrition label for the calories, fat, sodium, and other nutrients per serving of the product. Many frozen dinners and entrees are relatively high in sodium or fat, even the low-calorie types.

- When you look at the nutrition label, think how the amount of fat or sodium compares to the amounts that are right for you for the whole day. Also think about what else you will be eating at that meal or that day that can help you moderate your total fat and sodium intake. If you choose a high-fat or high-sodium entree for one meal, make an effort to choose foods low in fat or sodium for the next meal.

- The name and the picture can also provide clues to product composition. For example, "beef dinner" will generally have more beef than "beef with vegetables in sauce." The picture on the package should show the contents of the product too.

2. Decide what else to eat with the frozen dinner or entree. Most frozen dinners or entrees provide only 300 to 500 calories. They usually include about 2 to 2-1/2 ounces of meat, 1 to 1-1/2 servings of vegetables, and less than 1 serving of grain products such as rice or noodles. Large serving types—"for big appetites"—provide somewhat more. If the product is your main meal of the day, you'll probably want to eat something else with it.

Try these easy, healthy additions:

- a large whole-grain roll

- a small salad or ½ cup of frozen vegetables (microwave it along with your dinner in a covered container with 2 teaspoons of water)

- milk as your beverage, or yogurt or milk pudding for dessert

- fresh or canned sliced fruit—which can top the yogurt or pudding

If your frozen dinner or entree is high in fat or sodium, choose lower fat or sodium foods to go with it. Go easy on fatty spreads and dressing, and don't add salt at the table.

3. Make your own frozen meals—it's a great way to use leftovers and save money as well as time. Cook extra when you have time, and divide cooked meat or other main dishes into single portions on a microwave or oven-safe plate. (Plain sliced meat should have a lowfat gravy or other liquid to moisten it.) Add a serving or two of frozen vegetables with 2 teaspoons of water. Cover tightly and freeze promptly. For best quality, use your home-prepared dinners within 2 months.

Focus on Food Safety

Older people are more vulnerable to food-borne illness, so it's important to handle foods safely:

Check your food safety practices.

Do You—

- Always wash hands with warm soapy water before handling food?

- Thaw frozen foods in the refrigerator, not on the kitchen counter? Or thaw them in the microwave, following the oven manufacturer's directions?

- Cook raw meats, poultry, fish and eggs thoroughly?

- Keep hot foods hot and cold foods cold until serving time?

- Refrigerate or freeze leftover foods promptly? Don't let perishable foods sit out at room temperature for more than 2 hours.

For answers to your safety questions, contact:

- a County Extension Home Economist (look in your phone book under county government, Cooperative Extension Service, or your State university)

- USDA's Meat and Poultry Hotline (1-800-535-4555), weekdays, 10-4 Eastern time (in Washington, DC area, call 202-720-3333)

Maintaining a Healthy Weight

Many Americans are overweight. Being overweight can increase your risk for high blood pressure, diabetes, heart disease and certain cancers. Recent research suggests that people can be a little heavier as they grow older without added risk to health, although just how much heavier is not yet clear. Talk with your doctor to determine if your weight is right for you.

As people age, they usually need fewer calories to maintain a healthy weight. Older people may become less active too. Achieving and maintaining a healthy weight should be an ongoing part of caring for your health. If you need to lose some weight, don't try to lose weight too fast and avoid extreme approaches. Remember, quick weight loss plans often deprive the body of important nutrients and usually don't keep weight off.

Be Physically Active

Physical activity can help reduce and control weight by burning up calories and should be part of a healthy lifestyle at any age. Moderate exercise that places weight on your bones, such as walking, helps maintain and possibly even increases bone strength in older adults—another good reason to exercise. Scientists looking into the benefits of exercise for older adults agree that appropriate exercise improves overall health at any age. Regular exercise can improve the functioning of the heart and lungs, increase strength and flexibility, and contribute to a feeling of well-being.

You don't have to jog or do aerobics to benefit from exercise. Any regular physical activity is good. Regular brisk walking is an easy and enjoyable form of exercise that helps control weight, but you will benefit from any form of gentle exercise, even light gardening. Use your common sense to prevent injury when you exercise, and check with your doctor before beginning a vigorous exercise program or if you haven't exercised in a while.

Did You Know?

Starchy foods such as breads, cereals, rice, pasta, corn and potatoes are usually low in fat and provide fiber, as well as vitamins and minerals. Yet many people don't want to eat more breads and potatoes, because they think these foods are fattening. Actually, more calories are likely to come from the fat you put on these foods—butter, sour cream, or gravy—than from the "starch" itself. Eating more starchy foods is a good way to satisfy your appetite while watching your weight. Just go easy on the toppings!

Reduce Calories, Not Vitamins and Minerals

To lose weight you need to reduce the amount of calories you eat. But, you need to do this without giving up important nutrients. A weight reduction diet will be difficult to follow if you always feel hungry. Choosing lowfat foods allows you to cut calories without sacrificing important vitamins and minerals. For example, 1 cup of skim milk has about the same amount of calcium as 1 cup of whole milk, but only traces of fat and half the number of calories. On the other hand, fatty spreads and dressings, sugary foods such as candy or soft drinks, and alcoholic beverages such as beer, wine, and liquors add calories to your diet but little or no nutrients. Limiting your intake of fats, sweets, and alcoholic beverages will help keep the calories in your diet down, without sacrificing nutrients.

Some Advice About Diet Claims and Dieting

Our society's preoccupation with weight loss has created a multi-million-dollar industry that abounds with diet plans and claims. Some diet plans simply don't work at all, and others are harmful. Always seek the advice of your doctor or dietitian before you begin any special diet.

Beware of diets that—

*   make unrealistic promises—for example, dramatic weight loss in a short period of time.

*   include fasting.

*   eliminate one food group completely or include only one or two food groups

*   have a daily caloric intake that exceeds your usual caloric intake.

*   do not allow you to have a favorite food on occasion.

*   include foods that are expensive or difficult to find.

*   require costly fees.

*   do not address changing your eating habits.

The **best advice** for weight loss is not contained in any one diet, but simply follows some common sense ideas:

- Consult your doctor.

- Eat a well-balanced diet with a variety of foods from each food group.

- Make a long-term commitment to healthy eating habits.

- Include regular exercise.

- Create or choose a plan that fits your food preferences.

- Remember that radical changes are hard to make. Instead, begin to modify your intake by eating smaller portions and reducing fat, sugar, and, if you drink, alcoholic beverages.

What If I'm Underweight?

Though discussions of diet usually focus on losing weight, some people have trouble maintaining enough weight. This sometimes happens to older people when they find themselves living alone. People who are underweight are often more susceptible to illnesses and don't recover from them as well as others. If you are concerned about weighing too little, try to—

- eat three balanced meals every day, with foods from each food group.

- increase portion sizes of the foods you eat at each meal.

- try new foods and ingredients to perk up your appetite.

- eat when you feel hungry. Keep healthy snacks handy for munching and don't skip meals.

- try milk, cocoa, or soup instead of coffee and tea, which have few calories.

- add milk, cheeses, and crumb toppings to casseroles, soups, stews, or side dishes.

Food Choice Challenges

Some situations pose special challenges for making healthy food choices, especially snacktime, dessert time, and eating out.

Snacking

Americans, in general, are snackers and often substitute snacks for meals because they are quick and easy. Eating too many snacks that are high in sugar, fat, and salt can add calories without giving you important nutrients you need. On the other hand, nutritious snacks can help you get needed nutrients, especially if you find it easier to eat only small amounts of food at meals.

Ten Ideas for Healthy Snacking

- plain popcorn, without added butter or oil
- whole-grain crackers
- unsalted pretzels
- lowfat yogurt
- lowfat cheeses and spreads
- unsweetened fruit juices
- tomato juice
- fruit slices with peels (for more fiber)
- raw vegetable strips and pieces
- sparkling water flavored with a slice of lemon or lime

Limit the amount of food you eat at snacktime, so you won't be tempted to skip meals. For instance, take several crackers and eat them slowly—don't take a whole box of crackers to munch on. If you need to make your snack a mini-meal, try eating "meal foods"— half a sandwich and a glass of milk or a cup of soup. If you're limiting calories, choose lowfat dairy products and clear soups.

Desserts Can Be Nutritious Too

For many people, desserts are another source of "empty calories"— foods that add a lot of calories without many nutrients. You don't have to cut out desserts; many recipes for baked desserts can be modified to be lower in salt, fat, cholesterol, and sugar. Ingredients with dietary fiber, such as whole grains and dried fruits, can be added too. There are also low-calorie or lower fat substitutes available for ice cream, sour cream, and whipped cream

---

Hints for Reducing Fat, Saturated Fat, Cholesterol, Sugar, and Sodium in Your Baking

For...	Use...
whole egg	2 egg whites
whole milk	skim or lowfat milk
sugar	½ cup of sugar per cup of flour in cakes
	1 tablespoon of sugar per cup of flour in yeast breads
	Hint: when reducing sugar, add more flavoring such as vanilla
baking chocolate, 1 oz.	3 tablespoons of cocoa (if fat is needed, use 1 tablespoon or less of oil)
fat	minimum for muffins and quick breads is 1 to 2 tablespoons of fat per cup of flour
	minimum for cakes is 2 tablespoons of fat per cup of flour
	Hint: soft drop cookies generally contain less fat than rolled cookies

For . . .	Use . . .
sodium	¼ teaspoon of salt per cup of flour in yeast breads; half the amount
	of salt called for in other baked products
	1-1/4 teaspoons of baking powder per cup of flour in muffins, biscuits, waffles
	1 teaspoon of baking powder per cup of flour in cakes
sour cream	lowfat sour cream or yogurt
butter	margarine or vegetable oil (total fat will be the same, but saturated fat and cholesterol will be reduced)

Some Tips for Making Desserts More Nutritious:

TRY—

- fruit breads made with whole-wheat flour.

- fresh fruit, baked or broiled, spiced with cinnamon, nutmeg, or mint.

- pudding made with lowfat milk and less sugar.

- unsweetened fresh fruit topped with lowfat yogurt.

- rolled oat toppings for fruit crisps, instead of flour/sugar/butter crumb toppings.

- cookie recipes with less sugar and fat.

- single-crust pies—try a crust made with 1 cup of graham cracker crumbs and 3 tablespoons of soft margarine.

- ice milk, frozen yogurt, sherbets, sorbet, or flavored ices. When you do eat ice cream, try regular varieties rather than the rich super premium types, which are much higher in fat.

Did You Know?

Sugar means more than just white table sugar. It means all forms of caloric sweeteners, including brown sugar, raw sugar, corn syrup, honey and molasses. All contain calories but relatively few nutrients. It's okay to enjoy a sweet now and then—but if you're trying to cut calories, go easy.

Eating Better When Eating Out

More and more Americans are eating out, and older Americans are no exception. While you can't control the ingredients in the foods you eat in restaurants, you can choose wisely and eat moderate amounts.

The type of restaurant you eat in will determine what choices you can make. For example, cafeterias and buffets offer a variety of foods but no options for ordering foods prepared as you like. And restaurants offering "all-you-can-eat" tempt you to eat too much! Fast-food restaurants also limit your choices because many items are deep-fat fried or contain a lot of sodium. However, many chains now have salad bars, offering a healthful alternative.

The key strategies to eating healthy in a restaurant are watching serving sizes so you don't overeat, choosing items that are low in fat, and asking for alternatives like lowfat milk and margarine when possible.

Some Tips for Eating Healthy at Restaurants:

- Choose steamed, grilled, stirfried, or baked meats and vegetables.

- Limit the amount of fried foods, heavy sauces, and gravies you eat. Choose tomato-based sauces and soups instead of creamed ones.

- Eat bread and potatoes with only small amounts of butter or margarine.

- Order sauces and salad dressings on the side, when possible, and then add them sparingly.

- When portion choices are available, order small or half portions; if they're not available, eat half and take the rest home.

- At the salad bar, limit heavy dressings; go easy on toppings like croutons and cheese and items made with mayonnaise, such as macaroni salad.

- Ask questions about what the menu terms mean if you don't understand them. Some terms can be misleading. If you're unsure, ask how the food is prepared or what the ingredients are.

- Don't be afraid to send something back to the kitchen if it tastes too fatty or salty. After all, you haven't paid for it yet!

- You don't have to skip dessert; split one and you give away half the calories too!

Catching on to Menu Clues

Some terms commonly used in menus can provide clues to higher fat or sodium content.

Some terms can signal lower fat. Foods that are grilled or broiled, stirfried, roasted, poached, or steamed need less fat in preparation than frying. Few terms guarantee low sodium. Even "fresh" or "homemade" foods can be high in sodium depending on their ingredients and the amounts used.

Fast Food on a Lowfat Budget

You can enjoy fast food without eating too many calories, or too much fat or sodium. Just follow these pointers:

The Main Dish:

- Try hamburgers with one regular patty rather than those with two patties, and plain types rather than those with lots of extras like cheese, bacon, or "special" sauces.

- Order roast beef or grilled chicken for a leaner alternative to most burgers or fried chicken.

173

- Breaded, deep-fat fried fish and chicken sandwiches (especially those with cheese, tartar sauce, or mayonnaise) have more fat and calories than a plain burger.

- When fixing your sandwich, load up on lettuce, tomato, and onion, but limit pickles, mustard, catsup, and other sauces. If you're having fried chicken, remove the skin and some of the breading before you eat. Try broiled chicken as an alternative.

On the Side:

- Skip the fries if you're also ordering a main dish that is deep-fried or made with a sauce or cheese.

- Order a small portion of fries rather than a large one.

- Specify no salt when possible and add a small amount yourself.

- Choose a plain baked potato or mashed potatoes instead of fries, and add butter or margarine and salt sparingly.

- Have a tossed salad instead of fries.

- Ask for a dinner roll instead of a biscuit to limit calories and fat.

Salads:

- Load up on fresh greens, fruits, and vegetables.

- Go easy on the dressings and creamy salads such as potato salad, coleslaw, and macaroni or pasta salads.

Beverages:

- Choose milk, preferably skim or lowfat, instead of a soda or shake.

- Be aware that commercially prepared milkshakes often include sodium in their ingredients as well as whole milk and sugar.

- Ask for water if milk isn't available.

Dessert:

- Skip it! Or make it an occasional treat. Many of the dessert items are high in calories, fat, and sugar.

- Choose fresh fruit from the salad bar, if available, as an alternative.

ASK YOURSELF . . .

- Do I exercise regularly?

- What exercise could I add to my activities?

- Have I tried several diets that don't succeed in keeping lost pounds off?

- What common sense practices could I follow to control my weight?

- Do I know the ingredients in my favorite snacks?

- What are my favorite desserts—the ones I eat most frequently?

- How can I change desserts to reduce calories and add nutrients?

- What foods can I eat at snack and dessert times to add nutrients I need to my diet?

- What kinds of restaurants do I eat in? How can I choose healthier foods from the menu?

- Are there other restaurants I can try that allow better choices?

Try these recipes for desserts and snacks

Pumpkin Cupcakes

Try these cupcakes unfrosted for a nutrient-plus desert. The pumpkin is high in vitamin A and the raisins add iron.

24 cupcakes

Per cupcake:

Calories	140
Total fat	5 grams
Saturated fatty acids	1 gram
Cholesterol	27 milligrams
Sodium	130 milligrams

Whole wheat flour	1-1/2 cups
All-purpose flour	1 cup
Sugar	¾ cup
Baking powder	2 tablespoons
Ground cinnamon	2 teaspoons
Ground nutmeg	½ teaspoon
Salt	¼ teaspoon
Eggs, slightly beaten	3
Skim milk	1 cup
Vegetable oil	½ cup
Canned pumpkin	1 cup
Raisins- chopped	¾ cup
Vanilla	1 tablespoon

1. Preheat oven to 350°F.
2. Place 24 paper baking cups in muffin tins.
3. Mix dry ingredients thoroughly.
4. Mix remaining ingredients; add to dry ingredients. Stir until dry ingredients are barely moistened.
5. Fill paper cups two-thirds full.
6. Bake about 20 minutes or until toothpick inserted in center comes out clean.
7. Remove from muffin tins and cool on rack.
8. Freeze cupcakes that will not be eaten in the next few days.

Oatmeal Applesauce Cookies

Applesauce adds moistness to this low-calorie, lowfat and low-sodium version of oatmeal cookies.

About 5 dozen cookies

Per cookie:

Calories	45
Total fat	2 grams
Saturated fatty acids	Trace
Cholesterol	0
Sodium	35 milligrams

All-purpose flour	1 cup
Baking powder	1 teaspoon
Ground allspice	1 teaspoon
Salt	1/4 teaspoon
Margarine	½ cup
Sugar	½ cup
Egg whites	2
Rolled oats, quick cooking	2 cups
Unsweetened applesauce	1 cup
Raisins, chopped	½ cup

1. Preheat oven to 375°F.
2. Grease baking sheet. Mix flour, baking powder, allspice, and salt.
3. Beat margarine and sugar until creamy. Add egg whites; beat well.
4. Add dry ingredients.
5. Stir in oats, applesauce, and raisins. Mix well.
6. Drop by level tablespoonfuls onto baking sheet.
7. Bake 11 minutes or until edges are lightly browned. Cool on rack.

Peanut Butter-Date Spread

The dates and juice make this peanut butter-date spread lower in fat and calories per tablespoon than plain peanut butter. However, it is still fairly high in fat, so balance it out with lower fat choices elsewhere.

About ¾ Cup

Per tablespoon:

Calories	80
Total fat	5 grams
Saturated fatty acids	1 gram
Cholesterol	0
Sodium	Trace

"No salt-added" Peanut butter	½ cup
Dates, chopped	1/3 cup
Orange juice	3 tablespoons
Orange rind, grated	¼ teaspoon

1. Mix all ingredients.
2. Use as a spread on melba toast or lowfat crackers.

Questions Older People Ask

New information about nutrition seems to come out each day. Often, the information does not address the concerns of older adults. This section answers some common questions older people ask about nutrition.

Are there any foods or vitamins that can help prevent memory loss?

As of now, there is no reliable evidence that any foods or vitamins can help prevent memory loss such as occurs in Alzheimer's disease. Choline and lecithin have been tried to treat Alzheimer's, but neither was successful. People with Alzheimer's are at a greater risk for developing nutritional deficiencies, which can cause additional problems. Other kinds of severe memory loss and confusion are caused by excessive alcohol intake or by a deficiency of vitamin B-12 or folate. A

B-12 deficiency can sometimes be reversed by injections of this vitamin. It's important for anyone showing signs of memory loss and confusion to have a complete checkup, including a nutritional evaluation. Ask your health care provider.

Is there such a thing as "good cholesterol"?

You may have heard the terms "good cholesterol" and "bad cholesterol." These terms refer to substances called lipoproteins, which are "transport vehicles" that carry cholesterol in the blood. There are several kinds of lipoproteins. High-density lipoprotein (HDL) is often called the "good" kind because it removes cholesterol from the bloodstream, carrying it to the liver. The "bad" kind of cholesterol is transported by low-density lipoprotein (LDL). This is the cholesterol that gets deposited inside the arteries, where it may build up over time and eventually block the flow of blood. High levels of LDL increase your risk of heart disease, while high HDL levels lower your risk.

Diet can affect levels of LDL and HDL in the blood, but there are no foods that contain these substances. A cholesterol screening usually tells you the total amount of cholesterol circulating in your blood, but not how much of it comes from HDL and LDL. If your total cholesterol level is over 200 mg/dl and you have other risk factors for heart disease, your doctor may request another blood test to find out what your HDL and LDL levels are. This test must be done after you fast for 12 hours. Talk with your doctor about how the various components of blood cholesterol affect your risk.

I have trouble with my teeth and gums and have difficulty eating raw vegetables. How can I get enough fiber?

Cooked vegetables and fruits also supply fiber in your diet, as do cooked cereals and baked goods that contain whole grains. These will be much easier to chew. See your dentist or ask for a referral to one who specializes in dental problems of older adults. Much can be done to help your teeth and gums to make eating a variety of foods more enjoyable.

Things just don't taste good to me, so I have no interest in eating. What can I do to perk up my appetite?

People often find that their senses of taste and smell get duller as they age. As a result, they may overload their food with salt or even lose interest in food. Be creative with herbs, spices and lemon juice. They all add flavor that can perk up your taste again. Experiment with different spices to see what appeals to you. You may even want to try growing fresh herbs, either in your garden or in a pot on a sunny windowsill. Trying new recipes and choosing colorful foods in a variety of textures may also add interest to your meals.

I hate eating alone and as a result, I often skip meals. How can I make eating interesting?

Eating alone can be boring and sometimes even depressing. Many people don't want to spend time preparing meals just for themselves. Make an effort to make meals enjoyable. Try some of these ideas:

- Plan meals, set the table, light candles, play music, or eat when a television show you like is on. You deserve the same effort and care in preparing your own meals as the guests you might serve for a dinner party.

- Invite friends over for meals. You could each bring a part of the meal or trade portions of "planned leftovers."

- Eat out once a week or so. Many restaurants have lower prices and smaller portions at lunchtime. Some may offer reduced prices for older adults. Plan a daytime outing with a friend—go to lunch and visit a museum or attend an afternoon concert or theater performance. (See above for hints on making healthy food choices when you eat out.)

- Visit a senior center at lunchtime; participate in meals offered through your local agency on aging.

- Form a gourmet club with others who eat alone.

I've never liked eating breakfast. Do I need to eat breakfast to have a healthy diet?

It's not necessary to eat a big meal first thing in the morning. The important goal is to eat a balanced diet that includes foods from all the food groups each day. Set an eating pattern that works for you. For example, perhaps you like a mid-morning snack instead of a formal breakfast. Just be sure to make it a healthy snack, such as fruit and a muffin or toast. Often, people who skip meals eat too many snacks filled with empty calories.

What can I eat to help my arthritis?

Unfortunately, there is no food that relieves the pain of arthritis, but scientists are doing a lot of research in this area. You may see advertisements for food products or supplements that promise relief, but in truth they won't help you. A balanced diet will contribute to your overall good health, and avoiding too much weight will put less strain on your joints. There are also many simple tools such as jar openers that you can use to help you with everyday tasks. Contact your local chapter of the Arthritis Foundation, listed in the telephone book, for more information.

Can I always believe what I read in the newspaper?

New research about diet and health often gets in the newspaper or appears on the evening news, but no matter how promising or discouraging this news may be, making changes in your diet based on a single report is not wise. Government agencies and health organizations, such as the U.S. Departments of Agriculture and of Health and Human Services (USDA and DHHS), the National Academy of Sciences, and the American Heart Association, base their recommendations on dozens of studies carried out over many years. These groups continuously review new research findings and make recommendations only when there is widespread agreement among experts. Consult the resource list included in this chapter for sources of more information.

How do I know when a claim that a food product or supplement cures diseases is true?

These claims can be dangerous because they often prevent users from getting the medical help they need. They also create false hopes and waste money. In general, if it sounds too good to be true, it is. Suspect a product if it—

- makes outrageous claims, like curing a disease or reversing the aging process. No product or food has yet been proven to do either.

- promises immediate or fast results.

- does not list ingredients.

181

- cites only one study or a preliminary study as proof of results.

- does not give information about possible side effects.

- claims to be a secret formula.

- is available only from one source.

I don't eat many dairy products. How can I get enough calcium?

People who have trouble digesting milk can usually drink it in small amounts or can drink milk to which the enzyme lactase has been added (see above for suggestions). Buttermilk, yogurt, or cheese are good alternatives and are easier to digest. Other people simply don't like milk or dairy products. Calcium can be found in other foods. It's found naturally in leafy green vegetables like kale and broccoli. It's also added to some products such as fruit juice. It's best to get as much calcium as you can from the food you eat. If you feel you are not getting enough from foods, discuss whether you should take a calcium supplement (and what kind) with your doctor or dietitian.

I take diuretics; how can I get enough potassium?

First of all it's important to know if the diuretic you take is one that depletes potassium or one that has little effect on it. Generally, the more potent diuretics produce significant potassium losses. You should discuss the specific drug you are taking with the doctor who prescribed it for you. Most people's diets do not provide enough potassium to make up for what is lost due to the diuretic. However, proper choice of foods can effectively replace potassium losses.

Most foods provide some potassium. Fruits, vegetables, milk, and yogurt are among the best sources. Some meats, poultry, and fish are good sources too. Here are some common foods that are good sources of potassium:

- bran cereals

- cooked dried fruit such as apricots, peaches, prunes

- bananas

- potatoes, baked or boiled

- sweet potatoes, pumpkin, winter squash

- stewed tomatoes

- lima beans

- cooked dry beans, peas, lentils

- milk and yogurt (all types)

Did You Know?

One baked potato (even without the skin) has 610 mg of potassium; one banana (well-known as a good source of potassium) has 450 mg.

Tips and Recipes

You don't have to eliminate all of the fat, sugar, and sodium from the foods you eat to follow a healthy diet. Balance is the key. Think about how you can cut down on the fat, sugar, and sodium in the foods you prepare and eat. Consider also how you can get more whole grains, fruits, and vegetables. Simple changes make a difference. The following pages contain tips on preparing foods with less fat, sugar, and sodium as well as recipes to help you eat in a more healthful way.

Some Ideas for Better Eating

Make some simple changes in your recipes, using the recipes in this section as examples.

Notice that—

- Many of the recipes are prepared without added salt. Some use ingredients that already contain salt such as canned tuna, cereal, cheese, and soy sauce, while others are seasoned with herbs or spices.

- Lower fat ingredients are used instead of similar ingredients that are higher in fat. For example, water-packed tuna instead of oil-packed tuna, reduced-calorie salad dressing instead of regular salad dressing, skim milk instead of whole milk, and chicken breast without skin rather than chicken breast with skin.

- The desserts and quick bread are prepared with less sugar than most similar recipes.

- Whole-grain products are used in place of some or all of the all-purpose flour.

Make some simple changes at the table, too. See if you can take the salt shaker away or cut down the number of times you use it. Do you usually add a dab of butter or margarine to vegetables when you put them on the table? Try a low-calorie spread instead. Are there other changes you can make?

Tips About Breads, Cereals, Rice, and Pasta...

- Choose products made with whole grains often; for example, whole-wheat, oatmeal, oat-bran, pumpernickel, and rye breads, and cornmeal products, such as corn tortillas.

- Cook pasta and rice without salt or fats. Try using unsalted broth or tomato juice to add flavor.

- Try flavored pastas now available at many grocery stores, such as whole-wheat, spinach, or herb pasta

- Try brown rice; it has more flavor and more fiber.

- Make a pasta salad for dinner or lunch. It's easy to make and puts leftovers to good use. Just go easy on the mayonnaise or use reduced-calorie mayonnaise or salad dressing.

Tuna Pasta Salad

This salad is a tasty change from a typical tuna salad. It provides a serving of cooked pasta and half a serving of fruit in addition to the tuna.

4 servings, about 1 cup each

Per serving:

Calories	195
Total fat	2 grams
Saturated fatty acids	Trace
Cholesterol	13 milligrams
Sodium	170 milligrams

Elbow macaroni, uncooked	¾ cup
Tuna, water-pack, drained	6-1/2-ounce can
Celery, thinly sliced	½ cup
Seedless red grapes, halved	1 cup
Salad dressing, mayonnaise-type, reduced-calorie	3 tablespoons

- Cook macaroni according to package directions, omitting salt. Drain.
- Toss macaroni, tuna, celery, and grapes together.
- Mix in salad dressing.
- Serve warm or chill until served.

Menu Suggestion: Serve with broccoli spears, pumpernickel rolls, and ice milk topped with sliced strawberries.

Bran Apple Bars

Apples and bran cereal add dietary fiber. Using egg whites in place of a whole egg keeps cholesterol to a trace.

16 bars
4 servings, ½ cup each

Per bar:

Calories	110
Total fat	4 grams
Saturated fatty acids	1 gram
Cholesterol	Trace
Sodium	110 milligrams

Whole bran cereal (see Note)	1 cup
Skim milk	½ cup
Flour	1 cup
Baking Powder	1 teaspoon
Ground cinnamon	½ teaspoon
Ground nutmeg	¼ teaspoon
Margarine	1/3 cup
Brown sugar, packed	½ cup
Egg whites	2
Apple, pared, chopped	1 cup

1. Preheat oven to 350 F.
2. Grease 9- by 9-inch baking pan.
3. Soak bran in milk until milk is absorbed.
4. Mix dry ingredients thoroughly.
5. Beat margarine and sugar until creamy. Add egg whites; beat well. Stir in apples and bran mixture. Add dry ingredients; mix well.
6. Pour into pan.
7. Bake 30 minutes or until a toothpick inserted in center comes out clean.
8. Cool on rack.
9. Cut into 16 bars.

Note: Check the nutrition label of cereals for sodium content. Some whole-bran cereals contain almost twice as much sodium as others.

Zucchini Bread

This quick bread contains less fat, cholesterol, and sodium than many traditional squash breads. Use for dessert in place of an iced cake.

1 loaf, 18 slices, about ½-inch thick

Per slice:

Calories	110
Total fat	4 grams
Saturated fatty acids	1 gram
Cholesterol	0
Sodium	90 milligrams

Whole wheat flour	1 cup
All-purpose flour	1 cup
Baking powder	1 ½teaspoons
Ground cinnamon	1 teaspoon
Baking soda	¼ teaspoon
Salt	¼ teaspoon
Egg whites	3
Sugar	½ cup
Vegetable oil	1/3 cup
Vanilla	1 ½teaspoons
Zucchini squash, coarsely shredded lightly packed	2 cups

1. Preheat oven to 350 F.
2. Grease 9 by 5 by 3 inch loaf pan.
3. Mix dry ingredients, except sugar.
4. Beat egg whites until frothy. Add sugar, oil, and vanilla. Continue beating for 3 minutes.
5. Stir in zucchini; mix lightly.
6. Add dry ingredients. Mix just until dry ingredients are moistened.
7. Pour into loaf pan.
8. Bake 40 minutes or until toothpick inserted in center comes out clean.
9. Cool on rack. Remove from pan after 10 minutes.
10. To serve, cut into 18 slices about 1/2-inch thick.

Tips About Vegetables. . .

- Both raw vegetables and cooked vegetables provide dietary fiber. The less they are cooked, the more vitamins remain in the vegetables. Try steaming them just to the point that they are tender but crisp.

- Eat potatoes with their skins for more fiber.

- Season vegetables with herbs, yogurt, and lemon juice. Limit butter, margarine, heavy dressing, honey, salt and soy sauce.

- Canned vegetables are often high in sodium. Try some of the special low-sodium or "no-salt-added" versions.

- Add beans, split peas, and lentils to your diet; they're an inexpensive source of protein and fiber. Add them to soups, stews, salads, and rice dishes.

Herbed Vegetable Combo

These steamed vegetables with herb seasonings add color and flavor to a meal without adding fat or salt.

4 servings, about ¾ cup each

Per serving:

Calories	25
Total fat	Trace
Saturated tatty acids	Trace
Cholesterol	0
Sodium	10 milligrams

Water	2 tablespoons
Zucchini squash, thinly sliced	I cup
Yellow squash, thinly sliced	1 ¼cups
Green pepper, cut into 2-inch strips	½ cup
Celery, cut into 2-inch strips	¼ cup
Onion, chopped	¼ cup
Caraway seed	½ teaspoon
Garlic powder	1/8 teaspoon
Tomato, cut into 8 wedges	I medium

1. Heat water in large frypan.
2. Add squash, green pepper, celery, and onion.
3. Cover and cook over moderate heat until vegetables are tender-crisp—about 4 minutes.
4. Sprinkle seasonings over vegetables. Top with tomato wedges. Cover and cook over low heat until tomato wedges are just heated—about 2 minutes.

Tips About Fruits...

- Fruits offer natural sweetness with the added benefits of fiber, vitamins, and minerals.

- Use fresh or canned fruit slices as a colorful garnish for main dishes, salads, and cereals.

- Blend fresh, plain frozen, or canned fruit with milk for a fruitshake.

- Add dried fruit to muffins and quick breads.

- Eat fresh fruits topped with yogurt and sprinkled with cinnamon

- Bake or broil apples, pears, or bananas with cinnamon and nutmeg; fruit tastes even sweeter when eaten while warm.

Apple Crisp

Whole-wheat flour and rolled oats add dietary fiber. Using less sugar and fat than an old-fashioned apple crisp recipe means lower sugar and fat content per serving.

4 servings, 1/2 cup each

Per serving:

Calories	235
Total fat	9 grams
Saturated fatty acids	2 grams
Cholesterol	0
Sodium	105 milligrams
Tart apples, pared, sliced	4 cups

Water	¼ cup
Lemon juice	1 tablespoon
Brown sugar, packed	¼ cup
Whole-wheat flour	¼ cup
Old-fashioned rolled oats	¼ cup
Ground cinnamon	½ teaspoon
Ground nutmeg	¼ teaspoon
Margarine	3 tablespoons

1. Place apples in 8-by 8-by 2-inch baking pan.
2. Mix water and lemon juice, pour over apples.
3. Mix sugar, flour, oats, and spices.
4. Add margarine to dry mixture; mix until crumbly.
5. Sprinkle crumbly mixture evenly over apples.
6. Bake at 350º F until apples are tender and topping is lightly browned, about 40 minutes.

Tips About Milk, Yogurt, and Cheese . . .

These foods are an important source of calcium but can add fat and extra sodium to your diet.

-   Choose lower fat and lower sodium versions often, such as:

    * skim milk

    * evaporated skim milk

    * lowfat or nonfat plain yogurt

    * whipped cottage cheese for dips and dressings

    * part skim ricotta or mozzarella

    * lowfat process cheeses

    * lower sodium cheeses

-   If you don't like to drink milk, try using it in soups and puddings (see the following recipe for broccoli soup).

Broccoli Soup

This recipe has less sodium and fat than canned broccoli soup. Using unsalted broth and adding 1/4 teaspoon salt results in less sodium than using a salted broth and no salt.

4 servings, about 1 cup each

Per Serving:

Calories	110
Total fat	3 grams
Saturated fatty acids	2 grams
Cholesterol	9 milligrams
Sodium	250 milligrams

Broccoli, chopped (see Note)	1-1/2 cups
Celery, diced	1/4 cup
Onion, chopped	1/4 cup
Chicken broth, unsalted	1 cup
Skim milk	2 cups
Cornstarch	2 tablespoons
Salt	1/4 teaspoon
Pepper	Dash
Ground thyme	Dash
Swiss cheese, shredded	1/4 cup

1. Place vegetables and broth in saucepan. Bring to boiling, reduce heat, cover, and cook until vegetables are tender—about 8 minutes.
2. Mix milk, cornstarch, salt, pepper, and thyme; add to cooked vegetables. Cook, stirring contantly, until soup is slightly thickened and mixture just begins to boil.
3. Remove from heat. Add cheese and stir until melted.

Note: A 10-ounce package of frozen chopped broccoli can be used in place of fresh broccoli. The soup will have about 120 calories and 260 milligrams of sodium per serving.

Tips About Meat, Poultry, and Fish . . .

- You don't have to eliminate red meat, or any one meat, from your diet. Lean, trimmed beef is low in fat and supplies important amounts of minerals such as iron and zinc.

- Choose leaner types of meat:

  * beef—round, loin, sirloin, and chuck arm steaks or roasts, especially "select" grade cuts (often labeled in supermarkets as "lean")

  * pork—tenderloin, center loin roasts and chops

  * veal—roasts and chops

  * lamb—leg, loin roasts and chops, and foreshanks

  * chicken and turkey, especially light meat

  * most fish; choose tuna canned in water when available

  * shellfish

- Try substituting ground turkey or chicken for ground beef in casseroles and other dishes.

- Try dishes made with dry beans and peas as occasional alternatives. Dry beans and peas are low in fat and provide protein and minerals similar to lean meat, poultry, and fish. They also provide dietary fiber.

- Limit your use of processed meats such as hotdogs, sausage, and luncheon meats. They are usually high in both sodium and fat. Choose more lowfat or lower salt versions.

- Keep the fat and sodium content low when you prepare meats:

  * trim visible fat and remove the skin from poultry

  * broil and bake instead of fry

  * place meat on a rack when cooking so fat can drain away from the meat

  * cook with no added fat in nonstick pans

* baste meats with unsalted broth, tomato juice, or fruit juice instead of fatty drippings, or marinate before cooking

* cool stews and soups before serving so you can skim fat off the top

* limit sauces and gravies that are high in saturated fats, such as cream sauce

* use onion or garlic powder instead of seasoned salts

* season with herbs and spices

* use commercially prepared sauces sparingly; they are usually high in sugar or sodium or both

• Modify recipes so you use smaller amounts and leaner cuts of meat and more of other ingredients like potatoes, rice, noodles, grains, or vegetables.

Beef & Vegetable Stirfry

Using a lean meat cut, round steak, and only 1 teaspoon of oil keeps the fat lower than in a traditional stirfry.

4 servings, about 3/4 cup each

Per Serving:

Calories	145
Total fat	4 grams
Saturated fatty acids	1 gram
Cholesterol	44 milligrams
Sodium	300 milligrams

Beef round steak	3/4 pound (12 ounces)
Vegetable oil	1 teaspoon
Carrots, sliced	1/2 cup
Celery, sliced	1/2 cup
Onion, sliced	1/2 cup
Soy sauce	1 tablespoon
Garlic powder	1/8 teaspoon
Pepper	Dash
Zucchini squash, cut in thin strips	2 cups
Cornstarch	1 tablespoon
Water	1/4 cup

1. Trim all fat from steak. Slice steak across the grain into thin strips about 1/8-inch wide and 3 inches long. (Partially frozen meat is easier to slice.)
2. Heat oil in frypan. Add beef strips and stirfry over high heat, turning pieces constantly, until beef is no longer red—about 3 to 5 minutes. Reduce heat.
3. Add carrots, celery, onion, and seasonings. Cover and cook until carrots are lightly tender—3 to 4 minutes.
4. Add squash; cook until vegetables are tender-crisp—3 to 4 minutes.
5. Mix cornstarch and water until smooth. Add slowly to beef mixture, stirring constantly.
6. Cook until thickened and vegetables are coated with a thin glaze.

Chicken & Vegetable Stirfry

VARIATION

Per serving:

Calories	140
Total fat	2 grams
Saturated Fatty acids	Trace
Cholesterol	51 milligrams
Sodium	320 milligrams

Use 3 chicken breast halves without bone or skin (about 12 ounces of raw chicken) in place of beef. Slice into thin strips. Chicken should be cooked until thoroughly done or no longer pink in color.

Chicken Italiano

This colorful chicken main dish is quick and easy to prepare. All ingredients are cooked together in a single pan.

4 servings, 1 chicken breast half and 3/4 cup of spaghetti mixture each

Per serving:

Calories	280
Total fat	3 grams
Saturated fatty acids	1 gram
Cholesterol	68 milligrams
Sodium	320 milligrams

Chicken breast halves, skinned boned	4
Vegetable oil	1 teaspoon
Thin spaghetti, broken into fourths	4 ounces (about 1-1/2 cups dry)
Onion, cut in wedges	1 small
Green pepper, cut in strips	1 small
Instant minced garlic	1/8 teaspoon
Oregano leaves	1 teaspoon
Salt	1/8 teaspoon
Pepper	1/8 teaspoon
Bay leaf	1

Tomatoes	16-ounce can
Water	1/4 cup
Parsley, chopped	1 tablespoon, if desired

1. Pound chicken breasts with a metal mallet between sheets of plastic wrap until about 1/2-inch thick.
2. Heat oil in frypan. Brown chicken breasts on each side.
3. Add spaghetti, onion, and pepper strips around chicken. Spinkle with seasonings.
4. Break up large pieces of tomatoes. Pour tomatoes and water over top of chicken.
5. Bring to boiling. Reduce heat, cover, and cook until chicken and spaghetti are done, about 15 minutes.
6. Remove bay leaf. Garnish with parsley.

Menu Suggestion: Serve with spinach-mandarin orange salad with re-duced-calorie dressing and garlic bread (small amount of soft margarine and garlic powder).

Turkey Italiano

VARIATION

Per serving:

Calories	275
Total fat	3 grams
Saturated fatty acids	Trace
Cholesterol	70 milligrams
Sodium	305 milligrams

Use 1 pound raw turkey breast fillets or tenderloins in place of chicken. (Bone and skin are already removed.)

Broiled Sesame Fish

For a quick, lowfat main dish, try this fish recipe. It takes about 15 minutes to prepare and contains very little fat.

4 servings, about 2-1/2 ounces each

Per serving:

Calories	110
Total fat	3 grams
Saturated fatty acids	Trace
Cholesterol	46 milligrams
Sodium	155 milligrams

Cod fillets, fresh or frozen	1 pound
Margarine, melted	1 teaspoon
Lemon juice	1 tablespoon
Dried tarragon leaves	1 teaspoon
Salt	1/8 teaspoon
Pepper	Dash
Sesame seed	1 tablespoon
Parsley, chopped	1 tablespoon

1. Thaw frozen fish in refrigerator overnight or defrost briefly in a microwave oven. Cut fish into four portions.
2. Place fish on a broiler pan lined with aluminum foil. Brush margarine over fish.
3. Mix lemon juice, tarragon leaves, salt, and pepper. Pour over fish.
4. Sprinkle sesame seeds evenly over fish.
5. Broil until fish flakes easily when tested with a fork—about 12 minutes.
6. Garnish each serving with parsley.

Dilled Fish Fillets

Using dill weed and lemon juice for flavor in place of butter or margarine keeps the fat low.

4 servings, about 2-1/2 ounces each

Per serving:

Calories	90
Total fat	1 gram
Saturated fatty acids	Trace
Cholesterol	45 milligrams
Sodium	130 milligrams

Frozen haddock or cod fillets	1 pound
Lemon juice	1 tablespoon
Dried dill weed	1/8 teaspoon
Salt	1/8 teaspoon
Pepper	Dash

1. Thaw frozen fish in refrigerator overnight or thaw in microwave oven. Separate into four fillets or pieces.
2. Place fish in heated frypan. Sprinkle with lemon juice and seasonings.
3. Cover and cook over moderate heat until fish flakes when tested with a fork. about 5 minutes.

Menu Suggestion: Serve with braised carrots and celery, new potatoes boiled in skin, and applesauce muffins made from mix.

MICROWAVE INSTRUCTIONS: Place fish in a glass baking dish. Cover with wax paper. Cook at "medium" power for 3 minutes. Remove cover, turn fish over, and sprinkle with lemon juice and seasonings. Cover and continue cooking at "medium" power for 3 minutes or until fish flakes with a fork.

Modifying Your Recipes

Here's an example of how to use these tips. The recipe below shows simple adjustments in a typical beef stroganoff recipe that can help you moderate fat and cholesterol.

Changes from typical recipe:

- Use a less fatty meat cut—round steak in place of sirloin—and trim fat from meat.

- Use buttermilk in place of sour cream.

- Use a nonstick pan and no butter to cook the meat.

- Prepare gravy with buttermilk instead of butter.

Light Beef Stroganoff

4 servings, 1/2 cup of stroganoff and ½ cup of noodles each

Per serving:

Calories	275
Total fat	6 grams
Saturated fatty acids	2 grams
Cholesterol	71 milligrams
Sodium	325 milligrams

Beef round steak, boneless, trimmed	3/4 pound
Fresh mushrooms	1/4 pound
Onion sliced	1/2 cups
Beef broth, condensed	1/2 cup
Water	1/2 cup
Catsup	I tablespoon
Pepper	1/8 teaspoon
Flour	2 tablespoons
Buttermilk	1 cup
Noodles, cooked, unsalted	2 cups (about 2 ½ cups un-cooked)

199

1. Slice steak across the grain into thin strips, about 1/8-inch wide and 3 inches long. (It is easier to cut thin slices of meat if it is partially frozen.)
2. Wash and slice mushrooms.
3. Cook beef strips, mushrooms. and onion in nonstick frypan until beef is lightly browned.
4. Add broth, water, catsup, and pepper. Cover and simmer until beef is tender, about 45 minutes.
5. Mix flour with about ¼ cup of the buttermilk until smooth; add remaining buttermilk. Stir into beef mixture. Cook, stirring constantly, until thickened.
6. Serve over noodles.

For each serving, these changes result in savings of 240 calories, 24 grams total fat, 15 grams saturated fatty acids, and 62 milligrams cholesterol.

Adapt Your Staples for Better Health...

You can reduce fat and sodium in the boxed products you use, such as macaroni and cheese. just follow the chart below:

Mix	Changes	Serving size (cup)	Fat saved per serving (grams)	Sodium saved per serving (milligrams)
Macaroni and cheese	• Omit salt when cooking macaroni • Use lowfat milk • Reduce added margarine by half	3/4	6	265
Seasoned rice and rice/pasta mixtures	• Reduce added margarine by half	1/2	2	20
Bread stuffing	• Reduce added margarine by half	1/2	4	45
Scalloped and au gratin potatoes	• Use lowfat milk • Reduce added margarine by half	1/2	2	20

Note: Savings for macaroni and cheese and potatoes are for products made with 2 percent fat milk in place of whole milk. Reduce fat even further by using 1 percent fat or skim milk.

Want More Information?

For assistance in answering your questions about nutrition and health, contact the following organizations. If they cannot answer your questions directly, they will refer you to someone who can.

Administration on Aging
330 Independence Avenue, S.W.
Washington, DC 20201
(202) 619 0774
U.S. Government agency that provides information on health and aging programs, offered through State and area agencies on aging.

Alzheimer's Association
Suite 1000
919 N. Michigan Avenue
Chicago, IL 60611
(312) 335-8700 1-(800) 272-3900 toll-free hotline

Offers a hotline that provides information and assistance for families coping with Alzheimer's disease.

American Association of Retired Persons
1909 K Street, N.W.
Washington, DC 20049
(707) 434-7777

Membership organization for people over age 50, offering publications and volunteer-run programs on a variety of economic, social, and health issues.

American Dietetic Association
Suite 800
216 West Jackson Boulevard
Chicago, IL 60606
(312) 899-0040

Professional organization offering assistance in locating a registered dietitian in your community.

American Geriatrics Society
Suite 300
770 Lexington Avenue
New York, NY 10021
(212) 308-1414

Professional organization of physicians with geriatric training, offering assistance in locating a doctor in your community with special training in treating older adults.

Arthritis Foundation
1314 Spring Street, N.W.
Atlanta, GA 30309
(404) 872-7100

Provides information and programs on arthritis, including treatment options and self-help materials for those with arthritis and their families.

Food and Drug Administration
Office of Consumer Affairs
5600 Fishers Lane, HFE 88
Rockville, MD 20857
(301) 443-3170

U.S. Government agency that answers questions about the safety of food additives, drugs, and medical devices.

Human Nutrition Information Service
USDA
6505 Belcrest Road
Hyattsville, MD 20782
(301) 436-5724

U.S. Government agency that provides information on using the Dietary Guidelines and preparing foods.

National Institute on Aging
Public Information Office

Federal Building, Room 6C12
9000 Rockville Pike
Bethesda, MD 20892
(301) 496-1752

U.S. Government agency that provides information on health and other issues of interest to older people.

National Cancer Institute
Office of Cancer Communications
Building 31, Room 10A24
9000 Rockville Pike
Bethesda, MD 20892
1 (800)422 6237 toll-free hotline

U.S. Government agency that provides information on cancer prevention and treatment.

National Heart, Lung, and Blood Institute
Information Office
Building 31, Room 4A21 9000 Rockville Pike
Bethesda, MD 20892
(301) 496-4236

U.S. Government agency that conducts research and provides information about heart, lung. and blood diseases.

Office of Disease Prevention and Health Promotion
National Health Information Center
P.O. Box 1133
Washington, DC 20013-1133
1 (800) 336-4797

U.S. Government agency that operates a clearinghouse and hotline to provide health information and referrals.

Chapter 10

Eating Better When Eating Out: Using the Dietary Guidelines

What Are The Dietary Guidelines For Americans?

The Dietary Guidelines for Americans are seven basic principles for developing and maintaining a healthier diet. The Guidelines represent the best thinking in the field of nutrition and health and are the basis for all Federal nutrition information and education programs for healthy Americans. They were developed by the U.S. Department of Agriculture and the U.S. Department of Health and Human Services.

The Dietary Guidelines emphasize balance, variety, and moderation in the overall diet. The seven Guidelines are:

- Eat a variety of foods

- Balance the food you eat with physical activity—maintain or improve your weight

- Choose a diet low in fat, saturated fat, and cholesterol

- Choose a diet with plenty of grain products, vegetables, and fruits

- Choose a diet moderate in sugars

- Choose a diet moderate in salt and sodium

- If you drink alcoholic beverages, do so in moderation

U.S Department of Agriculture Human Nutrition Information Service Home and Garden Bulletin No. 232-11

The U.S. Department of Agriculture has prepared a series of practical "how to" publications on choosing and preparing foods using the Guidelines. This chapter focuses on how to choose foods when eating out in the Dietary Guidelines style. Other topics in the series include how to shop for food, prepare foods and plan menus, prepare bag lunches, snacks, and desserts, and make "meals in minutes" using the Dietary Guidelines.

Trends in Eating Out

Americans are on the move. Busy lifestyles and tight work and travel schedules make eating out routine for many of us. According to recent surveys:

- Americans, excluding those who live in institutions, eat more than one of every five meals at away-from-home eating establishments.

- Fast-food places serve four out of 10 meals eaten at away-from-home eating establishments.

- Four out of 10 consumers say they have changed their eating out habits to reflect nutritional concerns.

- Adults eat roughly 30 percent of their calories away from home.

- Americans spend more than 40 cents of every food dollar on food eaten away from home.

Setting The Stage For Eating Out

The principles for eating in the Dietary Guidelines style are basically the same regardless of where food is eaten. It's true you may have less control over how foods are prepared and what ingredients are used when you eat out, but you can control which foods you choose and the amount. Keep in mind that it's your total diet that counts and that the principles of variety, moderation, and balance work best when practiced regularly over a period of time. Occasional splurges can be worked into a long-range eating plan. Here's what we mean by variety, moderation, and balance.

Variety. No one food supplies all of the protein, vitamins, and minerals you need for good health. That's why it's important to choose from a wide variety of foods. You also need to choose foods that provide adequate starch and fiber and supply enough (but not too many) calories to maintain desirable weight.

To help ensure such variety, choose foods daily from each of these major food groups:

- Breads, cereals, and other grain products

- Fruits

- Vegetables

- Meat, poultry, fish, and alternates (such as eggs, dry beans, and peas)

- Milk, cheese, and yogurt

You can easily balance lack of variety in one meal with the food selections you make the rest of that day. For example, if your lunch is short on vegetables, add an extra vegetable or salad to your evening meal.

Moderation. The Dietary Guidelines suggest moderation, or "avoiding too much" fat, saturated fat, cholesterol, sugars, sodium, and alcohol. They also emphasize the importance of maintaining desirable weight by not eating too many calories. Moderation does not mean cutting out all foods that are high in calories, fat, saturated fat, cholesterol, sugars, sodium, and alcohol. Moderation does mean choosing these foods less often and in smaller amounts. Some experts suggest that we limit the amount of fat we eat to one-third of our calories or less. (In a 2,000-calorie diet, that's about 74 grams of fat a day.) For sodium, some experts consider 1,100 to 3,300 milligrams a day to be a safe and adequate level for adults. (This is the amount of sodium in about ½ to 1½ teaspoons of salt. It includes the sodium present in foods as well as what's added during cooking and at the table.) Most of us have diets that contain more fat and sodium than these recommendations, and many overdo on sugars and calories, too.

Balance. Balance means putting it all together so that you get the variety of foods you need for essential nutrients and the calories you need to maintain desirable weight, without getting too much fat, saturated fat, cholesterol, sugars, sodium, and alcohol.

Making Choices

How does eating out affect your overall diet? That depends on where you eat, what and how much you order, and what extras you add to the foods you order—dressings, spreads, condiments, and so forth. Of course, how often you eat out is important, too.

Where You Eat

Where you eat out greatly affects the food choices available to you. It's a lot easier to follow Guidelines-style eating at some restaurants than at others. For example, a greater selection of menu items gives you the opportunity to choose for variety. And if foods are prepared to order, you can have more control over the calories, fat, sugars, and sodium in your meal. Here's how eating places compare:

Full-service restaurants usually provide the greatest variety and flexibility in types of foods and preparation methods. Items are often prepared to order, so you can ask that foods be prepared differently than the menu specifies. One drawback of having foods prepared to order is the time it takes . . .what and how much do you eat while waiting for your order?

Cafeterias, smorgasbords, and restaurant buffets also provide a wide variety of food selections. Since foods are prepared in advance, there's no wait, but you are not able to order foods the way you want them. You do, however, have some control over portion size and the amounts of sauces, gravies, and dressings served with foods. Watch out for "all you-can-eat" offers, though. You may be tempted to eat too much just to get your money's worth!

Steakhouses and fish houses generally offer fewer menu items, although different sizes and cuts of meat are often available. Most items are prepared to order, but preparation methods may be more limited. Fish and shellfish items are often breaded and fried; broiled and steamed versions are increasingly available. Side dishes usually include items high in fat—french fries, hush puppies, and creamy coleslaw, for example. Salad bars are sometimes featured.

Pizza parlors offer variety in toppings and crust types but an otherwise limited menu. Toppings vary in calories, fat, and sodium content. Some parlors feature salad bars.

Sub shops offer a varied selection of subs and sandwiches but usually little else. Items are prepared to order so the amount of high-calorie, high-fat spreads can be limited. Sometimes smaller servings are available. Many offer a variety of breads.

Fast-food restaurants offer an expanding but still rather limited menu. Many items are deep-fat fried including chicken and fish items, french fries, onion rings, and fruit pies. However, smaller servings are available for some sandwiches and side orders, and you can request that foods be prepared without sauces or other condiments. Salads, baked potatoes, and whole-grain rolls are now available at some fast-food restaurants, and lowfat milk and fruit juices are joining soft drinks and shakes as beverage options.

Convenience store "mini-meals" and vending machines are a growing source of food eaten away from home. Offerings include chili, hot dogs and Polish sausages, nachos with cheese sauce, prepackaged hamburgers and sandwiches, single serving canned foods, candy, and snack foods. Fat, calories, sugars, and sodium are high in many of these items, especially in processed, prepackaged, and canned foods. Some refrigerated vending machines offer alternatives—yogurt, fruit, and fruit juices, for example.

Other people's homes can provide a real challenge to eating in the Guidelines style. How much control you have (or are willing to take) may depend on several factors, including the risk of offending your host and/or hostess! Buffet arrangements and informal parties permit you to be selective in what and how much you choose. However, there is often a tempting array of food and drinks that are high in fat, sugars, sodium, or alcohol. Family-style dinners may make it more difficult to avoid certain food selections, but you can still control serving sizes. Of course, formal sit-down dinners, where you're served a prepared plate of food, provide you with the least control.

What You Order—And How Much

Eating out is a special treat for many of us. How can you moderate calories, fat, sodium, and sugars without giving up your favorite foods? Have your favorite restaurant meal. Then, balance it out over the next day or two with meals that are lower in calories, fat, sodium, sugars, or alcohol. Or select Guidelines-style meals wherever you eat. Here are some ideas.

Appetizers

Enjoy steamed seafood, raw vegetables, or fruit. Go easy on rich sauces, dips, and batter-fried foods (cheese sticks, vegetables, chicken pieces).

Calories, fat, and sodium from foods like chips, peanuts, and pretzels can add up quickly, especially if you are talking and not paying attention to how much you're eating. Try to limit how much you eat. Or, fill up on raw vegetables if they're available.

	Calories	Fat (grams)	Sodium (milligrams)
10 potato chips	105	7	95
1/4 cup salted peanuts	210	18	155
2/3 cup thin pretzel sticks	100	trace	480

If soup is your choice, order a cup rather than a bowl. Or for a lighter meal, order soup and a dinner salad instead of an entree. Broth- or tomato-based soups are lower in fat than creamed types. For added starch and fiber, choose soups made with lentils, beans, or split peas. Most soups are high in sodium.

	Calories	Fat (grams)	Sodium (milligrams)
1 cup chicken consommé	30	0	635
1 cup Manhattan clam chowder	80	2	1,810
1 cup New England (creamed) clam chowder	165	7	990

Note: Values are for canned soups.

210

Breads

Breads are an important part of a varied diet. They supply starch, fiber, and some vitamins and minerals. Whole-grain types such as wheat, bran, oat, and rye provide even more fiber.

Breads and other baked goods differ widely in the fat and sugars they contain. Croissants, biscuits, and hush puppies are much higher in fat than most other breads. Sweet rolls and sticky buns are much higher in sugars and fat than loaf bread.

	Calories	Fat (grams)	Sodium (milligrams)
1 dinner roll	85	2	55
1 croissant	235	12	450
1 sweet bun	280	8	290

Butter and other spreads can make even the plainest bread high in fat and calories. See "What You Add," below.

Many crackers are high in fat and sodium so enjoy just a few and limit amounts of spreads and dips. If a variety of crackers is served, choose whole-grain types for extra fiber.

Entrees

Choose meat, fish, or poultry that is broiled, grilled, baked, steamed, or poached rather than fried. Broiled or grilled entrees are often basted with large amounts of fat, however. Ask to have your entree prepared without added fat; or request that lemon juice, wine, or just a small amount of fat be used.

Sometimes fried foods are your only choice. If so, have a smaller helping. Remove the skin or breading to cut fat and calories. This may also decrease sodium.

	Calories	Fat (grams)	Sodium (milligrams)
3 ounces cooked chicken breast, meat only	140	3	65
3 ounces cooked chicken breast, meat and skin	165	7	60
3 ounces fried chicken breast, meat, breading, and skin	220	11	235

211

Select lean cuts of meat—steamship round of beef, for example, in place of prime rib or spareribs. Trim away visible fat.

	Calories	Fat (grams)	Sodium (milligrams)
3 ounces cooked round roast of beef (lean only)	155	6	50
3 ounces roast prime rib (lean only)	250	17	65
3 ounces roast prime rib (lean and fat)	360	31	55

Many restaurants serve portions much larger than 3 ounces— as much as 6 to 10 ounces, or more in some cases.

- If the portion served is larger than your usual serving, don't eat it all—ask for a take-home bag.

- Sometimes you have a choice of portion size—a "petite" filet mignon (about 4 ounces cooked) rather than a regular sized one (about 6 ounces cooked), for example.

- Ask if half-portions are available for certain entrees, or order an appetizer rather than an entree as your main course.

Choose dishes flavored with herbs and spices rather than with rich sauces, gravies, or dressings.

Try stir fried mixtures, which are traditionally prepared with very little oil.

When pizza's your choice, consider that vegetable toppings such as onions and green peppers are generally lower in fat and sodium, and higher in fiber than sausage, pepperoni, anchovies, and olives.

	Calories	Fat (grams)	Sodium (milligrams)
1 slice cheese pizza with vegetable toppings (1/8 of 13-inch thin-crust pizza)	165	5	400
1 slice cheese pizza with "everything" (1/8 of 13-inch thin-crust pizza)	240	12	605

Hungry for a sub? Choose lean deli meats, such as turkey or ham, instead of higher fat cold cuts, such as bologna or salami; include lettuce and tomato as fillings; choose whole-grain rolls if available; and go easy on additions like oil, mayonnaise, and pickles. Some sub shops offer small as well as regular-sized servings. Splitting a sub with a friend is another way to reduce the amount you eat.

Vegetables/Salads

Plain vegetables are high in fiber and other nutrients and low in calories, fat, and sodium. However, butter, margarine, and sauces can increase calories, fat, and sodium considerably.

Look for vegetables seasoned with lemon, herbs, or spices rather than fat and salt.

Be adventurous with your next salad bar creation. Start with a bowl of romaine, boston lettuce, or spinach, and add an assortment of fruits and vegetables: raisins, grapes, apples, cauliflower, cucumbers, broccoli, turnips, tomatoes, carrots, and celery, for example. Watch out for dressings and toppings that can add a lot of calories, fat, and sodium. For more information, see "What You Add," below.

Ask for a tossed salad or baked potato in place of fries or chips.

Go easy on prepared salads that contain a lot of mayonnaise, salad dressing, or oil—macaroni salad, potato salad, creamy coleslaw, and marinated vegetables, for example. Some pasta salads are made with large amounts of oily dressing.

Desserts

Fruits are a great dessert in the Guidelines style. If there are no fruit selections under "desserts," check the appetizer menu, or ask—fruits may be available because they're ingredients in other items.

Order a light dessert such as sherbet, fruit ice, or sorbet. Sorbet is lower in calories and fat than most ice creams, although it's fairly high in sugar.

	Calories	Fat (grams)	Sodium (milligrams)
1 cup sorbet	190	0	30
1 cup sherbet	270	4	90
1 cup regular ice cream	270	14	115
1 cup premium ice cream	350	24	110
1 cup premium ice cream topped with hot fudge sauce, nuts, and whipped cream	580	39	160

If you decide on a rich dessert such as pie, cake, or pastry, try splitting it with a friend.

While others in your party are having dessert, you can have a cup of tea or coffee.

Beverages

Have the ideal thirst quencher—water!
Ask if skim or lowfat milk is available.
Go easy on soft drinks and sweetened fruit drinks.

	Calories	Sugar (teaspoons)
12 ounces cola	160	9
12 ounces fruit drink, ade, or punch	185	12

For a nonalcoholic "cocktail," ask for fruit juice mixed with seltzer or mineral water, or a glass of tomato juice with a twist of lemon or lime.

If you drink alcoholic beverages, set limits on how much you will drink. To control calories and sugars, request liquor mixed with water or seltzer rather than sweetened mixers. Order a glass of wine rather than a carafe. Or, try a wine spritzer (wine and seltzer water) in place of wine. Though "light" beers vary in their calories and alcohol content, many are lower than regular brands.

Regular or decaffeinated coffee and tea have no calories, fat, or sugars unless you add them!

What You Add

Limit amounts of butter, margarine, and cheese spread you add to bread and crackers—calories, fat, and sodium add up quickly!

	Calories	Fat (grams)	Sodium (milligrams)
1 pat butter or margarine	35	4	40
Tablespoon crock-type cheese spread	50	4	180

Salad dressings are often high in fat, calories, and sodium. Use them sparingly. For a zippy salad dressing alternative, ask for lemon juice or vinegar with just a small amount of oil. Reduced-calorie salad dressings, which are also lower in fat, are available at some restaurants.

	Calories	Fat (grams)	Sodium (milligrams)
1 tablespoon creamy Italian dressing	70	8	175
1 tablespoon regular Italian dressing	70	7	115
1 tablespoon reduced-calorie Italian dressing	15	2	120
1 tablespoon vinegar and oil (2 parts vinegar to 1 part oil)	40	4	trace

Salad toppings may add calories, fat, and sodium.

	Calories	Fat (grams)	Sodium (milligrams)
1 tablespoon imitation bacon bits	30	2	125
1 tablespoon sunflower seeds (unsalted)	50	4	trace
1 tablespoon chopped egg	15	1	10
1 tablespoon grated process cheese	25	2	100
1 tablespoon seasoned croutons	5	trace	10

Ask if gravies, sour cream, cream sauces, salad dressings, and other toppings can be served "on the side." You might be surprised to see how little can make foods tasty!

	Calories	Fat (grams)	Sodium (milligrams)
1 tablespoon sour cream	25	3	5
1 tablespoon hollandaise sauce	70	7	65

Some condiments are high in fat—mayonnaise and tartar sauce, for example.

Limiting your use of soy sauce, steak sauce, catsup, mustard, pickles, and other condiments will help control sodium.

	Calories	Fat (grams)	Sodium (milligrams)
1 tablespoon soy sauce	10	0	1,030
1 tablespoon steak sauce	10	0	230
1 tablespoon catsup	15	0	155
1 dill pickle strip	3	0	430

Taste food before you salt it. If you still want salt, try one shake instead of two.

	Sodium (milligrams)
1/8 teaspoon salt	250

Ask if freshly ground pepper or an herb blend is available to use in place of salt.

Reading Menus

Terms used in describing menu items can provide clues to fat and sodium content. Here are some terms that signal . . .

Higher Fat
buttered or buttery
fried, french fried, deep
  fried, batter fried;
  pan fried
breaded
creamed, creamy, or
  in cream sauce
in its own gravy, with
  gravy, or pan gravy
hollandaise
au gratin or in
  cheese sauce
scalloped or escalloped
rich
pastry

Higher Sodium
smoked
pickled
barbecued
in broth
in cocktail sauce
in a tomato base
with soy sauce
teriyaki
Creole sauce
mustard sauce
marinated
Parmesan

Some terms can signal lower fat. Foods that are grilled or broiled, for example, are likely to be lower in fat than those that are deep-fat fried—providing that only small amounts of fat are used during preparation and that fat is drained. Other terms that usually mean lower fat include "stirfried," "roasted," "poached," or "steamed." Few terms guarantee lower sodium. Even "fresh" or "homemade" foods can be fairly high in sodium, depending on the types and amounts of ingredients used to prepare them.

Eating Smart

Have you ever gone out to dinner and felt full after eating your appetizer, salad, and bread—even before the entree was served? When the entree and the dessert were served, though, you ate every bite. After all, you ordered it—you can't waste food! To eat smart, order one course at a time rather than all courses at the beginning of the meal. If you are served more than you want to eat, ask for a take-home bag.

Having It Your Way When Eating Out

Many restaurants are changing their menus and cooking styles to suit health-conscious customers. To encourage this, go to restaurants that offer the healthful foods you prefer or that prepare food to order. Call ahead to find out if special requests will be honored. Remember that you are the customer—don't be afraid to ask for what you want. Study the menu carefully, then ask questions. Restaurants can't handle every type of special request, but most will do their best to make reasonable changes for their patrons. If managers get enough requests for a particular menu item or accompaniment, they may make it regularly available.

Ask about serving sizes. Are "petite" servings or half-portions available? Some ways to cut down on portion sizes: choose an appetizer as your main dish; order a la carte; share food with a friend.

Ask how menu selections are prepared and what ingredients are used. Are the meats, chicken, or fish broiled with butter or other fat? Served with sauces? Are vegetables buttered or creamed? Fresh or canned?

See if your special requests can be accommodated. Order fish, chicken, or meat broiled without added fat. Ask if chicken can be prepared without the skin. Request that food be served with dressings and sauces on the side. See if salt or other ingredients can be omitted when your food is prepared.

Ask about availability of food items not listed on the menu— lowfat or skim milk, fresh fruit, and so forth.

Test Your Skills

On the following two pages you will find a sample restaurant menu. It offers many options—including ways to dine in the Guidelines style. Pretend you're making menu selections. Using the tips given so far, identify foods in each menu section that are lower in calories, fat, sugars, and sodium. Then put together a meal or two. Of course, no food is off limits, so you might also want to make selections in which foods higher in calories, fat, sugars and sodium are balanced with those that are lower. What items would you include in your meals?

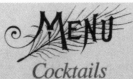

Cocktails

Mixed Drinks
Your choice
Frozen Strawberry Daiquiri
House special

Dry Table Wine
Burgundy and Chablis
Beer
Bottled and draft

Wine Spritzer
Fruit Juice Cocktail
Sparkling Water
with a Twist of Lime

Appetizers

Fresh Melon Wedge
with Lime Slice
Crispy Nachos
Smothered with melted Cheddar cheese, served with guacamole and sour cream
Fresh Fruit Medley
Served in a pineapple boat

Fried Wontons
Served with sweet and sour sauce
Chicken Liver Paté
Served with toasted croutons
Fried Potato Skins
Served with sour cream and chives
Split Pea Soup
Served with your choice of sour cream or sherry

Gazpacho
A crunchy soup of blended tomatoes, cucumbers, bell peppers, and celery, served chilled
Shrimp Cocktail
Served with a spicy cocktail sauce and lemon wedge

Main Course Salads
(Served with rye roll, whole-wheat bread sticks, or croissant)

All-You-Can-Eat Salad Bar
Spinach Salad
Fresh spinach leaves, crispy bacon bits, grated Parmesan, and hard-cooked eggs served with a hot vinaigrette dressing
Garden Pasta Salad
Homemade pasta and fresh vegetables, lightly tossed with a dill dressing

Chef's Salad with Choice of Dressing
Seafood Salad
Tender shrimp, lump crabmeat, and bay scallops sprinkled with an herb dressing and served on a bed of mixed greens
Fresh Fruit Salad with Yogurt Dressing

For Lunch-Time Appetites

Hot Turkey Sandwich
Served open face with giblet gravy and french fries
Grilled Reuben
Fresh corned beef, swiss cheese, and sauerkraut with tangy russian dressing on thick rye bread
Charbroiled Burger
Your choice of cheese and assorted toppings, served with homemade onion rings or french fries
Turkey Cordon Bleu
Slices of ham, turkey, and swiss cheese baked in a buttery pastry shell

Pita Pocket Sandwich
Warm pita bread stuffed with a medley of garden fresh vegetables and chunks of tender cooked chicken, tossed with a light herb dressing
Tuna Salad
Served on a fresh-baked croissant
Veggie Delight
Pan pizza smothered with mushrooms, green peppers, and onions

Pizza Lover's Special
The ultimate in pizza, the crispiest crust in town—covered with sausage, pepperoni, olives, and anchovies
Spinach Quiche
Filled with fresh chopped spinach, onion, and Parmesan, baked in a flaky crust
Fluffy Western Omelette
Three fresh eggs mixed with minced ham, green pepper, and onion

Entrees
(Served with your choice of two vegetables and a garden salad)

Pasta Primavera
Ribbons of fettucini and fresh vegetables tossed in a light
yogurt sauce, sprinkled with Parmesan

Baked Chicken Breast
Boneless breast of chicken baked in a delicate
lemon-basil sauce

Southern-Style Chicken
Fried to a crispy golden brown

Chicken Teriyaki
Grilled strips of chicken marinated in a spicy teriyaki sauce

Beef en Brochette
Skewered cubes of beef round with fresh mushroom caps

London Broil
Delicately marinated and grilled strips of flank steak
served in their own juice

Porterhouse Steak (16 ounces)
Charbroiled the way you like it, topped with crispy
onion rings

Petite Filet Mignon
Broiled to perfection, topped with mushroom caps

Barbecued Baby Back Ribs
A hefty rack of broiled pork ribs smothered with our
own hickory-smoked barbecue sauce

Veal Tenderloins
Plump medallions of veal in a rich cream sauce with
mushrooms and capers

Burritos
Your choice of beef, chicken, or bean; served with rice
and fresh salsa

Fish and Chips
Fresh filet of sole dipped in a special beer batter and
deep-fat fried, served with french-fried potatoes

Crabmeat Au Gratin
Lump backfin crabmeat in a creamy cheese sauce, baked
to a delicate brown

Sweet and Sour Shrimp
Batter-fried shrimp coated with a tangy
sweet-and-sour sauce

Today's Special
Lemon-Broiled Haddock Filets
Served with steaming brown rice pilaf, green beans almondine, tomato halves broiled with fresh basil,
and crusty french bread

Vegetables

French-Fried Potatoes
Herbed New Potatoes
Cheese-Stuffed Baked Potato
Sliced Tomatoes with Basil
Creamy Coleslaw

Broccoli Spears
  with Hollandaise Sauce
Steamed Zucchini-Carrot Medley
Garden Fresh Peas
  with Pearl Onions
Corn-on-the-Cob

Beverages

Fresh Brewed Coffee
Hot Tea
Iced Tea
Assorted Soft Drinks

Milk
  Whole or lowfat
Freshly Squeezed Lemonade
  or Limeade
Chilled Apple Cider

Desserts

Fresh Fruit Sorbet
  Assorted flavors
Poached Pears
  with Raspberry Glaze
Blueberry Pie A La Mode
New York Style Cheese Cake

Carrot Cake
  Topped with a thick cream
  cheese frosting
Assorted Fresh Pastries
  Rich, flaky pastries with
  assorted fillings
Fresh Strawberries (in Season)

Apple Dumpling
  Whole apple baked in a flaky
  cinnamon pastry, topped with
  whipped cream and chopped pecans
Ice Cream Sundae
  A rich french vanilla, topped
  with fudge sauce, nuts and whipped
  cream, served with a cookie

12

In Looking Over the Menu, Did You See. . .

- dishes unfamiliar to you? Ask the waiter to describe how the dish is prepared—and try something new if it fits into the Guidelines style.

- preparation terms and ingredients that signal "low" or "high" fat and "low" or "high" sodium?

- menu selections that might fit nicely into a Guidelines-style meal if you could have dressing, sauces, or toppings on the side?

- selections you might ask to be prepared differently?

Look at the foods you chose for your meal. Did you include a variety of foods from the five food groups shown above? Were some foods good sources of starch and fiber? Judging from what you've learned from this bulletin, does your meal appear to be moderate in calories, fat, sugars, sodium, and alcohol? If not, what food selections would you make the rest of the day to provide the balance needed to eat in the Guidelines style?

Here are some options within each menu section that tend to be lower in fat, sugars, sodium, or alcohol than others. Generally, they provide fewer calories, too.

Cocktails
Sparkling water with a twist of lime, fruit juice cocktail, or wine spritzer. Dry table wines have about half the calories of sweet table wines.

Appetizers
Melon wedge, fresh fruit medley, split pea soup (sour cream or sherry on the side), gazpacho, or shrimp cocktail (go easy on the sauce).

Main Course Salads
Rye roll or whole-wheat breadsticks to accompany main course salads (watch out for spreads); fresh fruit salad, garden pasta salad, or seafood salad (provided they're light on dressing). For some tips on making salad bar selections, see above.

Lunch-Time Appetites
Veggie delight or pita sandwich. If you choose a sandwich such as the tuna salad, lower the fat by having it on a french roll or bagel

rather than a croissant. Choose whole-grain bread for additional fiber and nutrients. Watch added cheeses and condiments if you choose the hamburger.

Entrees
Baked chicken breast, beef en brochette, burritos (bean filling for added fiber), pasta primavera (lots of vegetables and the yogurt sauce is lower in fat than traditional cream sauces). If you're ordering a steak, keep in mind that the petite filet is a smaller portion than the porterhouse.

Today's Special
You can't miss here. All the items are foods in the Guidelines style.

Vegetables
Herbed new potatoes, sliced tomatoes, zucchini and carrots, peas with pearl onions, or corn-on-the-cob (watch added butter and salt).

Beverages
Lowfat milk, lemonade or limeade, apple cider. If coffee or tea is your choice, drink it plain or limit the sugar and cream you add.

Desserts
Fresh fruit sorbet, poached pears, strawberries (with only a small amount, if any, of whipped cream). Alternative: either fruit item listed under Appetizers.

Getting hungry? The menu clearly shows that eating in the Guidelines style need not be dull. It doesn't mean giving up your favorite foods either. If you're really hungry for nachos smothered with cheese, order them. Balance the higher fat and sodium with other menu items that are lower. Or choose lower fat and sodium foods at other meals.

Worth Noting

Sometimes menu names or descriptions send mixed messages. In chicken teriyaki, for example, grilled chicken suggests lower fat, but teriyaki sauce suggests higher sodium. When making choices, you need to consider both the ingredients used and the preparation method. Menu items made with nutritious foods can be quite high in fat and calories—fried potato skins with sour cream, or apple dumpling, for example.

Restaurants are featuring more menu selections that can fit into a nutritious and healthful eating style. Study the foods carefully, however, before you decide. Don't be fooled by the title, "For Lunch-Time Appetites." Some of these selections provide just as much, or more, food (not to mention fat and calories) than the dinner entrees. Also, watch out for menu selections termed "light fare." "Light" may or may not mean that a menu item is lower in calories or fat.

Did you Know?

A typical "diet plate" may be higher in calories and fat than many other selections on the menu. Below is the calorie, fat and sodium content of a typical "diet plate."

	Calories	Fat (grams)	Sodium (milligrams)
Beef Patty (4 ounces)	325	24	95
Cottage Cheese (1/2 Cup)	110	4	425
Hard-Cooked Egg	80	6	70
Tomato Slices	10	Trace	5
Rye Crackers (4)	110	2	230
Totals	635	36	825

Eating On-the-go

Chances are your idea of "eating out" is a relaxing dinner at your favorite restaurant. If so, you might be surprised how often you "eat out" at other times. For example, how often do you find yourself eating. . .

- during a break at the shopping mall?

- watching a movie at the theater?

- as a midmorning or midafternoon pick-me-up at the office?

- at a sports or recreational event?

- at social functions and celebrations—weddings, birthday parties, showers, retirement farewells?

• in your car—on a long trip, commuting to and from work, running errands?

Should you be concerned about on-the-go eating? Maybe and maybe not. Any eating pattern can be adapted to the Dietary Guidelines, whether it's three meals a day, several small meals or snacks, or something in between. If you find yourself eating on-the-go on a regular basis, think about how the foods you select fit into your overall diet pattern. Are they often foods high in fat, sodium, or sugars, and too high in calories? Could you bring foods from home that have more nutrients, fewer calories, and less fat, sodium, and sugars? It's your total diet that counts in the long run, no matter when or where you eat. Concentrate on improving your overall diet through variety, moderation, and balance.

Snacking At The Shopping Mall

Snacks can be an enjoyable part of a shopping trip, and shopping malls offer a variety of foods and places to eat. How do these snacks fit into your total diet? Take a look at the calorie, fat and sodium content of some popular items below:

	Calories	Fat (grams)	Sodium (milligrams)
Frozen yogurt, 1 cup	210	4	100
Ice cream cone, single dip	190	9	55
Popcorn, with salt and butter, 1 cup	105	8	145
Soft pretzel with cheese	275	8	1,175
Chocolate chip cookie, 1 large	190	8	160
Hotdog, with mustard, relish, and onion	240	14	835
Bran muffin, 1 large	140	7	210
Danish pastry	220	12	220
Mixed nuts, ¼ cup	225	21	240

Parties

Occasions like birthday parties, cocktail parties, and receptions often mean a wide variety of tasty foods high in fat, sugars, sodium, and calories. Plan ahead to cut down before and after a big occasion.

- Fresh fruit and vegetable platters are great Guidelines-style party foods. Indulge, but watch the dips!

- Hors d'oeuvres such as fancy finger sandwiches, fried chicken drummettes, and swedish meatballs are high in calories, fat, and sodium.

- Have your birthday cake and eat it too. Just choose a small piece.

- For a mixed drink with fewer calories and less alcohol, try a wine spritzer made with wine and seltzer water; mineral water or tonic with a twist of lemon or lime; or fruit juice with club soda.

Business Functions

At business functions where food and beverages are served, you may feel you have to eat what's offered. You do have some control, however. For example, while talking business, you can make an effort to eat fewer snacks and drink fewer alcoholic beverages, if you drink. Also, most menus include some lower calorie and lower fat items.

Car Trips

When you're on a long trip, you may not have much choice about where you eat out. You probably stop whenever and wherever you happen to be when you're ready for a break. Taking a few foods along in the car can help. A small cooler will come in handy for items that need refrigeration. Here are some good snack choices:

- Small cans or cartons of fruit juice.

- All types of fresh fruit.

- Raw vegetables, such as cherry tomatoes, radishes, and cut-up cucumbers, carrots, celery, green pepper, broccoli, and cauliflower.

- Crackers and peanut butter or cheese.

- Small boxes or bags of raisins or dried fruit mix.

- A snack mix made with plain popcorn, unsweetened cereals, bite-size pretzels, and seasonings such as paprika, hot pepper sauce, and onion or garlic powder.

Picnicking

Picnics conjure up thoughts of all-American favorite foods, such as fried chicken, hotdogs, hamburgers, potato salad, cakes, cookies, etc. How can you eat in the Guidelines style when so many picnic foods are high in fat, sodium, sugars, and calories? Here are some suggestions:

- Grill chicken instead of frying it; remove the skin. If fried chicken is served, skip the skin.

- Grill hamburgers and steaks so the fat runs off during cooking.

- Trim visible fat from steaks.

- Go easy on salt and butter or margarine added to corn-on-the-cob.

- Load up on mixed green salad or vegetable relishes. Have smaller helpings of coleslaw, potato salad, and macaroni salad made with lots of mayonnaise.

- Liven up your hamburger with lettuce, tomatoes, onions, or other vegetables. Go easy on barbecue sauce, catsup, mustard, relishes, and pickles.

- Enjoy fresh melons, bananas, grapes, cherries, peaches, plums, berries, and other fresh fruits.

- Choose fruit juices or unsweetened iced tea rather than soft drinks.

Breakfast Fare

According to recent marketing surveys, more and more people are eating breakfast away from home. Two trends contributing to breakfast's new popularity are "breakfast bars" (at both full-service and fast-food restaurants) and the wide variety of breakfast sandwiches now available at fast food restaurants. Just as at other meals, following the Dietary Guidelines at breakfast doesn't mean eliminating all favorite foods from your diet. You can eat in the Guidelines style by choosing foods high in calories, fat, sodium, and sugars less often and by eating smaller portions.

Following are examples of typical restaurant breakfast offerings.

Cereals

Most are low in fat, except for granolas.

Presweetened cereals provide large amounts of added sugars—often more than you would add to unsweetened types.

1 oz. sugar-coated corn flakes = 1 oz. corn flakes + 2 tsps. sugar

Whole-grain varieties such as bran, shredded wheat, and oatmeal provide more fiber than corn and rice cereals.

	Calories	Fat (grams)	Sodium (Milligrams)	Fiber* (grams)
1 ounce bran flakes	90	trace	245	4.4
1 ounce shredded wheat	100	trace	2	2.8
1 ounce rice crinkles	110	trace	335	0.3

*Preliminary Data

Eggs

Yolks are high in cholesterol (274 milligrams each). Poaching or boiling eggs minimizes added fat and calories. Frying or scrambling with fat and other ingredients (breakfast meats, cheeses) adds calories, fat and sodium.

Meats

Most breakfast meats are fairly high in fat; ham and Canadian bacon are leaner than regular bacon and sausage. Most are relatively high in sodium.

	Calories	Fat (grams)	Sodium (milligrams)
3 slices bacon	110	9	305
2 slices Canadian bacon	85	4	710
3-inch sausage patty	200	17	420

Pancakes, French Toast, Waffles

Traditional toppings (butter/margarine, syrups, whipped cream) add calories, fat, and sugars.

If available, try fruit toppings such as fresh berries, pineapple, or applesauce.

Whole-grain varieties are higher in fiber than those made with white flour.

Gravies and Sauces

Creamed dishes (creamed chipped beef), gravies, and sauces provide extra fat, calories, and sodium.

Potatoes

Hash browns and home fries are high in calories and fat.

1 hashed brown potato patty =1 medium potato +1 1/2 teaspoons fat

Fruits and Juices

All provide vitamins and minerals for few calories.

None contain fat or cholesterol.

Most fruits provide fiber, especially those with edible seeds and skins.

Fruits canned in water or juice are low in added sugars; those packed in syrups are higher.

Most are low in sodium, except for tomato and vegetable blends.

	Calories	Fat (grams)	Sodium (milligrams)
6-ounce glass orange juice	80	0	2
6-ounce glass tomato juice	30	0	660

Milk

Skim and lowfat milks provide the same nutrients but fewer calories and less fat than whole milk.

Coffee and Tea

Both dairy and nondairy creamers add considerable amounts of fat and calories
Sugar adds calories.

The Truth About Fast Foods

Fast-food meals are more popular than ever in the United States. Some reasons we are eating more often at fast-food restaurants are obvious: convenience, relatively low cost, quick service, and predictable products. At the same time, we are more interested than ever before in the nutritional value of our food.

The statements below look at the challenge of making nutritious meal selections at fast-food restaurants. Are the following statements fact or fiction?

Fast foods are really "junk" foods.

FICTION. Most fast foods *do* provide essential nutrients, including protein, and certain vitamins and minerals. However, few foods that are rich in calcium and vitamins A and C available at fast-food restaurants. Many fast foods are also low in fiber and high in calories, fat, and sodium relative to the nutrients they provide. This is changing as many fast-food places add salad bars and other options that make it easier to follow the Dietary Guidelines. Balance fast-food choices with other selections during the day to get all the nutrients you need for good health, while moderating calories, fat, and sodium.

Many fast-food meals are high in sodium.

FACT. Many fast-food selections provide large amounts of sodium from salt and other ingredients. Furthermore, it isn't always easy to predict which foods provide the largest amounts. The sodium content of some items may surprise you! Balancing fast-food selections with lower sodium choices the rest of the day may be the best way to moderate sodium intake.

	Sodium (milligrams)
Quarter-pound hamburger with cheese	1225
French fries (regular size order)	150
Milkshake (10 ounces)	230
Fried chicken (2 pieces)	800

Fried fish and chicken sandwiches are lower in fat than hamburgers.

FICTION. Although poultry and fish have less fat than ground beef, the poultry and fish in fast-food sandwiches are usually breaded and fried. The fat and calorie content of these sandwiches can be the same or higher than a quarter-pound hamburger. Of course, the amount of meat in each sandwich and its toppings also affect fat and calorie content.

	Calories	Fat (grams)
Quarter-pound hamburger	445	21
Fish sandwich (with cheese)	420	23
Chicken sandwich	650	36

Baked potatoes and salad bar selections provide more nutrients and fewer calories than other fast-food entrees.

FACT AND FICTION. Potatoes and raw fruits and vegetables are good sources of vitamins, minerals, starch, and fiber. However, salad dressings and added toppings, especially in generous amounts, can quickly push calories and fat content to the level of other menu entrees—sometimes higher. Figures below show how plain baked potatoes and cheese-stuffed potatoes from fast food restaurants compare in calories and fat to a quarter-pound hamburger.

	Calories	Fat (grams)
Quarter-pound hamburger	445	21
Plain baked potato	250	2
Cheese-stuffed potato	590	34

Menus at fast-food restaurants change in response to consumer demand.

FACT. Restauranteurs are constantly adapting their menu choices to reflect consumers' desires for foods that are tasty, convenient, affordable, and nutritious. In recent years, foods lower in calories, fat, and sodium have been introduced as a result of consumers' rising interest in the nutritional value of foods. Many fast-food restaurants make free nutrition information on their products available to consumers who request it.

Calories, fat, and sodium can add up quickly in a fast-food meal. For example, take a look at the grand tally for a meal consisting of a quarter-pound cheeseburger, a large serving of fries, and a vanilla shake—quite a lot for one meal!

Calories	=	1,205
Fat	=	59 grams
Sodium	=	1,655 milligrams

Fast Food Tips

How can you enjoy fast foods without going overboard? Here are a few pointers. . .

The Main Selection

Choose regular sandwiches rather than doubles, and plain types rather than those with lots of extras, such as cheese, bacon, and "special" sauces. Order roast beef for a leaner option than most burgers. Breaded, deep-fat-fried fish and chicken sandwiches (especially with cheese and/or tartar sauce or mayonnaise) have more fat and calories than a plain burger. When "fixing" your sandwich, load up on lettuce, tomato, and onion, and go easy on pickles, mustard, catsup, and other sauces. If you're having fried chicken, remove some of the breading before eating.

On the Side

Skip the fries if you're ordering a sandwich that is deep-fat fried or made with sauce or cheese. Order a small rather than a large portion, specify no salt, and add just a small amount yourself. Or choose a plain baked potato or mashed potatoes instead of fried, and add butter/margarine and salt sparingly. Have a tossed salad instead of fries. When ordering chicken, have a dinner roll rather than a biscuit to save calories and fat.

Salads

Load up on fresh greens, fruits, and vegetables, but go easy on dressings and creamy salads—potato salad, macaroni salad, and coleslaw.

Beverages

Choose milk (preferably lowfat or skim) instead of a soda or shake. Ask for water if milk isn't available.

Dessert

Skip it or make it an occasional treat. Most options are loaded with calories, fat, and sugars.

For More Information

- Read the other bulletins in this series:

  Nutrition and Your Health: Dietary Guidelines for Americans, HG-232. This bulletin describes basic principles for developing and maintaining a healthier diet—the seven Dietary Guidelines developed by the U.S. Department of Agriculture and the U.S. Department of Health and Human Services. [*Editor's note: see Chapter 1 of this volume.*]

Dietary Guidelines and Your Diet, HG-232-1 through 7. Eacg bulletin focuses on one of the Dietary Guidelines, giving practical tips on how to implement that Guideline in the diet.

Dietary Guidelines and Your Diet, HG-232-8 through 11. These bulletins focus on using all of the Dietary Guidelines together in preparing foods and planning menus; making bag lunches, snacks, and desserts; shopping for food and making meals in minutes; and eating out.

Contact the Human Nutrition Information Service (HNIS) for information on ordereing the above bulletins and for a list of other current publications on Dietary Guidelines topics. The address is U.S. Department of Agriculture, HNIS, Room 325A, 6505 Belcrest Road, Hyattsville, Maryland 20782.

- Contact your local county extension agent (Cooperative Extension System), public health nutritionist, or dietician in hospitals or other community organizations.

Part Three

Current Issues in Nutrition

Chapter 11

Artificial Sweeteners: Sweetness Minus Calories = Controversy

Of the four artificial sweeteners that have whet the palates of millions of Americans over the years, the one souring ingredient common to them all has been controversy.

Saccharin, which has no calories yet is 300 times sweeter than sugar, aspartame, which has the same amount of calories as sugar (four per gram) yet is 180 to 200 times as sweet, and acesulfame K, which has no calories yet is 200 times sweeter than sugar, are currently available to help satisfy Americans' twin cravings for sweets and slimness. Cyclamate, calorie-free yet 30 times sweeter than sugar, was banned by the Food and Drug Administration in 1970 because of concerns over its safety. That ban is currently being reconsidered.

Some 93 million Americans 18 and over are now consuming products containing saccharin, aspartame, or acesulfame K, according to the Calorie Control Council, a trade group of manufacturers of dietary foods and beverages. That's an increase of more than 34 percent since 1984, and the number would be even higher if consumers under 18 were included.

The introduction of diet soft drinks in the 1950s provided the spark for the widespread use of artificial sweeteners today. Howard Roberts, vice president of science and technology for the National Soft Drink Association in Washington, D.C., has reported that the share of the soft drink market held by diet beverages rose from 15 percent in 1982 to more than 28 percent in 1989. "That whole market has taken off since 1982 and may represent 50 percent of total sales in the next

DHHS Publication No. (FDA) 91-2205 (May, 1991)

few years," he said. (Soft drinks of all kinds are now the nation's No. 1 beverage, according to the U.S. Department of Agriculture.)

A regular 12-ounce soft drink has about 150 calories, compared to none in most diet beverages. However, there is little documented evidence that consumption of artificially sweetened foods has contributed to weight loss among Americans.

Besides dieters, diabetics are regular users of artificial sweeteners. The American Diabetes Association says that although aspartame had not been tested extensively in diabetic patients, they could use the sweetener as long as consumption is not excessive. The association also supports moderate use of saccharin as a sugar substitute for diabetics.

Over the years, each of the artificial sweeteners has undergone long periods of review and debate. Controversy surrounding the sweeteners has tended to cloud public understanding of the complex issues involved. Here is some background on the tangled legal and scientific histories of saccharin, cyclamate, aspartame, and acesulfame K.

Saccharin

What puzzles many people is how a food additive may suddenly be branded as unsafe after many years of seemingly safe use. The case of saccharin is a good example of how the shifting requirements of the law, the progress of science, and new trends in food uses can change a substance's status from "safe" to "unsafe."

Americans have been consuming saccharin for more than 100 years. Produced by the Sherwin-Williams Co., it is—like so many other food additives—made from petroleum-based materials. Discovered by a Johns Hopkins University scientist in 1879, it was used initially as an antiseptic and food preservative. Its use in foods developed gradually after the turn of the century, surging during World Wars I and II because of sugar shortages and rationing.

The Food, Drug, and Cosmetic Act provides, in the now-famous Delaney Clause, that no new food additive can be used if animal feeding studies or other appropriate tests showed that it caused cancer. The Delaney Clause, however, does not apply to additives that were generally recognized by experts as safe for their intended uses. Saccharin, cyclamate, and a long list of other substances were being used in foods before passage of the Delaney Clause in 1958 and were considered "generally recognized as safe"—or what is known today as GRAS. (Aspartame, on the other hand, became the first artificial sweetener to fall under the 1958 amendment's requirement for pre-marketing proof of safety because the first petition to FDA for its approval was filed in 1973.)

In 1968, the Committee on Food Protection of the National Academy of Sciences said in a report that, although an adult's daily consumption of one gram of saccharin or less probably was not a health hazard, available studies on the cancer-causing potential of saccharin were inadequate. It urged additional studies and repeated that recommendation two years later. In 1972, with new studies under way, FDA decided to take saccharin off the GRAS list and establish interim limits that would permit its continued use until various studies were completed.

Two of the studies that followed only increased public health concerns. One was done in 1972 by the Wisconsin Alumni Research Foundation, the other in 1973 by FDA. In both tests, male and female rats were fed doses of saccharin from the time of weaning. The offspring of those rats were given saccharin for their entire lives. In both tests, the incidence of bladder tumors in the animals fed saccharin was considered significant. However, arguments were made that an impurity, not saccharin itself, was causing the tumors.

In February 1974, Canada's Health Protection Branch— FDA's counterpart there—began a major rat study to resolve the scientific uncertainties surrounding saccharin. The Canadian project, in which parent rats and their offspring were exposed to saccharin, focused on the effects of the suspect impurity in saccharin, orthotoluenesulfonamide (OTS). In early 1977, the study demonstrated that neither OTS nor other alleged culprits—bladder parasites and bladder stones—were causing the tumors. The substance responsible, the study showed, was saccharin.

Despite clamorous public protests, Canada prohibited all uses of saccharin except as a table-top sweetener to be sold only in pharmacies, and then only with a warning label. With the Canadian study now confirming the Wisconsin and FDA studies, FDA proposed on April 15, 1977, to revoke its 1972 sanction for the sweetener' s continued use in foods and beverages. FDA did propose to allow the sale of saccharin as an over-the-counter drug in the form of a table-top sweetener.

Public clamor over the proposed ban erupted at once, fueled by mention in the agency's announcement that the rats in the Canadian study were fed the equivalent of 800 cans of diet soda a day. High doses of suspect carcinogens are used in feeding studies to produce readily detectable rates of cancer, and the statement was intended simply to describe this testing method. Taken out of context, however, it was ripe for ridicule, and critics pounced on it.

The storm of protest led Congress, in November 1977, to pass the Saccharin Study and Labeling Act, which imposed a two-year moratorium against any ban of the sweetener. While permitting saccharin's continued availability, the law mandated that warning labels be used to advise consumers that saccharin caused cancer in animals. The law also directed FDA to arrange further studies of carcinogens and toxic substances (including saccharin) in foods and to determine whether there were any health benefits resulting from nonnutritive sweeteners.

FDA contracted with the National Academy of Sciences for these studies. The first NAS report, in November 1978, concluded that saccharin was a carcinogen in animals, although of low potency; that it was a potential cancer-causing agent in humans; that the impurities in saccharin were not the carcinogenic agents; and that saccharin seemed to promote the cancer-causing effects of other carcinogenic agents that might be consumed with it. NAS's second report, in March 1979, called for an overhaul of the entire food safety law—changes that might give FDA a range of options in regulating substances like saccharin. The issue is now before Congress. Since 1977, Congress has repeatedly extended the original moratorium.

Although various studies since the proposed 1977 ban have led to varying interpretations of the risks posed by saccharin, FDA's basic position remains that the substance should not be used in food and beverages except as a table-top sweetener.

Cyclamate

A cigarette placed almost unthinkingly on a pile of crystal powder led to the discovery of cyclamate by a University of Illinois scientist in 1937. When the scientist put the cigarette back in his mouth, he found that the powder, a derivative of cyclohexylsulfamic acid, had a sweet and pleasant taste. In the years that followed, the sweetener has endured both the sweet smell of success and the bitter taste of rejection.

Cyclamate was introduced into beverages and foods in the early 1950s, and it dominated the artificial sweetener market through most of the 1960s. But in 1968, the National Academy of Sciences (NAS) told FDA that, although consumption of reasonable quantities of cyclamate probably posed no hazard to humans, additional studies were needed to resolve various aspects of cyclamate's safety.

Further questions arose in 1969 after bladder tumors developed in rats and mice that were fed a mixture of cyclamate and saccharin. That prompted FDA to remove cyclamate from its GRAS list and to propose phasing it out of general food use.

Its continued availability to diabetics was suggested, but after an NAS medical advisory group concluded that cyclamate should not even be available as a drug under medical supervision, FDA imposed a total ban effective Sept. 11, 1970.

Abbott Laboratories, North Chicago, Ill., the sole U.S. producer of cyclamate, sought FDA's permission to re-market the artificial sweetener in November 1973, for use only in special dietary foods and for specific technological purposes. Abbott's petition included more than 400 toxicological reports, all completed after 1970, with assessments of cyclamate's carcinogenicity, mutagenicity (capability of producing genetic damage), and metabolism. In March 1976, the National Cancer Institute told FDA that Abbott's evidence did not establish or refute the cancer-causing potential of cyclamate. FDA concurred and informed the company that its evidence did not demonstrate "to a reasonable certainty" that cyclamate was safe for human consumption.

In effect, FDA was saying that the law placed the burden on the company to prove cyclamate was safe before it could be sold, rather than on FDA to prove it unsafe to keep it off the market. The 1958 Food Additives Amendment contains "general safety" provisions that apply not only to carcinogenicity but to any type of adverse health effect.

The fate of Abbott's 1973 petition was not resolved until Sept. 4, 1980, when then FDA commissioner Jere E. Goyan issued a final negative decision reaffirming an earlier ruling by an administrative law judge. In brief, Goyan's position was that the safety of cyclamate had not been demonstrated, that it had not been shown that cyclamate would not cause cancer and would not cause inheritable genetic damage. Essentially, the Goyan decision was based on what the company's evidence did not show. In saying that safety had not been adequately demonstrated, Goyan did not say the product causes cancer. The decision, in fact, noted that the evidence submitted "does not conclusively establish that cyclamate is a carcinogen."

Abbott filed again in 1982, asking FDA to permit expanded use of cyclamate and its use in combination with other artificial sweeten-

241

ers. Before its ban, cyclamate generally was used in combination with saccharin. Industry spokesmen say that combining artificial sweeteners enhances the sweetness of each, increases a product's stability (or shelf life), mitigates the bitter aftertaste of saccharin, and cuts costs. FDA said its review of the petition would include 59 new studies and other data supplied by Abbott.

The job of reviewing the information on carcinogenesis went to the Cancer Assessment Committee of FDA's Center for Food Safety and Applied Nutrition. The committee was to review the pertinent studies to determine whether cyclamate or its primary metabolite, cyclohexylamine (which some scientists believe may be more toxic than cyclamate itself), were potentially cancer-causing.

Noting that "current scientific thinking about carcinogenesis [had] undergone considerable evolution in the past several years," the committee concentrated its review on some 24 chronic feeding studies in which cyclamate or cyclohexylamine was given to laboratory animals. Although some of the studies preceded the 1970 ban, most were completed during the 1970s, before the 1980 Goyan decision. Particular emphasis was given by the FDA committee to the evaluation of data that seemed to implicate cyclamate as a cause of tumors in the urinary bladders of rats and in the lungs, liver and lymphoreticular tissues of mice. Other studies indicated that consumption of cyclamate could cause testicular atrophy and chromosome breakage, but the committee's evaluation was limited only to whether cyclamate caused cancer.

The committee concluded, in a report issued in April 1984, that the evidence did not indict cyclamate as a cancer-causing agent. Citing the studies with mice, the report stated: "There exists no credible evidence for the carcinogenicity of ingested cyclamate or cyclohexylamine on the basis of all studies on these substances using mice as experimental subjects." On the key rat studies, the committee also stated that there was "no credible case to be made for the association between the administration of high dietary levels of cyclamates and cancer of the bladder in rats. In addition, no neoplasms [tumors] observed at any other sites [of the animals' bodies] were considered to be induced by treatment with cyclamate."

At FDA's request, the National Academy of Sciences/National Research Council then undertook an independent review of the carcinogenicity data. On June 10, 1985, the NAS panel of scientists issued a report that concluded that the scientific evidence did not indicate that cyclamate or its major derivative, cyclohexylamine, was carcinogenic. However, the NAS committee recommended repeating animal studies that suggested that cyclamate may act as a tumor promoter—that is, as a substance that may cause the development of tumors when used with a carcinogen. The NAS panel acknowledged, however, that scientists were uncertain about how such findings might apply to humans. "If the findings [of tumor promotion] are confirmed, uncertainty would still exist about the assessment of risk of cyclamate use for humans . . . ," the NAS report noted.

In the meantime, FDA continues its review of cyclamate, including resolution of such safety issues as to whether cyclamate may cause genetic damage and testicular atrophy.

Aspartame

Like cyclamate, aspartame was discovered accidentally—in 1965 during research for ulcer drugs. Aspartame has been described by FDA and its manufacturer, G.D. Searle & Co., of Skokie, Ill., as one of the most thoroughly tested and studied additives ever approved by the agency.

Searle first sought FDA approval of aspartame in dry foods and as a table-top sweetener in March 1973. FDA approved that petition in July 1974, but challenges over the substance's safety and the validity of the company's data kept aspartame from being marketed. To resolve the safety issues, the contesting parties agreed to put the matter in the hands of a scientific board of inquiry. Before the board could meet, however, FDA had to resolve the challenge to the validity of various studies conducted for Searle. Their validity was affirmed by an outside panel of pathologists in a December 1978 report to FDA.

The board of inquiry held its hearings in early 1980. In a report to FDA the following October, the board concluded that the evidence did not support charges that aspartame consumption posed an increased risk of brain damage that could result in mental retardation or endocrine dysfunction. However, the board did recommend that aspartame's approval be withheld until more long-term animal tests were conducted on the possibility that aspartame might cause brain tumors.

With that, final action on the Searle petition rested with then FDA commissioner Arthur Hull Hayes Jr. On July 24, 1981, Hayes approved the use of aspartame in dry foods. Stating that Searle had "met its burden of proving that aspartame is safe," as required by law, Hayes said that aspartame consumption at even the "maximum projected" levels of daily consumption would "not pose a risk of brain damage resulting in mental retardation, endocrine dysfunction, or both." Hayes also noted that both he and FDA's Center for Food Safety and Applied Nutrition disagreed with the inquiry board's recommendation for further safety studies on the risk of brain tumors. In effect, Hayes ruled that both he and the center's food experts were satisfied that the data submitted demonstrated the safety of aspartame on that issue, as well. To ensure that public consumption levels of aspartame products remained below what might be considered toxic to humans, the decision required Searle to monitor and report consumption levels to FDA.

Approval of aspartame for use in carbonated beverages followed in July 1983. By the end of 1990, FDA had approved aspartame's use as a sweetener in 21 food categories. Breath mints, ready-to-drink iced tea, gelatin desserts, and fruit toppings are just a few of the products in which aspartame may be found. Aspartame's use as an "inactive ingredient" in human drug products was approved by FDA in January 1987.

Foods, beverages and drugs containing aspartame are required by FDA to include a statement for individuals suffering from a rare genetic disease called phenylketonuria (PKU). The warning notes that phenylalanine, an amino acid whose intake must be restricted by PKU victims, is present in the product. Phenylalanine is an essential nutrient for humans. However, when it increases to very high levels in body fluids, those who cannot metabolize it normally can suffer brain damage and mental retardation. Those most susceptible to brain damage from PKU are infants, and all states require newborn children to be screened for the disease. A person not born with PKU does not develop it later.

Following the 1983 approval for carbonated beverage use, some scientists and consumer groups charged that aspartame was a health hazard because it broke down and exposed consumers to excessive levels of methanol. At high enough levels, methanol is a poison and can cause blindness. It also is metabolized into formaldehyde, a "known carcinogen," the critics charged. (Some inhalation tests in animals show that formaldehyde produces nasal tumors.)

The critics maintained that decomposition of aspartame could occur—and expose consumers to possibly high levels of methanol and formaldehyde—if a beverage containing the sweetener was stored for long periods at high temperatures. FDA evaluated the charges and concluded "that the levels of methanol resulting from the use of aspartame in carbonated beverages did not pose any safety issues because they were well below levels of exposure expected to produce toxicity." It was also noted that other foods—including juices, fruits and vegetables—exposed consumers to higher amounts of methanol without adverse effects.

Aspartame's widely publicized approval for use in carbonated drinks also was accompanied by an increasing number of complaints from consumers about headaches, dizziness, and a wide variety of other symptoms they attributed to consuming aspartame-containing products.

In February of 1984, FDA asked the Centers for Disease Control in Atlanta to evaluate the consumer complaints received by the agency, Searle and others. FDA furnished CDC with the results of interviews conducted by its investigators with 517 of the 592 people who had reported complaints up to mid-April 1984.

After evaluating the complaints, CDC reported in November of 1984, that, although some individuals may have an "unusual sensitivity" to aspartame products, the data obtained "do not provide evidence for the existence of serious, widespread, adverse health consequences attendant to the use of aspartame." Although a wide variety of symptoms were reported, CDC said most were mild and the kind that would be "common to the general populace." Few complainants, the report said, went to a doctor with their symptoms.

CDC noted that investigations of this type are "unlikely to establish any cause-and-effect relationship" between the consumption of aspartame and the occurrence of symptoms. It acknowledged that some segments of the population might be sensitive to the sweetener but this could only be clearly established with additional clinical studies.

Acesulfame K

Like the new kid on the block, acesulfame K ("K" is the chemical symbol for potassium), the latest artificial sweetener on the market, was approved by FDA in July 1988 as a calorie-free sugar substitute in packets or tablets and as an ingredient in chewing gum, dry drink mixes, gelatins, puddings, and nondairy creamers.

Acesulfame K is not metabolized—that is "burned" or changed in the human body—so it contributes no calories. Soluble in water, it is stable at normal temperatures.

Beginning in 1982, Hoechst Celanese Corporation, the manufacturer of acesulfame K, submitted to FDA animal feeding studies on the safety of the sweetener. The agency was provided with data from four long-term studies—a two-year toxicity study in beagle dogs, a carcinogenicity study in mice, and two long-term rat studies.

In its evaluation of all the data, FDA found that the safety studies did not show any toxic effects that could be attributed to the sweetener. The agency applied a 100-fold safety factor in making its safety assessment—that is, the agency found that the maximum amount consumed by humans would be less than one-hundredth of the amount that caused no toxic effect when fed to animals.

Concern was expressed to FDA by consumer groups that tumors found in some rats fed acesulfame K may have been caused by the sweetener. FDA's detailed analysis of all the data, however, including data from other studies using these strains of animals, showed that any tumors found were typical of what could routinely be expected and were not due to feeding with acesulfame K.

At the time of the initial approval of acesulfame K's use, FDA deferred action on the company's request that the sweetener be permitted for use in confections, including hard and soft candy. In the past, FDA has interpreted the Food, Drug, and Cosmetic Act as barring the use of non-nutritive sweeteners in candies. Currently, FDA is reviewing petitions for other food uses for acesulfame K, including soft drinks and nonalcoholic beverages.

Chapter 12

Calcium and Osteoporosis: Maintaining a Strong Skeleton

Approximately 95 percent of our skeleton is developed during the first 18 years of life. Periods of rapid growth occur during the first year of life and during the adolescent growth spurt. After adult height is achieved, our bones continue to become more dense as minerals are deposited. This is the consolidation phase. An additional 5-percent increase in bone mass is accumulated by age 30 to 35. At this age, our bones are the most dense and we are in a period of peak bone mass. After age 40, we experience an age-related phase of slow bone loss. The most rapid loss of bone mass for women occurs during the first 4 to 8 years after menopause. This chapter discusses the consequences of bone loss and also the lifestyle factors that protect the skeleton.

Osteoporosis

When enough bone mass is lost that bones become vulnerable to fracture, the individual has developed osteoporosis. Osteoporosis is a debilitating disease that affects over 24 million Americans. Each year in the United States, 1.3 million fractures are attributable to osteoporosis. The most common fractures occur at the wrist, the spine, and the hip. Hip fractures alone result in annual health-care costs of $10 billion. This figure will continue to increase with the increase of the elderly population. Between 15 and 25 percent of persons with a

---

Excerpt from *Nutrition: Eating for Good Health*, U.S. Department of Agriculture, Agricultural Information Bulletin 685

hip fracture enter long-term-care institutions. Hip fractures are as-sociated with a high mortality rate due to surgical deaths and to com-plications such as thromboembolism, fat embolism, and pneumonia.

Treatment of Osteoporosis

A number of drugs are being investigated for their efficacy in the treatment of osteoporosis. These include calcitonin, bisphosphonates, and 1,25-dihydroxyvitamin D3. These drugs slow bone resorption but have little effect on the stimulation of bone formation. Other agents being researched are fluoride and parathyroid hormone; these may stimulate bone formation but are not proven to reduce the rates of fracture.

Because of the lack of a cure for osteoporosis, the prevention of excessive bone loss is the current focus. Approximately 80 percent of bone mass is genetically determined. The other 20 percent can be modified by lifestyle factors. Adequate calcium intake, weight-bear-ing exercise, and estrogen-replacement therapy for women who have entered menopause are the primary lifestyle factors associated with reducing the risk of osteoporosis. Factors associated with increased risk of osteoporosis include smoking and abuse of alcohol and caffeine. Thin, small-framed women are more vulnerable to osteoporosis, and Caucasians and Asians are at higher risk than African-Americans. Women are at greater risk than men by a ratio of 4 to 1. Women have less bone mass, experience accelerated loss of bone mass following menopause, and ingest less calcium than do men.

A researcher at the USDA Human Nutrition Research Center at Tufts University (Boston, MA), Bess Dawson-Hughes, has shown that calcium supplements can prevent the usual bone loss associated with aging in women who consume less than 400 milligrams (mg) of cal-cium per day. Furthermore, two studies have reported that the risk of hip fracture is reduced by as much as 60 percent on higher calcium intakes.

Other nutrients that are important to the skeleton are protein, vitamins C and D, phosphorus, magnesium, manganese, copper, zinc, and boron.

Estrogen-replacement therapy can also prevent or retard bone loss in perimenopausal and postmenopausal women as long as the therapy is continued and the dietary calcium intake is sufficient. Calcium supplementation in combination with estrogen replacement has synergistic positive effects on bone loss; that is, the effectiveness of each treatment is enhanced.

Early-Life Steps To Prevent Osteoporosis

Building bone mass in early life may be the most effective way to prevent osteoporosis in later life. If this opportunity is missed, it probably cannot be made up. Even small increases in bone mass can have a great impact on the risk of fracture. For instance, a 5-percent increase in bone mass can reduce the risk of osteoporotic fracture by 40 percent.

A lifelong habit of drinking milk is associated with increased bone mass. Researchers at the Indiana University School of Medicine in Indianapolis have shown that calcium supplements increase the bone mass in preadolescent children, compared to that in their identical twins who received placebos during a 3-year study.

Getting Enough Calcium

In the American diet, almost 75 percent of dietary calcium comes from dairy products. Few other foods are concentrated sources of absorbable calcium. At Purdue University (West Lafayette, IN) and Creighton University (Omaha, NE), plant foods are being screened for calcium absorption. These include broccoli, bok choy, kale, and tofu made with calcium salts. Calcium is well absorbed from these vegetables and from all dairy products—that is, milk, yogurt, cheese, processed cheese, and their low-fat counterparts. Spinach is a concentrated source of calcium, but this calcium is poorly absorbed because it is complexed with oxalic acid and is therefore indigestible

Depending on their stage of growth, people need 2 to 5 cups of milk or the calcium equivalent each day. American females more than 12 years old typically consume less calcium than this recommended amount. Calcium intake in American women is 40 to 50 percent below that in men. A 1984 National Institutes of Health consensus-development conference recommended 1,000 mg of calcium per day for premenopausal women and 1,500 mg per day for postmenopausal women. However, 25 percent of American women have an intake below 300 mg per day, which is the amount of calcium in one glass of milk. Calcium supplements are recommended for individuals who cannot get adequate calcium through diet. However, supplements do not contain all the nutrients necessary for building bones, and people often forget to take pills. An alternative source of calcium is the fortified beverages now on the market.

Exercise

Weight-bearing exercise has a positive impact on bone density. An effective exercise program applies weight loading to all parts of the skeleton. For example, the right arm of a right-handed tennis player has a higher bone density than does the left arm. Activities that are exclusively aerobic seem to be the least effective in building peak bone mass. Thus, weight lifters have higher bone density than do swimmers. We do not know if the positive effects of exercise on bone mass are retained when exercise is discontinued.

A partial explanation for bone loss in the elderly is the reduction in physical activity with age. The physical work of the average sedentary elderly adult is 30 percent less than that of the average younger adult. If immobilization occurs, bone loss is accelerated; but bone mass can increase when the individual again becomes ambulatory.

The Known and Unknown

Obtaining adequate dietary calcium, exercise, and estrogen-replacement therapy following menopause are three lifestyle choices for maintaining a strong skeleton. The interaction of these factors is not well understood. Nor do we know the residual positive effect after cessation of treatment. Research to determine the best food sources of absorbable calcium and the most effective exercise programs, in combination with education programs on behavior modification, can help reduce the suffering and the healthcare costs associated with bone loss.

Connie M. Weaver
Head, Department of Foods and Nutrition,
Purdue University, West Lafayette, IN

Chapter 13

A Consumer's Guide to Fats

Once upon a time, we didn't know anything about fat except that it made foods tastier. We cooked our food in lard or shortening. We spread butter on our breakfast toast and plopped sour cream on our baked potatoes. Farmers bred their animals to produce milk with high butterfat content and meat "marbled" with fat because that was what most people wanted to eat.

But ever since word got out that diets high in fat are related to heart disease, things have become more complicated. Experts tell us there are several different kinds of fat, some of them worse for us than others. In addition to saturated, monounsaturated and polyunsaturated fats, there are triglycerides, trans fatty acids, and omega 3 and omega 6 fatty acids.

Most people have learned something about cholesterol, and many of us have been to the doctor for a blood test to learn our cholesterol "number." Now, however, it turns out that there's more than one kind of cholesterol, too.

Almost every day there are newspaper reports of new studies or recommendations about what to eat or what not to eat: Lard is bad, olive oil is good, margarine is better for you than butter—then again, maybe it's not.

Amid the welter of confusing terms and conflicting details, consumers are often baffled about how to improve their diets.

FDA recently issued new regulations that will enable consumers to see clearly on a food product's label how much and what kind of fat the product contains. (See "A Little 'Lite' Reading" in Part IV.) Un-

Publication No. (FDA) 95-2286

derstanding the terms used to discuss fat is crucial if you want to make sure your diet is within recommended guidelines (see below).

Fats and Fatty Acids

Fats are a group of chemical compounds that contain fatty acids. Energy is stored in the body mostly in the form of fat. Fat is needed in the diet to supply essential fatty acids, substances essential for growth but not produced by the body itself.

There are three main types of fatty acids: saturated, monounsaturated and polyunsaturated. All fatty acids are molecules composed mostly of carbon and hydrogen atoms. A saturated fatty acid has the maximum possible number of hydrogen atoms attached to every carbon atom. It is therefore said to be "saturated" with hydrogen atoms.

Some fatty acids are missing one pair of hydrogen atoms in the middle of the molecule. This gap is called an "unsaturation" and the fatty acid is said to be "monounsaturated" because it has one gap. Fatty acids that are missing more than one pair of hydrogen atoms are called "polyunsaturated."

Saturated fatty acids are mostly found in foods of animal origin. Monounsaturated and polyunsaturated fatty acids are mostly found in foods of plant origin and some seafoods. Polyunsaturated fatty acids are of two kinds, omega-3 or omega-6. Scientists tell them apart by where in the molecule the "unsaturations," or missing hydrogen atoms, occur.

Recently a new term has been added to the fat lexicon: trans fatty acids. These are byproducts of partial hydrogenation, a process in

---

Fat Content Most Important

Percentage of people who said these food qualities were "very important" to them.

Low caffeine	31.2%
Low calorie	38.2%
Low sodium	41.3%
Low fat/Low cholesterol	58.6%

Note: Respondents could choose more than one answer.
(Source: Nielsen Marketing Research)

---

which some of the missing hydrogen atoms are put back into polyunsaturated fats. Some of the hydrogenated fatty acids take on a "straight" structure; these are the trans fatty acids. "Hydrogenated vegetable oils," such as vegetable shortening and margarine, are solid at room temperature because straightening fatty acids allows them to pack more tightly.

Cholesterol

Cholesterol is sort of a "cousin" of fat. Both fat and cholesterol belong to a larger family of chemical compounds called lipids. All the cholesterol the body needs is made by the liver. It is used to build cell membranes and brain and nerve tissues. Cholesterol also helps the body produce steroid hormones needed for body regulation, including processing food, and bile acids needed for digestion.

People don't need to consume dietary cholesterol because the body can make enough cholesterol for its needs. But the typical U.S. diet contains substantial amounts of cholesterol, found in foods such as egg yolks, liver, meat, some shellfish, and whole-milk dairy products. Only foods of animal origin contain cholesterol.

Cholesterol is transported in the bloodstream in large molecules of fat and protein called lipoproteins. Cholesterol carried in low-density lipoproteins is called LDL-cholesterol; most cholesterol is of this type. Cholesterol carried in high-density lipoproteins is called HDL-cholesterol. (See "Fat Words.")

A person's cholesterol "number" refers to the total amount of cholesterol in the blood. Cholesterol is measured in milligrams per deciliter (mg/dl) of blood. (A deciliter is a tenth of a liter.) Doctors recommend that total blood cholesterol be kept below 200 mg/dl. The average level in adults in this country is 205 to 215 mg/dl. Studies in the United States and other countries have consistently shown that total cholesterol levels above 200 to 220 mg/dl are linked with an increased risk of coronary heart disease. (See "Lowering Cholesterol" in the March 1994 FDA Consumer.)

LDL-cholesterol and HDL-cholesterol act differently in the body. A high level of LDL-cholesterol in the blood increases the risk of fatty deposits forming in the arteries, which in turn increases the risk of a heart attack. Thus, LDL-cholesterol has been dubbed "bad" cholesterol.

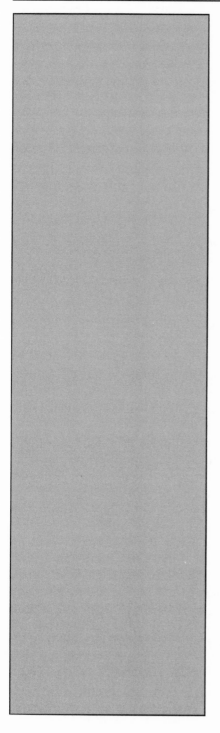

On the other hand, an elevated level of HDL-cholesterol seems to have a protective effect against heart disease. For this reason, HDL-cholesterol is often called "good" cholesterol.

In 1992, a panel of medical experts convened by the National Institutes of Health (NIH) recommended that individuals should have their level of HDL-cholesterol checked along with their total cholesterol.

According to the National Heart, Lung, and Blood Institute (NHLBI), a component of NIH, a healthy person who is not at high risk for heart disease and whose total cholesterol level is in the normal range (around 200 mg/dl) should have an HDL-cholesterol level of more than 35 mg/dl. NHLBI also says that an LDL-cholesterol level of less than 130 mg/dl is "desirable" to minimize the risk of heart disease.

Some very recent studies have suggested that LDL-cholesterol is more likely to cause fatty deposits in the arteries if it has been through a chemical change known as oxidation. However, these findings are not accepted by all scientists.

The NIH panel also advised that individuals with high total cholesterol or other risk factors for coronary heart disease should have their triglyceride levels checked along with their HDL-cholesterol levels.

Triglycerides and VLDL

Triglyceride is another form in which fat is transported through the blood to the body tissues. Most of the body's stored fat is in the form of triglycerides. Another lipoprotein—very low-density lipoprotein, or VLDL—has the job of carrying triglycerides in the blood. NHLBI considers a triglyceride level below 250 mg/dl to be normal.

It is not clear whether high levels of triglycerides alone increase an individual's risk of heart disease. However, they may be an important clue that someone is at risk of heart disease for other reasons. Many people who have elevated triglycerides also have high LDL-cholesterol or low HDL-cholesterol. People with diabetes or kidney disease—two conditions that increase the risk of heart disease—are also prone to high triglycerides.

Dietary Fat and Cholesterol Levels

Many people are confused about the effect of dietary fats on cholesterol levels. At first glance, it seems reasonable to think that eating less cholesterol would reduce a person's cholesterol level. In fact, eating less cholesterol has less effect on blood cholesterol levels than eating less saturated fat. However, some studies have found that eating cholesterol increases the risk of heart disease even if it doesn't increase blood cholesterol levels.

Another misconception is that people can improve their cholesterol numbers by eating "good" cholesterol. In food, all cholesterol is the same. In the blood, whether cholesterol is "good" or "bad" depends on the type of lipoprotein that's carrying it.

Polyunsaturated and monounsaturated fats do not promote the formation of artery-clogging fatty deposits the way saturated fats do. Some studies show that eating foods that contain these fats can reduce levels of LDL-cholesterol in the blood. Polyunsaturated fats, such as safflower and corn oil, tend to lower both HDL- and LDL-cholesterol. Edible oils rich in monounsaturated fats, such as olive and canola oil, however, tend to lower LDL-cholesterol without affecting HDL levels.

How Do We Know Fat's a Problem?

In 1908, scientists first observed that rabbits fed a diet of meat, whole milk, and eggs developed fatty deposits on the walls of their

255

arteries that constricted the flow of blood. Narrowing of the arteries by these fatty deposits is called atherosclerosis. It is a slowly progressing disease that can begin early in life but not show symptoms for many years. In 1913, scientists identified the substance responsible for the fatty deposits in the rabbits' arteries as cholesterol.

In 1916, Cornelius de Langen, a Dutch physician working in Java, Indonesia, noticed that native Indonesians had much lower rates of heart disease than Dutch colonists living on the island. He reported this finding to a medical journal, speculating that the Indonesians' healthy hearts were linked with their low levels of blood cholesterol.

De Langen also noticed that both blood cholesterol levels and rates of heart disease soared among Indonesians who abandoned their native diet of mostly plant foods and ate a typical Dutch diet containing a lot of meat and dairy products. This was the first recorded suggestion that diet, cholesterol levels, and heart disease were related in humans. But de Langen's observations lay unnoticed in an obscure medical journal for more than 40 years.

After World War II, medical researchers in Scandinavia noticed that deaths from heart disease had declined dramatically during the war, when food was rationed and meat, dairy products, and eggs were scarce. At about the same time, other researchers found that people who suffered heart attacks had higher levels of blood cholesterol than people who did not have heart attacks.

Since then, a large body of scientific evidence has been gathered linking high blood cholesterol and a diet high in animal fats with an elevated risk of heart attack. In countries where the average person's blood cholesterol level is less than 180 mg/dl, very few people develop atherosclerosis or have heart attacks. In many countries where a lot of people have blood cholesterol levels above 220 mg/dl, such as the United States, heart disease is the leading cause of death.

High rates of heart disease are commonly found in countries where the diet is heavy with meat and dairy products containing a lot of saturated fats. However, high-fat diets and high rates of heart disease don't inevitably go hand-in-hand.

Learning from Other Cultures

People living on the Greek island of Crete have very low rates of heart disease even though their diet is high in fat. Most of their dietary fat comes from olive oil, a monounsaturated fat that tends to lower levels of "bad" LDL-cholesterol and maintain levels of "good" HDL-cholesterol.

The Inuit, or Eskimo, people of Alaska and Greenland also are relatively free of heart disease despite a high-fat, high-cholesterol diet. The staple food in their diet is fish rich in omega-3 polyunsaturated fatty acids.

Some research has shown that omega-3 fatty acids, found in fish such as salmon and mackerel as well as in soybean and canola oil, lower both LDL-cholesterol and triglyceride levels in the blood. Some nutrition experts recommend eating fish once or twice a week to reduce heart disease risk. However, dietary supplements containing concentrated fish oil are not recommended because there is insufficient evidence that they are beneficial and little is known about their long-term effects.

Omega-6 polyunsaturated fatty acids have also been found in some studies to reduce both LDL- and HDL-cholesterol levels in the blood. Linoleic acid, an essential nutrient (one that the body cannot make for itself) and a component of corn, soybean and safflower oil, is an omega-6 fatty acid.

At one time, many nutrition experts recommended increasing consumption of monounsaturated and polyunsaturated fats because of their cholesterol-lowering effects. Now, however, the advice is simply to reduce dietary intake of all types of fat. (Infants and young children, however, should not restrict dietary fat.)

The available information on fats may be voluminous and is sometimes confusing. But sorting through the information becomes easier once you know the terms and some of the history.

The "bottom line" is actually quite simple, according to John E. Vanderveen, Ph.D., director of the Office of Plant and Dairy Foods and Beverages in FDA's Center for Food Safety and Applied Nutrition. "What we should be doing is removing as much of the saturated fat from our diet as we can. We need to select foods that are lower in total fat and especially in saturated fat." In a nutshell, that means eating fewer foods of animal origin, such as meat and whole-milk dairy products, and more plant foods such as vegetables and grains.

Government Advice

Dietary guidelines endorsed by the U.S. Department of Agriculture and the U.S. Department of Health and Human Services advise consumers to:

- Reduce total dietary fat intake to 30 percent or less of total calories.
- Reduce saturated fat intake to less than 10 percent of calories.
- Reduce cholesterol intake to less than 300 milligrams daily.

Glossary of Fat Words

Here are brief definitions of the key terms important to an understanding of the role of fat in the diet.

Cholesterol: A chemical compound manufactured in the body. It is used to build cell membranes and brain and nerve tissues. Cholesterol also helps the body make steroid hormones and bile acids.

Dietary cholesterol: Cholesterol found in animal products that are part of the human diet. Egg yolks, liver, meat, some shellfish, and whole-milk dairy products are all sources of dietary cholesterol.

Fatty acid: A molecule composed mostly of carbon and hydrogen atoms. Fatty acids are the building blocks of fats.

Fat: A chemical compound containing one or more fatty acids. Fat is one of the three main constituents of food (the others are protein and carbohydrate). It is also the principal form in which energy is stored in the body.

Hydrogenated fat: A fat that has been chemically altered by the addition of hydrogen atoms (see trans fatty acid). Vegetable shortening and margarine are hydrogenated fats.

Lipid: A chemical compound characterized by the fact that it is insoluble in water. Both fat and cholesterol are members of the lipid family.

Lipoprotein: A chemical compound made of fat and protein. Lipoproteins that have more fat than protein are called low-density lipoproteins (LDLs). Lipoproteins that have more protein than fat are called high-density lipoproteins (HDLs). Lipoproteins are found in the blood, where their main function is to carry cholesterol.

Monounsaturated fatty acid: A fatty acid that is missing one pair of hydrogen atoms in the middle of the molecule. The gap is called an "unsaturation." Monounsaturated fatty acids are found mostly in plant and sea foods. Olive oil and canola oil are high in monounsaturated fatty acids. Monounsaturated fatty acids tend to lower levels of LDL-cholesterol in the blood.

Polyunsaturated fatty acid: A fatty acid that is missing more than one pair of hydrogen atoms. Polyunsaturated fatty acids are mostly found in plant and sea foods. Safflower oil and corn oil are high in polyunsaturated fatty acids. Polyunsaturated fatty acids tend to lower levels of both HDL-cholesterol and LDL-cholesterol in the blood.

Saturated fatty acid: A fatty acid that has the maximum possible number of hydrogen atoms attached to every carbon atom. It is said to be "saturated" with hydrogen atoms. Saturated fatty acids are mostly found in animal products such as meat and whole milk. Butter and lard are high in saturated fatty acids. Saturated fatty acids tend to raise levels of LDL-cholesterol ("bad" cholesterol) in the blood. Elevated levels of LDL-cholesterol are associated with heart disease.

Trans fatty acid: A polyunsaturated fatty acid in which some of the missing hydrogen atoms have been put back in a chemical process called hydrogenation, resulting in "straighter" fatty acids that solidify at higher temperatures. Trans fatty acids are under study to determine their effects on cholesterol.

by Eleanor Mayfield

Eleanor Mayfield is a writer in Silver Spring, Md.

Chapter 14

Fiber: Something Healthy to Chew On

Our grandparents called it the "bulk" or "roughage" in their diet; the popular name today is "fiber"; and scientists prefer to describe it as "dietary fiber." But, as with the proverbial rose, by any name it seems the same—the stuff that puts the crunch in carrots, the bulk in salads, the chewiness in whole-meal bread, and the thickness in the stewed prunes and pea soup.

For many years, neither scientists nor the public appreciated fiber. It was classified by experts as a "nonessential" in the diet. Consumers overlooked it, even though it had been common knowledge for centuries that foods that provide bulk or roughage retain liquids and therefore help to relieve constipation and promote bowel regularity.

However, in recent years, scientists have taken a second look at dietary fiber and, as a result, fiber has become one of the "in things" in nutrition. In the 1960s and early 1970s, Dr. Denis Burkitt and other British physicians began promoting a theory about fiber and its effect on health. They noted that several diseases that are common in Western countries are virtually unknown in rural Africa but do occur among Africans who move to urban areas. The doctors theorized that these differences occur because the Africans changed from their native unrefined, high-fiber diet to the relatively low-fiber, more processed diet typical of urban areas.

The Burkitt theory was highly controversial in scientific circles, but it had the effect of stimulating scientific interest, and thus encouraging further research. While much more research is needed to clearly

DHHS Publication No. (FDA) 91-2206 (April, 1991)

define the role of fiber in the diet, some of the information uncovered recently about its functions in the digestive tract has been convincing enough for the U.S. Department of Health and Human Services and Department of Agriculture to advise the public to eat foods with adequate fiber.

In *Dietary Guidelines for Americans,* published by the two federal agencies in 1980 and recently reaffirmed, the following advice was offered about fiber:

> Eating foods with fiber is important for proper bowel function and can reduce symptoms of chronic constipation, diverticular disease, and hemorrhoids. Populations like ours with diets low in dietary fiber and complex carbohydrates and high in fat, especially saturated fat, tend to have more heart disease, obesity, and some cancers. Just how dietary fiber is involved is not yet clear.

Some of the benefit from a higher fiber diet may be from the food that provides the fiber, not from fiber alone. For this reason, it's best to get fiber from foods rather than from supplements. In addition, excessive use of fiber supplements is associated with greater risk for intestinal problems and lower absorption of some minerals.

Advice for today: Eat more vegetables, including dry beans and peas; fruits; and breads, cereals, pasta, and rice. Increase your fiber intake by eating more of a variety of foods that contain fiber naturally.

There were but seven pieces of advice in the publication, yet guidance about that "nonessential" of the not-too-distant past was among the seven. Just how fiber went from nonentity status to one of the basic elements for healthy eating is a comment on the flexibility of the scientific community when new information is discovered.

Fiber does its work in the digestive tract as part of a blended mixture. Although the fiber components lose their plant identity, they retain their water-binding, gel-forming, and other physical properties during the chewing and digestive processes.

Fiber's effect on the digestive system begins in the mouth. The considerable chewing that may be required for foods such as salad greens and whole-grain products stimulates saliva flow. This in turn starts the stomach's digestive juices flowing. Once swallowed, fiber contributes bulk and some swelling of stomach contents as water is absorbed. Soluble forms of fiber such as pectins and gums increase the viscosity, or thickness, of the stomach contents. These effects contribute to a feeling of fullness and also slow down emptying of the stomach.

Once past the stomach, the insoluble fibers, by increasing the bulk and weight of the food mass, cut down on transit time through the intestines. On the other hand, the increased viscosity resulting from pectin and other soluble fibers slows down the movement. This allows more time for digested food to be absorbed into the body, but the process also has it nutritional drawbacks: Some minerals, such as calcium and zinc, may be bound by fiber and, as a result, don't get absorbed; and fiber can bind bile acids, which aid in the digestive process.

Cellulose and other insoluble fibers are essentially unchanged as they pass through the intestines, but the pectins and gums are fermented by bacteria in the large intestine, producing gases and some fatty acids.

With new interest in fiber has come new information, indicating that fiber may offer some protection against conditions such as constipation, diverticulosis (a disorder of the large intestine), obesity, diabetes, cancer, and heart disease.

The firmest indication to date of fiber's beneficial effects involves constipation, which is no small health concern for many Americans. Folk knowledge has now been confirmed by science: Fiber, or roughage, in the diet can help relieve constipation and promote more frequent bowel movements. Particularly effective are the fibrous foods containing insoluble types of fiber, such as the coarse, tough parts of vegetables and wholegrain products.

Diverticulosis, a condition in which small sacs, or diverticula, bulge outward from the lining of the large intestine, may also be aided by dietary fiber. The National Institute of Arthritis, Diabetes, Digestive and Kidney Diseases says that studies indicate that 10 percent of those over 40 years of age and 50 percent over 60 have diverticulosis. There are no symptoms of diverticulosis, but if the sacs become infected, a condition known as diverticulitis develops and usually requires medical treatment.

The exact cause is unknown, but the combined pressure of food and gas on weak spots in the intestinal wall may lead to development of the sacs. Chronic constipation and the use of potent laxatives may also increase pressure in the intestines and may cause or aggravate the condition. Those with the condition are often put on a diet that includes plenty of fluids, fruits, coarse bread and cereals, and leafy, fibrous vegetables. Such a diet produces softer, bulkier stools.

Another condition that may be related to fiber is "irritable bowel syndrome." The syndrome is characterized by constipation or diarrhea or alternating periods of both. Some studies indicate that wheat bran, in particular, may be helpful in some cases of irritable bowel syndrome.

Fiber may also contribute to controlling obesity. Well-known for their low-calorie characteristics, foods such as celery, salad greens, and apples have other advantages for those who want to control their weight. These foods contain fibrous portions that require extra time to eat and provide bulk in the stomach, which may give a greater feeling of fullness than foods with less fiber. Further, by slowing down food leaving the stomach, they may delay the return of hunger.

Some evidence suggests that the physical properties of dietary fiber that slow down stomach emptying and transit time in the intestines can aid in controlling some types of diabetes. Diets high in starchy foods and adequate in fiber have been found to bring about desirable lowering of blood glucose and increases in insulin sensitivity.

The scientific detectives are still at work on the possible relationship between fiber consumption and cancer of the colon (the large intestine). Colon cancer is less common in countries where people eat more fiber than Americans do; however, their diets also contain less fat and protein than ours and differ in other ways. A 1983 report by the National Academy of Sciences concluded that the evidence was not yet conclusive that dietary fiber protects against colon cancer. The evidence does suggest that the insoluble components of fiber (cellulose, hemicelluloses and lignin) may protect against colon cancer through their dilution of bowel contents and removal of excess bile acids as well as through their bulking abilities.

Research also indicates that some water-soluble fiber components may help to reduce blood cholesterol levels, which can lessen the chances of coronary heart disease, and scientific judgment remains reserved on the role fiber may play.

Clearly, the scientific jury is still out with respect to fiber's relationship to several diseases. However, the evidence adds up to removing the "non" from the nonessential status fiber had not too many years ago. It is now clearly sensible to include healthy amounts of fiber in the foods we eat. But just how much is a "healthy amount?" The experts answer that question by advising individuals to eat several servings of food each day that contain fiber, preferably from different plant sources. That includes fruits and vegetables, whole-grain breads, cereals and other products made from whole grains, nuts, and legumes (beans and peas).

The types of fiber and the amounts present in those foods vary greatly. Fruits are general sources of pectins, particularly citrus fruits and apples. Cellulose is common in all plants, but there's more in the outer layers of cereal grains and the tough fibrous parts of fruits, vegetables and legumes.

Starchy foods, which contain desirable and substantial complex carbohydrates, usually are also good sources of fiber. Starchy foods from seeds, such as cereal and legumes, and those from roots and tubers, such as carrots and potatoes, contain many nutrients in addition to fiber. And for those struggling to control or reduce weight, starchy foods usually have fewer calories per serving than fatty foods.

Fiber is generally concentrated in one part of the plant, often in the outer layers, and some may be lost during processing in the home or by manufacturers. Some fiber is lost in paring fruits and vegetables, for example. And, in the process of making white and other extracted flours, the outer coats (bran) of grain are removed, decreasing the fiber content. Thus, wholegrain products are preferred by those who want the most fiber out of their food. Likewise, whole plant parts provide more fiber than products made from them; for example, the orange has more fiber than the juice extracted from it.

Soluble fiber, such as gums and pectins, may be added during processing as thickeners or for other purposes. The dietary contribution of such additions is highly variable, but it still adds to the total fiber intake. It's not necessary to take fiber tablets or other special fiber supplements unless recommended by a physician. Nature makes ample fiber available, and makes it available on a year-round basis.

Don't go overboard in consuming fiber. As noted earlier, fiber can bind some minerals—such as calcium, zinc, copper and selenium—preventing their absorption and use by the body. Too much dietary fiber may lead to deficiencies in these trace minerals. Any attempt to increase fiber consumption above usual levels should be undertaken gradually. Individual tolerances for fiber vary—an adequate amount for one person may produce distressing side effects in another.

What Is Dietary Fiber?

Scientific definitions of dietary fiber vary, but according to Dorland's Illustrated Medical Dictionary, it is: "That part of whole grain, vegetables, fruits, and nuts that resists digestion in the gastrointestinal tract."

It's the material in plant cell walls that's not digested or only partially digested by humans.

To chemists, fiber used to mean crude fiber—the residue left after treating a plant sample first with a weak acid and then with a weak alkali. It is this crude fiber that has been listed on food labels. However, scientists have come to realize that this laboratory treatment is much harsher than the treatment food gets from enzymes and other body secretions in the digestive tract. A new method for analyzing "dietary" fiber has been accepted for official use, and it is this dietary fiber that is now listed on some food labels.

The fiber in the diet is a diverse group of chemical compounds—cellulose, hemicelluloses, pectins, gums, and lignin. All are complex carbohydrates except lignin, a very tough substance found in many plants.

Cellulose, hemicelluloses and lignin are components of wood as well as edible plants. As might be expected, they are rough and fibrous. They're also insoluble in water. Pectins and gums are water-soluble and form gel-like, or viscous, textures. (Pectin is a familiar substance to those who make homemade jelly.) Pectins and gums are intermeshed in plants with other dietary components, mainly in cell walls.

All of the dietary fibers are found in varying combinations and amounts in plant leaves, stems, tubers, roots, flowers, and seeds. Cellulose, the most abundant fiber compound, forms the basic structural material of cell walls. Cotton is almost pure cellulose, and the outer layers of cereal grains contain large amounts of cellulose.

Fiber varies from plant to plant. The broccoli stalk, much of which we don't eat, contains more fiber than the flower parts, all of which we usually eat. The fiber in a carrot (a root) is quite different from that in broccoli, or cereal grain (seeds), or a lettuce leaf. That the amount of fiber may increase with the age of the plant is evident if you've eaten a stringy green bean that has grown beyond the young, tender stage.

by Marilyn Stephenson

Marilyn Stephenson is a registered dietitian with FDA's Center for Food Safety and Applied Nutrition.

Chapter 15

Illnesses and Injuries Associated With the Use of Selected Dietary Supplements

Products marketed as "dietary supplements" include a diverse range of products, from traditional nutrients, such as vitamins or minerals, to such substances as high-potency free amino acids, botanicals, enzymes, animal extracts, and bioflavanoids that often have no scientifically recognized role in nutrition.

There is currently no systematic evaluation of the safety of products marketed as dietary supplements. Dietary supplements routinely enter the marketplace without undergoing a safety review by FDA. Published studies on the safety of these products are extremely sparse. There is no systematic collection and review of adverse reaction reports for dietary supplements, as there is for drugs, and physicians rarely seek information about their patients' use of dietary supplements. Despite the lack of any system for gaining information about the risks of dietary supplements, an increased number of reports of adverse reactions to dietary supplement products has recently been recognized. Because of concern about these products, FDA has, in the last year, initiated an effort to collect and evaluate existing studies and case reports on safety problems associated with dietary supplements. As a result of that effort, FDA has begun to identify dietary supplements for which serious adverse reactions have been documented. A list of selected dietary supplements associated with serious safety problems follows. This list is not intended to include all hazardous ingredients in dietary supplements.

I. Herbals

Herbal and other botanical ingredients of dietary supplements include processed or unprocessed plant parts (bark, leaves, flowers, fruits, and stems), as well as extracts and essential oils. They are available in a variety of forms, including water infusions (teas), powders, tablets, capsules, and elixirs, and may be marketed as single substances or in combination with other materials, such as vitamins, minerals, amino acids, and non-nutrient ingredients. Although data on the availability, consumer use, and health effects of herbals are very limited, some herbal ingredients have been associated with serious adverse health effects.

A. *Chaparral* (Larrea tridentata)

Chaparral, commonly called the creosote bush, is a desert shrub with a long history of use as a traditional medicine by Native Americans. Chaparral is marketed as a tea, as well as in tablet, capsule, and concentrated extract form, and has been promoted as a natural antioxidant "blood purifier," cancer cure, and acne treatment. At least six cases (five in the United States and one in Canada) of acute non-viral hepatitis (rapidly developing liver damage) have been associated with the consumption of chaparral as a dietary supplement. Additional cases have been reported and are under investigation. In the majority of the cases reported thus far, the injury to the liver resolves over time, after discontinuation of the product. In at least two patients, however, there is evidence that chaparral consumption caused irreversible liver damage. One patient suffered terminal liver failure requiring liver transplant.

Most of these cases are associated with the consumption of single ingredient chaparral capsules or tablets; however, a few of the more recent cases appear to be associated with consumption of multi-ingredient products (capsules, tablets or teas) that contain chaparral as one ingredient. Chemical analyses have identified no contaminants in the products associated with the cases of hepatitis. Products from at least four different distributors and from at least two different sources have been implicated thus far.

After FDA's health warning, many distributors of chaparral products voluntarily removed the products from the market in December of 1992. Some chaparral products remain on the market, however, and other distributors who removed their products from the market are seeking to clarify the status of these products.

B. Comfrey (Symphytum officinale *(common comfrey)*, S. asperum *(prickly comfrey)*, or S. X uplandicum *(Russian comfrey))*

Preparations of comfrey, a fast-growing leafy plant, are widely sold in the United States as teas, tablets, capsules, tinctures, medicinal poultices, and lotions. Since 1985, at least seven cases of hepatic veno-occlusive disease—obstruction of blood from the liver with potential scarring (cirrhosis)—including one death, have been associated with the use of commercially available oral comfrey products.

Comfrey, like a number of other plants (e.g., *Senecio* species), contains pryrrolizidine alkaloids. The toxicity of pyrrolizidine alkaloids to humans is well-documented. Hepatic veno-occlusive disease, following ingestion of pyrrolizidine alkaloid-containing products, has been documented repeatedly throughout the world. Hepatic veno-occlusive disease is usually acute and may result in fatal liver failure. In less severe cases, liver disease may progress to a subacute form. Even after apparent recovery, chronic liver disease, including cirrhosis, has been noted. Individuals who ingest small amounts of pyrrolizidine alkaloids for a prolonged period may also be at risk for development of hepatic cirrhosis. The diagnosis of pyrrolizidine alkaloid-induced hepatic veno-occlusive disease is complex, and the condition is probably underdiagnosed.

The degree of injury caused by pyrrolizidine alkaloid-containing plants, like comfrey, is probably influenced by such factors as the age of the user, body mass, gender, and hepatic function, as well as the total cumulative dose digested and the type of exposure (i.e., whether exposure was to leaves or roots, infusions or capsules). Infants in general appear to be particularly susceptible to adverse effects of exposure to pyrrolizidine alkaloids; there are reports of infants developing hepatic veno-occlusive disease following acute exposure of less than one week. Transplacental pyrrolizidine poisoning has been suggested by the occurrence of hepatic disease in the newborn infant of a woman who consumed herbal tea during pregnancy.

Although liver damage is the major documented form of injury to humans from pyrrolizidine alkaloid-containing herbals, animal studies suggest that their toxicity is much broader. Animals exposed to pyrrolizidine alkaloids have developed a wide range of pulmonary, kidney and gastro-intestinal pathologies. Pyrrolizidine alkaloid-containing plants, including comfrey, have also been shown to cause cancer in laboratory animals.

Four countries (the United Kingdom, Australia, Canada and Germany) have recently restricted the availability of products containing comfrey, and other countries permit use of comfrey only under a physician's prescription.

C. *Yohimbe* (Pausinystalia yohimbe)

Yohimbe is a tree bark containing a variety of pharmacologically active chemicals. It is marketed in a number of products for body building and "enhanced male performance." Serious adverse effects, including renal failure, seizures and death, have been reported to FDA with products containing yohimbe and are currently under investigation.

The major identified alkaloid in yohimbe is yohimbine, a chemical that causes vasodilatation, thereby lowering blood pressure. Yohimbine is also a prescription drug in the United States. Side effects are well recognized and may include central nervous system stimulation that causes anxiety attacks. At high doses, yohimbine is a monoamine oxidase (MAO) inhibitor. MAO inhibitors can cause serious adverse effects when taken concomitantly with tyramine-containing foods (e.g., liver, cheeses, red wine) or with over-the-counter (OTC) products containing phenylpropanolamine, such as nasal decongestants and diet aids. Individuals taking yohimbe should be warned to rigorously avoid these foods and OTC products because of the increased likelihood of adverse effects.

Yohimbe should also be avoided by individuals with hypotension (low blood pressure), diabetes, and heart, liver or kidney disease. Symptoms of overdosage include weakness and nervous stimulation followed by paralysis, fatigue, stomach disorders, and ultimately death.

D. *Lobelia* (Lobelia inflata)

Lobelia, also known as Indian tobacco, contains pyridine-derived alkaloids, primarily lobeline. These alkaloids have pharmacological actions similar to, although less potent than, nicotine. There have been several reported cases of adverse reactions associated with consumption of dietary supplements containing lobelia.

Depending on the dose, lobeline can cause either autonomic nervous system stimulation or depression. At low doses, it produces bronchial dilation and increased respiratory rate. Higher doses result in respiratory depression, as well as sweating, rapid heart rate, hypotension, and even coma and death. As little as 50 milligrams of dried herb or a single milliliter of lobelia tincture has caused these reactions.

Because of its similarity to nicotine, lobelia may be dangerous to susceptible populations, including children, pregnant women, and individuals with cardiac disease. Lobelia is nevertheless found in dietary supplement products that are marketed for use by children and infants, pregnant women, and smokers.

E. Germander (Teucrium *genus*)

Germander is the common name for a group of plants that are contained in medicinal teas, elixirs and capsules or tablets, either singly or in combination with other herbs, and marketed for the treatment of obesity and to facilitate weight loss.

Since 1986, at least 27 cases of acute nonviral hepatitis (liver disease), including one death, have been associated with the use of commercially available germander products in France. These cases show a clear temporal relationship between ingestion of germander and onset of hepatitis, as well as the resolution of symptoms when the use of germander was stopped. In 12 cases, re-administration of germander was followed by prompt recurrence of hepatitis. Recovery occurred gradually in most cases, approximately two to six months after withdrawal of germander. Analyses of these cases does not indicate a strong relationship between the dosage or duration of ingestion and the occurrence of hepatitis.

Although the constituent in germander responsible for its hepatic toxicity has not been identified, germander contains several chemicals, including polyphenols, tannins, diterpenoids, and flavonoids.

On the basis of the 27 French hepatitis cases, the French Ministry of Health has forbidden the use of germander in drugs. Its use has been restricted in other countries.

F. Willow Bark (Salix *species*)

Willow bark has long been used for its analgesic (pain killing), antirheumatic, and antipyretic (fever-reducing) properties. Willow

271

bark is widely promoted as an "aspirin-free" analgesic, including in dietary supplement products for children. Because it shares the same chemical properties and the same adverse effects as aspirin, this claim is highly misleading. The "aspirin-free" claim is particularly dangerous on products marketed, without warning labels, for use by children and other aspirin-sensitive individuals.

The pharmacologically active component in willow bark is "salicin," a compound that is converted to salicylic acid by the body after ingestion. Both willow bark and aspirin are salicylates, a class of compounds that work by virtue of their salicylic acid content. Aspirin (acetylsalicylic acid) is also converted to salicylic acid after ingestion.

All salicylates share substantially the same side effects. The major adverse effects include irritation of the gastric mucosa (a particular hazard to individuals with ulcer disease), adverse effects when used during pregnancy (including stillbirth, bleeding, prolonged gestation and labor, and low-birth-weight infants), stroke, and adverse effects in children with fever and dehydration. Children with influenza or chickenpox should avoid salicylates because their use, even in small doses, is associated with development of Reye syndrome, which is characterized by severe, sometimes fatal, liver injury. Salicylate intoxication (headache, dizziness, ringing in ears, difficulty hearing, dimness of vision, confusion, lassitude, drowsiness, sweating, hyperventilation, nausea, vomiting, and central nervous system disturbances in severe cases) may occur as the result of over-medication, or kidney or liver insufficiency. Hypersensitivity, manifested by itching, bronchospasm and localized swelling (which may be life-threatening), can occur with very small doses of salicylates and may occur even in those without a prior history of sensitivity to salicylates. Approximately 5 percent of the population is hypersensitive to salicylates.

G. Jin Bu Huan

Jin Bu Huan is a Chinese herbal product whose label claims that it is good for "insomnia due to pain," ulcer, "stomachic [sic] neuralgia, pain in shrunken womb after childbirth, nervous insomnia, spasmodic cough, and etc." Jin Bu Huan has been recently reported to be responsible for the poisoning of at least three young children (ages 13 months to 2 ½ years), who accidentally ingested this product. The children were hospitalized with rapid-onset, life-threatening bradycardia (very low heart rate), and central nervous system and respiratory depression. One child required incubation (assisted breathing). All three ultimately recovered, following intensive medical care.

Although the product label identified the plant source for Jin Bu Huan as *Polygala chinensis*, this appears to be incorrect since preliminary analyses indicate the presence of tetrahydropalmatine (THP), a chemical not found in *Polygala*. THP is found, however, in high concentrations in plants of certain *Stephania* species. In animals, exposure to THP results in sedation, analgesia, and neuromuscular blockade (paralysis). The symptoms of the three children are consistent with these effects.

An additional case of THP toxicity, reported in the Netherlands, appears to be associated with the same product, and is being investigated.

H. Herbal products containing Stephania and Magnolia species

A Chinese herbal preparation containing *Stephania* and *Magnolia* species that was sold as a weight-loss treatment in Belgium has been implicated recently as a cause of severe kidney injury in at least 48 women. These cases were only discovered by diligent investigations by physicians treating two young women who presented with similar cases of rapidly progressing kidney disease that required renal dialysis. Once it was determined that both these women had used the herbal diet treatment, further investigation of kidney dialysis centers in Belgium found a total of 48 individuals with kidney injury who had used the herbal product.

At the time that a report of these adverse effects was published in February 1993, 18 of the 48 women had terminal kidney failure that will require either kidney transplantation or life-long renal dialysis.

I. Ma huang

Ma huang is one of several names for herbal products containing members of the genus *Ephedra*. There are many common names for these evergreen plants, including squaw tea and Mormon tea. Serious adverse effects, including hypertension (elevated blood pressure), palpitations (rapid heart rate), neuropathy (nerve damage), myopathy (muscle injury), psychosis, stroke, and memory loss, have been reported to FDA with products containing Ma huang as ingredients and are currently under investigation.

273

The *Ephedras* have been shown to contain various chemical stimulants, including the alkaloids ephedrine, pseudoephedrine and norpseudoephedrine, as well as various tannins and related chemicals. The concentrations of these alkaloids depends upon the particular species of Ephedra used. Ephedrine and pseudoephedrine are amphetamine-like chemicals used in OTC and prescription drugs. Many of these stimulants have known serious side effects. Ma huang is sold in products for weight control, as well as in products that boost energy levels. These products often contain other stimulants, such as caffeine, which may have synergistic effects and increase the potential for adverse effects.

II. Amino Acids

Amino acids are the individual constituent parts of proteins. Consumption of foods containing intact proteins ordinarily provides sufficient amounts of the nine amino acids needed for growth and development in children and for maintenance of health of adults. The safety of amino acids in this form is generally not a concern. When marketed as dietary supplements, amino acids are sold as single compounds, in combinations of two or more amino acids, as components of protein powders, as chelated single compounds, or in chelated mixtures. Amino acids are promoted for a variety of uses, including bodybuilding. Some are promoted for claimed pharmacologic effects.

The Federation of American Societies for Experimental Biology (FASEB) recently conducted an exhaustive search of available data on amino acids and concluded that there was insufficient information to establish a safe intake level for any amino acids in dietary supplements, and that their safety should not be assumed. FASEB warned that consuming amino acids in dietary supplement form posed potential risks for several subgroups of the general population, including women of childbearing age (especially if pregnant or nursing), infants, children, adolescents, the elderly, individuals with inherited disorders of amino acid metabolism, and individuals with certain diseases.

At least two of the amino acids consumed in dietary supplements have also been associated with serious injuries in healthy adults.

A. *L-tryptophan*

L-tryptophan is associated with the most serious recent outbreak of illness and death known to be due to consumption of dietary supplements. In 1989, public health officials realized that an epidemic of eosinophilia-myalgia syndrome (EMS) was associated with the ingestion of L-tryptophan in a dietary supplement. EMS is a systemic connective tissue disease characterized by severe muscle pain, an increase in white blood cells, and certain skin and neuromuscular manifestations.

More than 1,500 cases of L-tryptophan-related EMS have been reported to the national Centers for Disease Control and Prevention. At least 38 patients are known to have died. The true incidence of L-tryptophan-related EMS is thought to be much higher. Some of the individuals suffering from L-tryptophan-related EMS have recovered, while other individuals' illnesses have persisted or worsened over time.

Although initial epidemiologic studies suggested that the illnesses might be due to impurities in an L-tryptophan product from a single Japanese manufacturer, this hypothesis has not been verified, and additional evidence suggests that L-tryptophan itself may cause or contribute to development of EMS. Cases of EMS and related disorders have been found to be associated with ingestion of L-tryptophan from other batches or sources of L-tryptophan. These illnesses have also been associated with the use of L-5-hydroxytryptophan, a compound that is closely related to L-tryptophan, but is not produced using the manufacturing process that created the impurities in the particular Japanese product.

B. Phenylalanine

A number of illnesses, including those similar to the eosinophilia myalgia syndrome (EMS) associated with L-tryptophan consumption, have been reported to FDA in individuals using dietary supplements containing phenylalanine. There are also published reports of scleroderma/scleroderma-like illnesses, which have symptoms similar to EMS, occurring in children with poorly controlled blood phenylalanine levels, as well as in those with phenylketonuria (PKU), a genetic disorder characterized by the inability to metabolize phenylalanine.

III. Vitamins and Minerals

Vitamin and mineral dietary supplements have a long history of use at levels consistent with the Recommended Dietary Allowances

(RDAs) or at low multiples of the RDAs, and are generally considered safe at these levels for the general population. Intakes above the RDA, however, vary widely in their potential for adverse effects. Certain vitamins and minerals that are safe when consumed at low levels are toxic at higher doses. The difference between a safe low dose and a toxic higher dose is quite large for some vitamins and minerals and quite small for others.

A. Vitamin A

Vitamin A is found in several forms in dietary supplements. Preformed vitamin A (vitamin A acetate and vitamin A palmitate) has well-recognized toxicity when consumed at levels of 25,000 International Units (IU) per day, or higher. (Beta-carotene does not have the potential for adverse effects that the other forms of vitamin A do, because high intakes of beta-carotene are converted to vitamin A in the body at much lower levels.) The RDA for vitamin A is 1,000 retinol equivalents (RE) for men, which is equivalent to 3,300 IU of preformed vitamin A, and 80 percent of these amounts for women.

The adverse effects associated with consumption of vitamin A at 25,000+ IU include severe liver injury (including cirrhosis), bone and cartilage pathologies, elevated intracranial pressure, and birth defects in infants whose mothers consumed vitamin A during pregnancy. Groups especially vulnerable to vitamin A toxicity are children, pregnant women, and those with liver disease caused by a variety of factors, including alcohol, viral hepatitis, and severe protein-energy malnutrition.

There are some studies that suggest vitamin A toxicity has occurred at levels of ingestion below 25,000 IU. In addition, the severity of the injuries that occur at 25,000 IU suggests that substantial, but less severe and less readily recognized, injuries probably occur at somewhat lower intakes. Most experts recommend that vitamin A intake not exceed 10,000 IU for most adults or 8,000 IU for pregnant and nursing women.

B. Vitamin B$_6$

Neurologic toxicity, including ataxia (alteration in balance) and sensory neuropathy (changes in sensations due to nerve injury), is associated with intake of vitamin B$_6$ (pyridoxine) supplements at levels above 100 milligrams per day. As little as 50 milligrams per day has caused resumption of symptoms in an individual previously injured by higher intakes. The RDA for vitamin B_6 is 2 milligrams. Vitamin B_6 is marketed in capsules containing dosages in the 100-, 200- and 500-milligrams range.

C. Niacin (nicotinic acid and nicotinamide)

Niacin taken in high doses is known to cause a wide range of adverse effects. The RDA for niacin is 20 milligrams. Niacin is marketed in dietary supplements at potencies of 250 mg, 400 mg, and 500 mg, in both immediate and slow-release formulations. Daily doses of 500 mg from slow-release formulations, and 750 mg of immediate release niacin, have been associated with severe adverse reactions including gastrointestinal distress (burning pain, nausea, vomiting, bloating, cramping, and diarrhea) and mild to severe liver damage. Less common, but more serious (in some cases life-threatening), reactions include liver injury, myopathy (muscle disease), maculopathy of the eyes (injury to the eyes resulting in decreased vision), coagulopathy (increased bleeding problems), cytopenia (decreases in cell types in the blood), hypotensive myocardial ischemia (heart injury caused by too low blood pressure) and metabolic acidosis (increases in the acidity of the blood and urine).

Niacin (nicotinic acid) is approved as a prescription drug to lower cholesterol. Many of the observed adverse reactions have occurred when patients have switched to OTC formulations of niacin, and particularly when they have switched from immediate-release formulations to dietary supplements containing slow-release niacin formulations without the knowledge of their physicians.

D. Selenium

Selenium is a mineral found in dietary supplement products. At high doses (approximately 800 to 1,000 micrograms per day), selenium can cause tissue damage, especially in tissues or organs that concentrate the element. The toxicity of selenium depends upon the chemical form of selenium in the ingested supplement and upon the selenium levels in the foods consumed. Human injuries have occurred following ingestion of high doses over a few weeks.

IV. Other Products Marketed as Dietary Supplements

A. *Germanium*

Germanium is a nonessential element. Recently, germanium has been marketed in the form of inorganic germanium salts and novel organogermanium compounds as a "dietary supplement." These products are promoted for their claimed immunomodulatory effects or as "health-promoting" elixirs. Germanium supplements, when used chronically, have caused nephrotoxicity (kidney injury) and death. Since 1982, there have been 20 reported cases of acute renal failure, including two deaths, attributed to oral intakes of germanium elixirs. In surviving patients, kidney function has improved after discontinuation of germanium, but none of the patients have recovered normal kidney function.

One particular organogermanium compound, an azaspiran organogermanium, has been studied for its potential use as an anticancer drug. Forty percent of the patients in this study experienced transient neurotoxicity (nerve damage), and two patients developed pulmonary toxicity. Because of these side effects, medically supervised administration of this drug with monitoring for toxicity has been recommended for those using germanium chronically.

Chapter 16

Monosodium Glutamate (MSG)

Monosodium glutamate (MSG) has been used for many years as a flavor enhancer for a variety of foods prepared at home, in restaurants, and by food processors. The substance has become controversial because some people believe they suffer allergic-type reactions when they consume MSG. Because of MSG's common use in Chinese cuisine, these reactions have become known popularly as "Chinese restaurant syndrome."

FDA has studied adverse reaction reports and other data concerning MSG's safety for many years. The agency believes that some sensitive people can have mild and transitory reactions in some circumstances when they consume significant amounts of MSG (such as would be found in heavily flavor-enhanced foods). Nevertheless, the agency believes that MSG is a safe food ingredient for the general population. FDA continues to evaluate the regulatory status of MSG and plans to broaden the labeling requirement for the substance to include not only that it be listed when it is added as a separate ingredient (as is currently required) but also that it be listed when it is a functional component of other ingredients.

What Is MSG?

Asians have used MSG as a flavor enhancer for at least 2,000 years in the form of a broth made with the types of seaweed known as sea

---

HFI-40 October 1991 BG 91-7.1

tangle. Today, MSG is manufactured by a fermentation process using starch, sugar beets, sugar cane, or molasses.

MSG is the sodium salt of glutamic acid, an amino acid found naturally in our bodies. Other salts of glutamic acid, such as calcium glutamate and potassium glutamate, also have flavor-enhancing properties. Glutamic acid, or glutamate, is a major "building block" of many proteins in foods, such as cheese, meat, peas, mushrooms, and milk. Some glutamate is present in foods in a "free" form, not bound with other amino acids. It is only in this free form that glutamate can enhance a food's flavor. Part of the flavor-enhancing effect of tomatoes, certain cheeses, and fermented or hydrolyzed protein products is due to the presence of free glutamate.

Hydrolyzed proteins, or protein hydrolysates, are acid-treated or enzymatically-treated proteins from certain food sources. They contain salts of free amino acids, including glutamates, at levels of 5 to 20 percent. Hydrolyzed proteins are used in place of MSG as flavors and flavor enhancers in many foods, such as canned vegetables, canned tuna, and processed meats.

MSG, as sold in grocery stores, is a fine, white crystal substance, similar in apparent to salt or sugar. It does not have a distinct taste of its own. Precisely how MSG works to "wake up" or enhance the flavor of foods is not fully understood. Many Western scientists believe that MSG stimulates taste receptors in the tongue, while their Eastern counterparts believe the chemical has a unique fifth basic taste— beyond salty, sweet, sour, and bitter that they call "umami," derived from the Japanese word meaning "deliciousness."

Scientific Reviews of MSG

FDA is evaluating MSG's safety as part of an ongoing project initiated in 1970 to review safety data on the ingredients of processed foods that are listed as "generally recognized as safe" (GRAS) under the 1958 Food Additives Amendment to the Federal Food, Drug, and Cosmetic Act.

Until its evaluation is complete, MSG remains on the GRAS list with a requirement that it must be identified as "monosodium glutamate" on the ingredient label of any food to which it is added.

In 1980, as part of the GRAS review, an independent body of scientists, the Select Committee on GRAS Substances of the Federation of American Societies for Experimental Biology, concluded that MSG is safe at current use levels, but safety at significantly increased levels of consumption requires additional evaluation.

FDA's Advisory Committee on Hypersensitivity to Food Constituents also reviewed MSG and in 1986 concluded that MSG posed no threat to the general public, but that reactions might occur in a small percentage of the population. This position was later reinforced by a report from the FDA Center for Food Safety and Applied Nutrition's Adverse Reaction Monitoring System (ARMS).

The ARMS report, released in 1990, found that a small percentage of individuals have moderate reactions such as skin flushing, tightening of jaw and upper chest muscles, and headaches shortly after eating food containing MSG. No severe reactions were documented, but one investigator reported aggravation of asthma in some individuals after they had consumed MSG, in some cases many hours later. Because of the way the testing was conducted, it couldn't be determined whether MSG actually caused these asthmatic reactions.

One of the problems with the reports of adverse reactions that FDA has received is that it is difficult to link the reactions specifically to MSG. Most are cases in which people have had reactions after eating certain foods containing MSG and are not controlled studies.

A controlled study was conducted in 1972 by Richard A. Kenney, Ph.D., of George Washington University Medical Center, Washington, D.C. Dr. Kenney's study used placebos and orally administered MSG in a representative sample of humans. The study showed that one-third of those tested experienced symptoms when given large doses of MSG but, at amounts normally consumed with food, almost none did. In fact, some people who claimed to be sensitive to MSG reacted similarly when exposed to the placebo.

Scientists' concerns are not related to consumption of foods that naturally contain glutamates; the concern, rather, is that a diet extremely high in MSG used as a flavor enhancer could result in acute elevation of glutamate in the blood. Hypothetically, this could cause overstimulation of portions of the brain, adversely affecting the central nervous system and possibly leading to brain injury. However, no scientific evidence has surfaced to support the hypothesis that MSG, consumed at levels found in food products, can cause brain injury.

Unconfirmed cases of such injuries continue to be examined, however, as do reports by George Schwartz, M.D., a Santa Fe, N.M., physician. Dr. Schwartz alleges that even at low doses, glutamates can cause life-threatening reactions. He has published a book titled *Bad Taste: the MSG Syndrome,* and has made many public statements about his belief in the danger of MSG. A group known as "No MSG" also supports Dr. Schwartz's views.

Although reports such as Dr. Schwartz's may be of value in identifying a population for future investigation, without additional information they cannot lead to meaningful conclusions concerning MSG's potential role in provoking these reactions.

The most recent evaluation of MSG's safety came from the European Communities' Scientific Committee for Food. In a report released by the committee in June 1991, MSG was reaffirmed as safe, and its "acceptable daily intake" was established as "not specified," the most favorable designation for a food ingredient. In addition, the EC committee's report said, "Infants, including prematures, have been shown to metabolize glutamate as efficiently as adults and therefore do not display any special susceptibility to elevated oral intakes of glutamate."

The Joint Expert Committee on Food Additives of the United Nations Food and Agricultural Organization and the World Health Organization have also placed MSG in the safest category of food additives.

As part of its GRAS review, FDA is contracting with a third party to update a literature review of MSG's safety. When its own review is completed, FDA will publish a proposal in the Federal Register announcing its conclusions on the safety of MSG and will request written comments from the public before issuing a final decision.

Label Listing

There have been instances when MSG or some other form of glutamate has been added to foods as a component of a hydrolyzed protein without the requirement that it be specifically identified on the label. That has been a controversial issue, and FDA plans to change that provision of the regulations and require glutamate to be specifically listed in those cases as well. Currently, when hydrolyzed protein is an ingredient in a food, FDA's labeling regulations don't require that the glutamate component of the protein be listed separately on the label. (FDA does not usually require components of ingredients to be listed on the label unless there is a public health reason for doing so.) However, FDA has reconsidered this position and is now planning to require that the phrase "(contains glutamate)" be added to the label as part of the common or usual name for those hydrolyzed protein products that contain significant amounts of glutamate. For example, the label would state "hydrolyzed soy protein (contains glutamate)."

FDA's decision to make this change does not result from any public health concern about the safety of MSG. FDA is requiring the declaration of MSG because:

- MSG comprises a significant proportion (up to 20 percent) of hydrolyzed protein.

- At such levels, the MSG itself (and not just the hydrolyzed protein) functions as a flavor enhancer.

- Consumer interest in this issue has been high.

The "(contains glutamate)" declaration will be published as a tentative provision in a final rule on hydrolyzed protein labeling scheduled for publication in the Federal Register in mid-1992. The tentative final regulation will allow time for additional comments.

Chapter 17

Never Say Diet?

Considering that weight loss programs, pills and potions typically slim the wallet but not the dieter, and with research pointing to genetic and metabolic differences between stout and slim people, obesity experts are now debating whether dieting can achieve permanent weight loss.

Defining Obesity

Obesity is associated with such health problems as diabetes, gallstones, hypertension, and heart disease. Obesity is also linked to colorectal cancer and to breast, uterine and ovarian cancer in women and prostate cancer in men. But how many extra pounds does it take before a person crosses the line from overweight to obese? It depends on whom you ask: The definition of obesity is currently in a state of flux.

Traditionally, obesity was defined as 20 percent or more above an optimal weight for height derived from actuarial statistics that correlated with lowest death rates. Now, some health experts say that the weight-for-height yardstick is both imprecise and overly restrictive.

Recent research suggests that more important than the amount of extra weight a person carries is where it is located. "Rather than weight-for-height, obesity should be defined in terms of waist-to-hip ratio," says C. Wayne Callaway, MD, associate clinical professor of

FDA Consumer / October 1991

medicine at George Washington University in Washington, D.C., and a leading authority on obesity.

Waist-to-hip ratio can be calculated by dividing the number of inches around the waistline by the circumference of the hips. For example, someone who has a 27-inch waist and 38-inch hips would have a ratio of 0.71. A woman whose ratio is 0.8 or higher would be at high risk of weight-related health problems, as would a man whose ratio is 0.95 or above.

Numerous studies show that fat in the hips and thighs is less health-threatening than abdominal fat. While other fat cells empty directly into general circulation, the fatty acid contents of abdominal fat cells go straight to the liver, by way of the portil vein, before being circulated to the muscles. This process interferes with the liver's ability to clear insulin from the bloodstream. As blood levels of insulin increase, muscles and other cells become insulin-resistant, and blood glucose levels rise as a result. In response, the pancreas cranks out more insulin, prompting the autonomic nervous system (which controls heart rate, blood pressure, and other vital signs) to produce norepinephrine, an adrenalin-like chemical that raises blood pressure. This sets the stage for the development of diabetes, hypertension, and heart problems.

Callaway also points out that weight tables do not take age-related weight gain into account (as people age, fat cells become less metabolically active, so one can weigh more and still be healthy) and "arbitrarily" assign lower weights to women at a given height than to men. "There is no evidence showing that women live longer if they weigh less than men of equal stature," he says.

To be a more useful indicator of health risks, experts advocate broadening the definition of obesity to meet three criteria: weight for age and height rather than for gender and height, waist-to-hip ratio, and presence of such weight-related health problems as hypertension.

Food or Fate?

As researchers try to figure out why some people get fat and others don't, it is becoming increasingly apparent that obesity has a variety of causes—heredity, environment, metabolism, and level of physical activity—and, therefore, no single "cure."

Adipose tissue (fat cells) stores energy in the form of fat to meet the body's energy needs when other sources, such as glucose, are unavailable or depleted.

The body has an almost limitless capacity to store fat. Not only can each fat cell balloon to more than 10 times its original size, but should the available cells get filled to the brim, new ones will propagate. As the body stores more fat, weight and girth increase.

A number of studies have shown that genetics may be the most important determinant of how much you weigh. Some people are more prone to weight gain than others even when caloric intake is the same, according to a study of 12 pairs of identical male twins aged 19 to 27 conducted at Quebec's Laval University and reported in the May 24, 1990, issue of the *New England Journal of Medicine.* After eating an extra 1,000 calories six days a week for 100 days, some of the twins gained 9 pounds apiece while others gained as much as 29 pounds each—in some twin pairs, the extra calories were stored as fat while others used up the excess calories by building muscle tissue. The twins in each pair gained the same amount of weight and in the same places, suggesting that as-yet unidentified genetic factors influence the amount of weight gain and its distribution.

The same issue of the *New England Journal of Medicine* also reported on a study comparing the body mass of 673 pairs of identical and fraternal Swedish twins who had been raised together or apart to determine how much influence heredity had over obesity (identical twins have the exact same genetic makeup whereas fraternal twins do not: twins who were raised together were subject to the same environmental influences while those who were raised apart were not). Even if they had grown up together, the fraternal twins were less likely than the identical twins to share a similar pattern of body weight whereas identical twins—even when raised apart—did not vary significantly in weight. The researchers concluded that genetic factors, apart from diet or lifestyle, strongly influence how much a person weighs.

Previously, researchers at the University of Iowa found evidence of a recessive obesity gene (the child needs one copy of the gene from each parent to have the tendency towards overweight). A study of 277 schoolchildren and their families showed a pattern of obesity that followed the classic model for recessive inheritance.

However, it is likely that a number of genetic mechanisms exert influence on weight, among them genes that dictate metabolism and appetite. One that is being investigated actively is the gene that codes for lipoprotein lipase (LPL), an enzyme produced by fat cells to help store calories as fat. If too much LPL is produced, the body will be especially efficient at storing calories.

LPL is partly controlled by reproductive hormones (estrogen in women, testosterone in men), so gender-based differences in the activity of the enzyme also factor into obesity. In women, fat cells in the hips, thighs and breasts secrete LPL, while in men the enzyme is produced by fat cells in the midriff region. Fat cells in the abdominal area release their contents for quick energy, while fat in the thighs and buttocks are used for long-term energy storage. Thus, a man can often pare his paunch more readily than a woman can shed her saddlebags.

LPL also makes it easier to regain lost weight, according to a study conducted at Cedars-Sinai Medical Center in Los Angeles and reported in the April 12, 1990, issue of the *New England Journal of Medicine*. Nine people who lost an average of 90 pounds had their LPL levels measured before dieting and after maintaining their new weights for three months. The researchers found that levels of the enzyme rose after weight loss, and that the fatter the person was to start with, the higher the LPL levels were—as though the body was fighting to regain the weight. They believe that weight loss activated the gene producing the enzyme. This may be one reason why it is easier for a dieter to regain lost weight than for someone who has never been obese to put weight on.

Set for Life?

This study supports the much-debated "set point" theory, which holds that inner mechanisms set a person's weight at a predetermined level and if anything is done to change the weight, the body will adjust to restore fat content to the set point.

"I regard body temperature, which stays around 98.6 degrees F, to be a set point. Weight doesn't have a set point in that sense," says Xavier Pi-Sunyer, M.D., director of the Obesity Research Center at St. Luke's-Roosevelt Hospital Center in New York.

If there is a set point for weight, it generally seems to move in one direction—that is, the body will not make adjustments to counteract a large weight gain but will fight efforts to lose the weight. "When a person gains weight and stays at that weight a while, the body will defend that weight. It becomes the new 'set point'," explains Pi-Sunyer.

Aside from the action of LPL, the body uses other adaptive mechanisms when food intake is reduced. To cite just two of them: Dieting depresses the metabolic rate so that calories are burned more slowly, and as fat cells shrink, they become more responsive to the action of insulin and do not release their contents as readily.

"The body is very good at defending itself from the danger of underweight, but is not really equipped to handle overweight. Throughout the ages, people have not had a problem with having too much to eat. That's a modern problem," says Pi-Sunyer.

Though a definitive study has yet to be done in humans showing that weight gain becomes more likely after each successive diet (the so-called "yo-yo" syndrome), the Cedars-Sinai study strengthens this controversial hypothesis. However, in order to show conclusively that weight loss gets harder each time a person loses and regains weight, the subjects in the Cedars-Sinai study would have to be followed through several cycles of weight gain and loss to determine whether LPL levels kept rising after each diet.

Repeatedly losing and gaining weight may have other health consequences, according to a report in the June 27, 1991, *New England Journal of Medicine.* American and Swedish researchers analyzed weight fluctuations and later health problems over a period of 32 years in more than 3,000 women and men who participated in the Framingham (Mass.) Health Study. The researchers said that people who repeatedly lose and regain weight appear to have an overall higher death rate and to be at greater risk of heart disease and some cancers than those whose weight remains stable (even if overweight) or steadily increases.

Are All Calories Created Equal?

"The body will do what it was programmed to do even if that's not what you want it to do," notes Callaway. For this reason, restricting food intake to 1,000 or 1,200 calories in order to lose weight is "doomed to failure," he says. "For many people, going on one more diet isn't going to solve a weight problem in the long run."

Even well-established weight-loss programs are not individualized enough to account for genetics, past dieting attempts, and a person's activity level, he says.

While Pi-Sunyer agrees that putting everyone on the same prepackaged weight-loss regimen can be counterproductive, he believes that restricting caloric intake is an important weight-control tool. "You can easily cut caloric intake just by restricting the amount of fat and sugar you eat. This might be the only adjustment a moderately overweight person would need to make in order to lose weight."

Research indicates that obesity may be linked to the proportion of fat in the diet rather than to the amount of calories consumed, according to a survey of the diets and exercise habits of 107 men and 109 women reported in the September 1990 issue of *American Journal of Clinical Nutrition.* Researchers at Indiana University in Bloomington found that overweight subjects got 35 percent of their calories from fat and 46 percent from carbohydrates, compared to 29 percent of calories from fat and 53 percent from carbohydrates for their slender counterparts. A recent University of Vermont study suggests that limiting fat intake to about 20 percent of total calories enabled chronically obese patients who failed to lose weight on a variety of reducing programs to lose an average of 20 to 30 pounds over the course of a year.

Scientists used to think that all calories were created equal. That is, whether it came from fat, carbohydrates or protein, a calorie produced a certain amount of heat when the body burned it to fuel metabolic processes. Thus, according to "The Dieter's Law of Thermodynamics," mashed potatoes and milkshakes were no more culpable in promoting weight gain than pasta and peas—as long as caloric intake was limited to 1,000 or some other magic number.

Alas, further research has shown this to be an illusion. Calories from carbohydrates, fat and protein are used differently by the body. Virtually all fat calories are immediately stored in fat cells. Carbohydrates and protein are converted into glucose for fuel, with only those calories in excess of the body's energy needs being stored.

Compounding the problem, a gram of fat has 9 calories while an equal amount of carbohydrates or protein has 4. "For the same number of calories, a person can have a much bigger serving of a food that is primarily carbohydrate as one that is high in fat," observes Walter Glinsmann, M.D., associate director for clinical nutrition at the Food and Drug Administration's Center for Food Safety and Applied Nutrition. For instance, a 6.5-ounce baked potato has the same number of calories as 1.5 ounces of potato chips (about 225).

The type of fat in the diet is important as well. Currently, the National Cholesterol Education Program recommends that the diet be limited to 30 percent of calories from fat, with no more than 10 percent of those coming from saturated fats. "Unsaturated fats are precursors of such biologically active molecules as prostaglandins, which are involved in a variety of body processes, including blood pressure regulation and immune system function. Various types of fat have different roles in health maintenance and disease risk," says Glinsmann.

Exercise the Key

Rather than severely restricting caloric intake and depressing metabolic activity as a result, weight-loss specialists now advise moderate exercise as a means of achieving weight control. "A person not only burns calories while exercising, but if he or she is eating an adequate amount of food, calories will continue to be burned at a higher rate for up to several hours afterward," says Callaway.

"For most people, cutting fat intake and adding moderate exercise can work as well as a commercial weight control program," says Pi-Sunyer. Exercisers are also more likely than sedentary people to keep weight off, whether they use a "do-it-yourself" diet or attend a program.

Unfortunately, weight maintenance is a universal failing of all weight-loss programs, regardless of how expensive or well-established. "If you're going to evaluate weight-loss success, you can't just look at the number of pounds lost. You have to look at long-term weight maintenance," says Callaway.

"Diet programs make money on the weight-loss phase, not the weight maintenance phase. At the time when people need the most help in controlling their weight, many programs cut them off," says Pi-Sunyer. By various estimates, as many as 85 percent of dieters put the weight back on within two years after weight loss.

"Perhaps weight-loss programs should be less focused on weight control and more focused on identifying individual risk factors and dietary patterns associated with obesity, and to modify them where possible," suggests Glinsmann.

"Obesity is not yet well understood," concedes Pi-Sunyer, "and all we can do right now is to tell people to exercise and to cut down on fat intake." However, while genetic predisposition towards obesity can be mitigated by exercise and sensible eating habits, some people will have to work a lot harder at keeping weight at optimal levels than others. "It like jazz—there's a theme and rhythm and you've got to work within that framework, but you can improvise," say Callaway.

Product Bans and Controversies

In the wake of last year's House Committee on Small Business hearings on the $33 billion weight-loss industry, FDA and the Federal Trade Commission separately announced investigations into the safety and efficacy of diet pills and programs, and how they are promoted in advertising. FDA also moved to pull dangerous or ineffective products off store shelves.

In the fall of 1990, FDA proposed a ban on 111 ingredients in over-the-counter (OTC) diet products, including amino acids, cellulose, grapefruit extract, and kelp. The agency had given manufacturers of these products an opportunity to provide data from clinical tests showing they were effective in promoting weight loss, but did not receive adequate information to support advertising claims, according to William Gilbertson, Pharm. D., director of FDA's OTC Drug Review Program. Many of these ingredients had been marketed before 1962 [when an amendment to the 1938 Food, Drug, and Cosmetic Act was passed requiring drugs not only to be safe, but also effective] and had never been evaluated for efficacy, Gilbertson explains. He says that manufacturers wanting to market weight-loss drugs using the banned ingredients will have to get prior FDA approval—which means filling a new drug application and supplying data from clinical tests to support claims.

FDA also recalled Cal-Ban 3000, a heavily advertised diet pill containing guar gum (a vegetable gum that swells when it absorbs moisture, providing a feeling of fullness, according to advertising claims) after receiving a number of consumer complaints of adverse reactions. In a number of cases, the tablet caused gastric or esophageal obstruction, and one person died as a result of complications following surgery to remove the mass of gum blocking his throat.

The most widely used ingredient in OTC diet pills, phenylpropanolamine hydrochloride (PPA), an appetite suppressant that is chemically related to amphetamines, has been the subject of a decade-long medical dispute. Though clinical tests yielded conflicting results (often due to defects in study design), an FDA panel concluded in 1982 that enough data existed to support the efficacy of PPA in curbing the appetite to qualify it as an OTC weight-loss aid. However, a controversy developed over PPA's safety. The drug can cause small elevations of blood pressure at recommended doses, and there are a few reports of marked blood pressure elevation and intracranial bleeding associated with its use. Whether such events are truly drug-related and can occur at recommended doses is the subject of debate.

In May, FDA held a public meeting to explore such issues as whether PPA can cause such central nervous system damage as stroke when taken at (or over) the recommended dosage, whether the drug poses a health hazard to teenagers, and whether PPA is especially hazardous to those with eating disorders.

For its part, FTC has begun to look into advertising claims of 14 diet programs. "We are concerned with programs that go beyond promising weight loss and claim to be able to keep the weight off," says Richard Kelly, assistant director of FTC's division of service industry practices. Additionally, FTC is looking into whether diet companies are touting the safety of their programs while playing down such health risks as the development of gallstones or loss of muscle tissue. Kelly expects the FTC investigation to be completed by the end of the year.

FTC also monitors advertising claims for diet aids on an ongoing basis and takes legal action to get companies to stop making unfounded claims. Among the agency's recent targets: Fat-Magnet, a pill that claimed to break up into thousands of tiny fat-attracting particles that flush fat from the body, and FibreTrim, a high-fiber supplement that its manufacturer claimed could aid in weight reduction.

FDA's ban of ineffective diet drugs could make future FTC action easier.

"The FDA says these products are not efficacious, which is a good piece of evidence to have when we go to trial," says Judy Wilkenfeld, assistant director of FTC s advertising practices division.

by Ruth Papazian

Consumers can get a list of ineffective diet aids by writing to: FDA, HFE-20, 5600 Fishers Lane, Rockville, Md. 20857.

Chapter 18

The Facts About Weight Loss Products and Programs

The Weight-Loss Industry

Looking for a quick and easy way to lose weight? You're not alone. An estimated 50 million Americans will go on diets this year. And while some will succeed in taking off weight, very few —perhaps 5 percent—will manage to keep all of it off in the long run.

One reason for the low success rate is that many people look for quick and easy solutions to their weight problems. They find it hard to believe in this age of scientific innovations and medical miracles that an effortless weight-loss method doesn't exist.

So they succumb to quick-fix claims like "Eat All You Want and Still Lose Weight!" or "Melt Fat Away While You Sleep!" And they invest their hopes (and their money) in all manner of pills, potions, gadgets, and programs that hold the promise of a slimmer, happier future.

The weight-loss business is a booming industry. Americans spend an estimated $30 billion a year on all types of diet programs and products, including diet foods and drinks. Trying to sort out all of the competing claims—often misleading, unproven, or just plain false—can be confusing and costly.

This brochure is designed to give you the facts behind the claims, to help you avoid the outright scams, and to encourage you to consider thoroughly the costs and the consequences of the dieting decisions you make.

DHHS Publication No. (FDA) 92-1189 (1992)

The Facts About Weight Loss

Being obese can have serious health consequences. These include an increased risk of heart disease, stroke, high blood pressure, diabetes, gallstones, and some forms of cancer. Losing weight can help reduce these risks. Here are some general points to keep in mind:

- *Any claims that you can lose weight effortlessly are false.* The only proven way to lose weight is either to reduce the number of calories you eat or to increase the number of calories you burn off through exercise. Most experts recommend a combination of both.

- *Very low-calorie diets are not without risk and should be pursued only under medical supervision.* Unsupervised very low-calorie diets can deprive you of important nutrients and are potentially dangerous.

- *Fad diets rarely have any permanent effect.* Sudden and radical changes in your eating patterns are difficult to sustain over time. In addition, so-called "crash" diets often send dieters into a cycle of quick weight loss, followed by a "rebound" weight gain once normal eating resumes, and even more difficulty reducing when the next diet is attempted.

- *To lose weight safely and keep it off requires long-term changes in daily eating and exercise habits.* Many experts recommend a goal of losing about a pound a week. A modest reduction of 500 calories per day will achieve this goal, since a total reduction of 3,500 calories is required to lose one pound of fat. An important way to lower your calorie intake is to learn and practice healthy eating habits.

In Search of the "Magic Bullet"

Some dieters peg their hopes on pills and capsules that promise to "burn," "block," "flush," or otherwise eliminate fat from the system. But science has yet to come up with a low-risk "magic bullet" for weight loss. Some pills may help control the appetite, but they can have serious side effects. (Amphetamines, for instance, are highly addictive and can have an adverse impact on the heart and central nervous system.) Other pills are utterly worthless.

The Federal Trade Commission (FTC) and a number of state Attorneys General have successfully brought cases against marketers of pills claiming to absorb or burn fat. The Food and Drug Administration (FDA) has banned 111 ingredients once found in over-the-counter diet products. None of these substances, which include alcohol, caffeine, dextrose, and guar gum, have proved effective in weight-loss or appetite suppression.

Beware of the following products that are touted as weight-loss wonders:

- Diet patches, which are worn on the skin, have not been proven to be safe or effective. The FDA has seized millions of these products from manufacturers and promoters.

- "Fat blockers" purport to physically absorb fat and mechanically interfere with the fat a person eats.

- "Starch blockers" promise to block or impede starch digestion. Not only is the claim unproven, but users have complained of nausea, vomiting, diarrhea, and stomach pains.

- "Magnet" diet pills allegedly "flush fat out of the body." The FTC has brought legal action against several marketers of these pills.

- Glucomannan is advertised as the "Weight Loss Secret That's Been in the Orient for Over 500 Years." There is little evidence supporting this plant root's effectiveness as a weight-loss product.

- Some bulk producers or fillers, such as fiber-based products, may absorb liquid and swell in the stomach, thereby reducing hunger. Some fillers, such as guar gum, can even prove harmful, causing obstructions in the intestines, stomach, or esophagus. The FDA has taken legal action against several promoters of products containing guar gum.

- Spirulina, a species of blue-green algae, has not been proven effective for losing weight.

Phony Devices and Gadgets

Phony weight-loss devices range from those that are simply ineffective to those that are truly dangerous to your health. At minimum, they are a waste of your hard-earned money. Some of the fraudulent gadgets that have been marketed to hopeful dieters over the years include:

- Electrical muscle stimulators have legitimate use in physical therapy treatment. But the FDA has taken a number of them off the market because they were promoted for weight loss and body toning. When used incorrectly, muscle stimulators can be dangerous, causing electrical shocks and burns.

- "Appetite suppressing eyeglasses" are common eyeglasses with colored lenses that claim to project an image to the retina which dampens the desire to eat. There is no evidence these work.

- "Magic weight-loss earrings" and devices custom-fitted to the purchaser's ear that purport to stimulate acupuncture points controlling hunger have not been proven effective.

Diet Programs

Approximately 8 million Americans a year enroll in some kind of structured weight-loss program involving liquid diets, special diet regimens, or medical or other supervision. In 1991, about 8,500 commercial diet centers were in operation across the country, many of them owned by a half-dozen or so well-known national companies.

Before you join such a program, you should know that according to published studies relatively few participants succeed in keeping off weight long-term. Recently, the FTC brought action against several companies challenging weight-loss and weight-maintenance claims. Unfortunately, some other companies continue to make overblown claims. The FTC stopped one company from claiming its diet program

---

Clues to Fraud

It is important for consumers to be wary of claims that sound too good to be true. When it comes to weights-loss schemes, consumers should be particularly skeptical of claims containing words and phrases like:

• easy	• new discovery
• effortless	• mysterious
• guaranteed	• exotic
• miraculous	• secret
• magical	• exclusive
• breakthrough	• ancient

---

caused rapid weight loss through the use of tablets that would "burn fat" and a protein drink mix that would adjust metabolism. The FTC also took action against three major programs using doctor-supervised, very low-calorie liquid diets, and they agreed to stop making the claims they had been making unless they could back them up with hard data.

Before you sign up with a diet program, you might ask these questions:

- What are the health risks?

- What data can you show me that proves your program actually works?

- Do customers keep off the weight after they leave the diet program?

- What are the costs for membership, weekly fees, food, supplements, maintenance, and counseling? What's the payment schedule? Are any costs covered under health insurance? Do you give refunds if I drop out?

- Do you have a maintenance program? Is it part of the package or does it cost extra?

- What kind of professional supervision is provided? What are the credentials of these professionals?

- What are the program's requirements? Are there special menus or foods, counseling visits, or exercise plans?

Sensible Weight Maintenance Tips

Losing weight may not be effortless, but it doesn't have to be complicated. To achieve long-term results, it's best to avoid quick-fix schemes and complex regimens. Focus instead on making modest changes to your life's daily routine. A balanced, healthy diet and sensible, regular exercise are the keys to maintaining your ideal weight. Although nutrition science is constantly evolving, here are some generally-accepted guidelines for losing weight:

- Consult with your doctor, a dietician, or other qualified health professional to determine your ideal healthy body weight.

- Eat smaller portions and choose from a variety of foods.

- Load up on foods naturally high in fiber: fruits, vegetables, legumes, and whole grains.

- Limit portions of foods high in fat: dairy products like cheese, butter, and whole milk; red meat; cakes and pastries.

- Exercise at least three times a week.

For Help and Information

The Federal Trade Commission has jurisdiction over the advertising and marketing of foods, non-prescription drugs, medical devices, and health care services. The FTC can seek federal court injunctions to halt fraudulent claims and obtain redress for injured consumers.

The Food and Drug Administration has jurisdiction over the content and labeling of foods, drugs, and medical devices. The FDA can take law enforcement action to seize and prohibit the sale of products that are falsely labeled.

Most state Attorneys General have authority under state consumer protection statutes to investigate and prosecute unfair or deceptive acts and practices. Many have the power to seek consumer restitution, civil fines, and revocation of a company's authority to do business.

To get more information or to file complaints about weight-loss products or programs, write:

Federal Trade Commission
Correspondence Branch
Washington, D.C. 20580

or

Food and Drug Administration
Consumer Affairs and Information
5600 Fishers Lane, HFC-110
Rockville, MD 20857

or

Your State Attorney General
Office of Consumer Protection
Your State Capital

Chapter 19

Vegetarian Diets: the Pluses and the Pitfalls

Many people are attracted to vegetarian diets. It's no wonder. Health experts for years have been telling us to eat more plant foods and less fat, especially saturated fat, which is found in larger amounts in animal foods than plant foods.

C. Everett Koop, M.D., former surgeon general of the Public Health Service, in his 1988 Report on Nutrition and Health, expressed major concern about Americans' "disproportionate consumption of foods high in fats, often at the expense of foods high in complex carbohydrates and fiber—such as vegetables, fruits, and whole-grain products—that may be more conducive to health."

And, while guidelines from the U.S. Departments of Agriculture and Health and Human Services advise 2 to 3 daily servings of milk and the same of foods such as dried peas and beans, eggs, meat poultry and fish, they recommend 3 to 5 servings of vegetables, 2 to 4 of fruits, and 6 to 11 servings of bread, cereal, rice, and pasta—in other words, 11 to 20 plant foods, but only 4 to 6 animal foods.

It's wise to take precautions, however, when adopting diets that entirely exclude animal flesh or dairy products.

"The more you restrict your diet, the more difficult it is to get all the nutrients you need," says Marilyn Stephenson, R.D., of the Food and Drug Administration's Center for Food Safety and Applied Nutrition. "To be healthful, vegetarian diets require very careful, proper planning. Nutrition counseling can help you get started on a diet that is nutritionally adequate."

FDA Consumer/May 1992

Certain people, such as Seventh-day Adventists, choose a vegetarian diet because of religious beliefs. Others give up meat because they feel that eating animals is unkind. Some people believe it's a better use of the Earth's resources to eat low on the food chain; the North American Vegetarian Society notes that 1.3 billion people could be fed with the grain and soybeans eaten by U.S. livestock. On the practical side, many people eat plant foods because animal foods are more expensive.

"I'm a vegetarian because I just plain enjoy the taste of vegetables and pasta," says Judy Folkenberg of Bethesda, Md. Reared on a vegetarian diet that included eggs and dairy products, Folkenberg added fish to her diet five years ago. "I love crab cakes and shrimp," she says.

Just as vegetarians differ in their motivation, their diets differ as well. In light of these variations, it's not surprising that the exact number of vegetarians is unknown. In a National Restaurant Association Gallup Survey in June 1991, 5 percent of respondents said they were vegetarians, yet 2 percent said they never ate milk or cheese products, 3 percent never ate red meat, and 10 percent never ate eggs.

Vegetarian Varieties

The Institute of Food Technologists, in the July 1991 issue of its journal, *Food Technology*, describes six types of vegetarians. They are listed here by degree of exclusion of animal foods and by the foods included in the diet:

- semi-vegetarian—dairy foods, eggs, chicken, and fish, but no other animal flesh

- pesco-vegetarian—dairy foods, eggs, and fish, but no other animal flesh

- lacto-ovo-vegetarian—dairy foods and eggs, but no animal flesh

- lacto-vegetarian—dairy foods, but no animal flesh or eggs

- ovo-vegetarian—eggs, but no dairy foods or animal flesh

- vegan—no animal foods of any type.

Risks

Vegetarians who abstain from dairy products or animal flesh face the greatest nutritional risks because some nutrients naturally occur mainly or almost exclusively in animal foods.

Vegans, who eat no animal foods (and, rarely, vegetarians who eat no animal flesh but do eat eggs or dairy products), risk vitamin B_{12} deficiency, which can result in irreversible nerve deterioration. The need for vitamin B_{12} increases during pregnancy, breast-feeding, and periods of growth, according to Johanna Dwyer, D.Sc., R.D., of Tufts University Medical School and the New England Medical Center Hospital, Boston. Writing in 1988 in the *American Journal of Clinical Nutrition*, Dwyer reviewed studies of the previous five years and concluded that elderly people also should be especially cautious about adopting vegetarian diets because their bodies may absorb vitamin B_{12} poorly.

Ovo-vegetarians, who eat eggs but no dairy foods or animal flesh, and vegans may have inadequate vitamin D and calcium. Inadequate vitamin D may cause rickets in children, while inadequate calcium can contribute to risk of osteoporosis in later years. These vegetarians are susceptible to iron deficiency anemia because they are not only missing the more readily absorbed iron from animal flesh, they are also likely to be eating many foods with constituents that inhibit iron absorption—soy protein, bran, and fiber, for instance. Vegans must guard against inadequate calorie intake, which during pregnancy can lead to low birth weight, and against protein deficiency, which in children can impair growth and in adults can cause loss of hair and muscle mass and abnormal accumulation of fluid.

According to the Institute of Food Technologists and the American Dietetic Association, if appropriately planned, vegan diets can provide adequate nutrition even for children. Some experts disagree.

Gretchen Hill, Ph.D., associate professor of food science and human nutrition at the University of Missouri, Columbia, believes it's unhealthy for children to eat no red meat.

"My bet is those kids will have health problems when they reach 40, 50 or 60 years of age," she says, "mostly because of imbalances with micronutrients [nutrients required only in small amounts], particularly iron, zinc and copper." While meat is well-known as an important source of iron, Hill says it may be even more valuable for copper and zinc. Copper not only helps build the body's immunity, it builds red blood cells and strengthens blood vessels. "A lot of Americans are marginal in this micronutrient," she says, "and, as a result, are more susceptible to diseases. Children can't meet their zinc needs without eating meat."

Also, vegetarian women of childbearing age have an increased chance of menstrual irregularities, Ann Pedersen and others reported last year in the *American Journal of Clinical Nutrition*. Nine of the study's 34 vegetarians (who ate eggs or dairy foods) missed menstrual periods, but only 2 of the 41 non-vegetarians did. The groups were indistinguishable when it came to height, weight and age at the beginning of menstruation.

Can Veggies Prevent Cancer?

The National Cancer Institute states in its booklet *Diet, Nutrition & Cancer Prevention: The Good News* that a third of cancer deaths may be related to diet. The booklet's "Good News" is: Vegetables from the cabbage family (cruciferous vegetables) may reduce cancer risk, diets low in fat and high in fiber-rich foods may reduce the risk of cancers of the colon and rectum, and diets rich in foods containing vitamin A, vitamin C, and beta-carotene may reduce the risk of certain cancers.

Part of FDA's proposed food labeling regulations, published in the Nov. 27, 1991, Federal Register, states, "The scientific evidence shows that diets high in whole grains, fruits, and vegetables, which are low in fat and rich sources of fiber and certain other nutrients, are associated with a reduced risk of some types of cancer. The available evidence does not, however, demonstrate that it is total fiber, or a specific fiber component, that is related to the reduction of risk of cancer."

As for increasing fiber in the diet, Joanne Slavin, Ph.D., R.D., of the University of Minnesota, in 1990 in *Nutrition Today*, gives this advice: "Animal studies show that soluble fibers are associated with the highest levels of cell proliferation, a precancerous event. The current interest in dietary fiber has allowed recommendations for fiber supplementation to outdistance the scientific research base. Until we have a better understanding of how fiber works its magic, we should recommend to American consumers only a gradual increase in dietary fiber from a variety of sources."

FDA acknowledges that high intakes of fruits and vegetables rich in beta-carotene or in vitamin C have been associated with reduced cancer risk. But the agency believes the data are not sufficiently con-

vincing that either nutrient by itself is responsible for this association.

Pointing out that plant foods' low fat content also confers health
benefits, FDA states in its proposed rule that diets low in fat give
protection against coronary heart disease and that it has tentatively
determined, "Diets low in fat are associated with the reduced risk of
cancer."

FDA notes that diets high in saturated fats and cholesterol increase
levels of both total and LDL cholesterol, and thus the risk for coronary heart disease, and that high-fat foods contribute to obesity, a
further risk factor for heart disease. (The National Cholesterol Education Program recommends a diet with no more than 30 percent fat,
of which no more than 10 percent comes from saturated fat.)

For those reasons, the agency would allow some foods to be labeled
with health claims relating diets low in saturated fat and cholesterol
to decreased risk of coronary heart disease and relating diets low in
fat to reduced risk of breast, colon and prostate cancer. "Examples of
foods qualifying for a health claim include most fruits and vegetables;
skim milk products; sherbets; most flours, grains, meals, and pastas
(except for egg pastas); and many breakfast cereals," the proposed rule
states.

Dwyer, in her article, summarizes these plant food benefits:

> "Data are strong that vegetarians are at lesser risk for obe-
> sity, atonic [reduced muscle tone] constipation, lung cancer,
> and alcoholism. Evidence is good that risks for hyperten-
> sion, coronary artery disease, type II diabetes, and gall-
> stones are lower. Data are only fair to poor that risks of
> breast cancer, diverticular disease of the colon, colonic can-
> cer, calcium kidney stones, osteoporosis, dental erosion, and
> dental caries are lower among vegetarians."

Death rates for vegetarians are similar or lower than for non-vegetarians, Dwyer reports, but are influenced in Western countries by
vegetarians' "adoption of many healthy lifestyle habits in addition to
diet, such as not smoking, abstinence or moderation in the use of alcohol, being physically active, resting adequately, seeking ongoing
health surveillance, and seeking . . . guidance when health problems
arise."

Slow Switching

It's generally agreed that to avoid intestinal discomfort from increased bulk, a person shouldn't switch to foods with large amounts of fiber all at once. A sensible approach to vegetarian diets is to first cut down on the fattiest meats, replacing them with cereals, fruits and vegetables, recommends Jack Zeev Yetiv, M.D., Ph.D., in his book *Popular Nutritional Practices: A Scientific Appraisal.* "Some may choose to eliminate red meat but continue to eat fish and poultry occasionally, and such a diet is also to be encouraged."

Changing to the vegetarian kitchen slowly also may increase the chances of success.

"If you suddenly cut out all animal entrees from your diet, it's easy to get discouraged and think there's nothing to eat," says lifelong veggie-eater Folkenberg. "I build my meals around a starchy carbohydrate such as pasta or potatoes. Even when I occasionally cook seafood, I center on the carbohydrate, making that the larger portion. Shifting the emphasis from animal to plant foods is easier after you've found recipes you really enjoy."

Because vegans and ovo-vegetarians face the greatest potential nutritional risk, the Institute of Food Technologists recommends careful diet planning to include enough calcium, riboflavin, iron, and vitamin D, perhaps with a vitamin D supplement if sunlight exposure is low. (Sunlight activates a substance in the skin and converts it into vitamin D.)

For these two vegetarian groups, the institute recommends calcium supplements during pregnancy, infancy, childhood, and breast-feeding. Vegans need to take a vitamin B_{12} supplement because that vitamin is found only in animal food sources. Unless advised otherwise by a doctor, those taking supplements should limit the dose to 100 percent of the National Academy of Sciences' Recommended Dietary Allowances.

Vegans, and especially children, also must be sure to consume adequate calories and protein. For other vegetarians, it is not difficult to get adequate protein, although care is needed in small children's diets.

Nearly every animal food, including egg whites and milk, provides all eight of the essential amino acids in the balance needed by humans and therefore constitutes "complete" protein. Plant foods contain fewer of these amino acids than animal foods.

The American Dietetic Association's position paper on vegetarian diets, published in its journal in 1988 and co-authored by Dwyer and Suzanne Havala, R.D., states that a plant-based diet provides adequate amounts of amino acids when a varied diet is eaten on a daily basis. The mixture of proteins from grains, legumes, seeds, and vegetables provides a complement of amino acids so that deficits in one food are made up by another. Not all types of plant foods need to be eaten at the same meal, since the amino acids are combined in the body's protein pool.

Frances Lappe, in *Diet for a Small Planet* writes that to gain the greatest use of all the amino acids, it's best to consume complementary proteins within three to four hours. High amounts of complete proteins can he gained by combining legumes with grains, seeds or nuts.

Also available are various protein analogs. These substitute "meats"—usually made from soybeans—are formed to look like meat foods such as hot dogs, ground beef, or bacon. Many are fortified with vitamin B_{12}.

The following section lists sources of the nutrients of greatest concern for vegetarians who don't eat animal foods.

As with any diet, it's important for the vegetarian diet to include many different foods, since no one food contains all the nutrients required for good health. "The wider the variety, the greater the chance of getting the nutrients you need," says FDA's Stephenson.

The American Dietetic Association recommends:

- minimizing intake of less nutritious foods such as sweets and fatty foods

- choosing whole or unrefined grain products instead of refined products

- choosing a variety of nuts, seeds, legumes, fruits, and vegetables, including good sources of vitamin C to improve iron absorption

- choosing low-fat varieties of milk products, if they are included in the diet

- avoiding excessive cholesterol intake by limiting eggs to two or three yolks a week

307

- for vegans, using properly fortified food sources of vitamin B_{12} such as fortified soy milks or cereals, or taking a supplement

- for infants, children and teenagers, ensuring adequate intakes of calories and iron and vitamin D, taking supplements if needed

- consulting a registered dietitian or other qualified nutrition professional, especially during periods of growth, breast-feeding, pregnancy, or recovery from illness

- if exclusively breast-feeding premature infants or babies beyond 4 to 6 months of age, giving vitamin D and iron supplements to the child from birth or at least by 4 to 6 months, as your doctor suggests

- usually, taking iron and folate (folic acid) supplements dur - ing pregnancy.

With the array of fruits, vegetables, grains, and herbs available in U.S. grocery stores and the availability of vegetarian cookbooks, it's easy to devise tasty vegetarian dishes.

People who like their entrees on the hoof also can benefit from adding more plant foods to their diets. You don't have to be a vegetarian to enjoy dishes from a vegetarian menu.

Replacing Animal Sources of Nutrients

Vegetarians who eat no meat, fish, poultry or dairy foods face the greatest risk of nutritional deficiency. Nutrients most likely to be lacking and some non-animal sources are:

- vitamin B_{12}—fortified soy milk and cereals

- vitamin D—fortified margarine and sunshine

- calcium—tofu, broccoli, seeds, nuts, kale, bok choy, legumes (peas and beans), greens, calcium-enriched grain products, and lime-processed tortillas

- iron—legumes, tofu, green leafy vegetables, dried fruit, whole grains, and iron-fortified cereals and breads, especially whole-wheat (absorption is improved by vitamin C, found in citrus fruits and juices, tomatoes, strawberries, broccoli, peppers, dark-green leafy vegetables, and potatoes with skins)

- zinc—whole grains (especially the germ and bran), whole-wheat bread, legumes, nuts, and tofu.

As all plant foods—including fruit, contain some protein, by eating a variety of fruits, vegetables and grains, even vegans probably can get enough of this nutrient. To improve the quality of protein and ensure getting enough:

Combine

legumes such as black-eyed peas, chickpeas, peas, peanuts, lentils, sprouts, and black, broad, kidney, lima, mung, navy, pea, and soy beans

with

grains such as rice, wheat, corn, rye, bulgur, oats, millet, barley, and buckwheat

Part Four

The Food Label

Chapter 20

Answers To Consumer Questions About The Food Label

Randy Sager of Potomac, Md., turns a box of croutons from side to side, looking for the "Nutrition Facts" panel. Like millions of Americans, she has come to value the information about serving size, calories and nutrients.

The croutons are missing a Nutrition Facts panel and so is a package of baked goods in Sager's grocery cart. Saying she doesn't usually buy foods without nutrition labeling, she adds, "But I'm hungry, so I'm buying it."

Sager is not alone in having come to depend on the Nutrition Facts panel and making decisions based on its presence. According to an FDA Consumer poll, missing nutrition information is one of consumers' chief labeling concerns.

It's been about a year since the new food label made its debut on many foods, and with it, mandatory nutrition labeling and a new format for presenting information. Manufacturers had until Aug. 8, 1994, to include the Nutrition Facts panel on labels of packaged food. Food packaged before that date still may be on the shelves, and this may be one explanation for the lack of nutrition information on some labels.

To find out what issues most concerned consumers after the label started appearing on foods, FDA Consumer polled four nutrition-related consumer inquiry programs: FDA's Office of Consumer Affairs, the FDA Seafood Hotline, the U.S. Department of Agriculture's Meat and Poultry Hotline, and the American Dietetic Association's Consumer Nutrition Hot Line.

FDA Consumer / June 1995

Here are the questions that the poll showed perplexed consumers the most, along with the answers

Where can I get more information to help me understand the new food label?

There are several sources for labeling information:

FDA's Office of Consumer Affairs
HFE-88
Rockville, MD 20856

FDA Seafood Hotline
(1-800) FDA-4010
(202) 205-4314 in the Washington, D.C., area 24 hours a day

USDA Meat and Poultry Hotline
(1-800) 535-4555
(202) 720-3333 in the Washington, D.C., area
Recorded messages available 24 hours a day. Home economists and registered dietitians available 10 a.m. to 4 p.m. Eastern time, Monday through Friday.

National Center for Nutrition and Dietetics
American Dietetic Association's Consumer Nutrition Hot Line
(1-800) 366-1655
Recorded messages available 9 a.m. to 9 p.m. Eastern time, Monday through Friday. Registered dietitians available 10 a.m. to 5 p.m. Eastern time, Monday through Friday.

These sources will provide written information, as well as answer specific labeling questions.

For information on food labeling educational materials, contact:

FDA/USDA Food Labeling Education Information Center
National Agricultural Library
10301 Baltimore Blvd., Room 304
Beltsville, MD 20705-2351
(301) 504-5719; facsimile (301) 504-6409

Can a product be labeled "fat-free," "sugar-free," or "sodium-free" and still contain those nutrients?

Under FDA and USDA regulations, "free" for various nutrients is defined as:

- sugar-free: less than 0.5 grams (g) per serving

- sodium-free: less than 5 milligrams (mg) per serving

- fat-free: less than 0.5 g of fat per serving

- cholesterol-free: less than 2 mg of cholesterol and 2 g or less of saturated fat per serving

- saturated fat free: less than 0.5 g of saturated fat per serving and less than 0.5 g trans fatty acids per serving

- calorie-free: fewer than 5 calories per serving.

FDA and USDA chose these limits because they are the lowest points at which detection of calories or a nutrient can be made. These and lower levels are of no dietary significance.

How can I use the food label to help me follow a low-fat, low-sodium, or other prescribed or modified diet?

If your doctor has prescribed a diet that limits the amount, usually in grams or milligrams, of certain nutrients—for example, a 2,000-mg sodium diet—look at the Nutrition Facts panel, usually on the side or back of the food package. It lists the amount by weight of specific nutrients in a serving of the food. Use these numbers, given in grams or milligrams, to track your daily intake of nutrients.

If you're trying to follow the Dietary Guidelines for Americans by restricting fat, sodium and cholesterol and increasing fiber to recommended levels, use the % Daily Values. For example, the Dietary Guidelines recommend that fat intake be limited to 30 percent or less of calories. For a 2,000-calorie diet. this amounts to 65 g, the Daily Value for fat used in food labeling. Even though your calorie intake may be higher or lower, you still can use the % Daily Values in a relative way to see how a serving of food contributes to your overall diet.

For specific diet information, you may want to refer to these articles in the FDA Consumer series "The New Food Label":

- "Making It Easier to Shed Pounds " July-August 1994

- "Scouting for Sodium and Other Nutrients Important to Blood Pressure," September 1994

- "Coping with Diabetes," November 1994

- "Help in Preventing Heart Disease," December 1994

- "Better Information for Special Diets," January-February 1995.

[Editor's note: These articles are also reprinted in Part IV of this volume.]

For further help, see a registered dietitian or nutritionist.

Why is it that the calories I calculate based on protein, carbohydrate and fat amounts don't match the total calories per serving listing on the food label?

The difference is probably due to rounding rules. Food labeling regulations require manufacturers to round as follows:

- nearest 5-calorie increment up to and including 50 calories. (If it's less than 5, a listing of zero is OK.)

- nearest 10-calorie increment above 50 calories.

So, the calorie declaration for a food with 12 g of fat that would furnish 108 calories is rounded to 110, while one with 116 calories is rounded to 120.

This is true for "total calories" and "calories from fat."

The amount by weight of nutrients also is rounded. This can cause some discrepancy between your calculations and the label's values, too, because the manufacturer may use the precise numbers to calculate calories.

Overall, though, your figures should come close to the labeled ones.

Why are African American women excluded from the claim on the association between reduced calcium intake and increased risk for osteoporosis?

Based on scientific research, FDA concluded that the general population is not at a significant risk for developing osteoporosis, a bone disease. For example, studies show that despite their generally lower calcium intake, African Americans have higher bone mass at maturity and a very low incidence or osteoporosis-related bone fracture. Thus, the final claim targets those at greatest risk: teen and young adult white and Asian American women. However, calcium is a nutrient everyone needs

What does "total fat" on the Nutritional Facts panel include?

Total fat refers to all the fat in the food: saturated, polyunsaturated and monounsaturated. Only total fat and saturated fat information is required on the label because high intakes of both are linked to high blood cholesterol, which in turn is linked to increased risk of coronary heart disease. Listing the amount of polyunsaturated and monounsaturated fats in the food is voluntary.

Also, the amounts of saturated, polyunsaturated and monounsaturated fats may not always add up to the full amount declared for total fat because the government-established definitions for those subcategories of fat do not include fatty acids in the trans form. So the label value for total fat may be higher than the sum of the subcategories.

Cholesterol is sort of a "cousin" to fat. Both fat and cholesterol belong to a larger family of chemical compounds called lipids. Lowering cholesterol intake, along with saturated fat, may reduce the risk of heart disease. That's why the amount of cholesterol in a food is required on the label.

Explain the 2,000-calorie basis cited on the food label.

This is the calorie level used to calculate % Daily Values on the label for nutrients whose recommended intakes are based on calorie intake.

In deciding on this number, FDA and USDA referred to the National Academy of Sciences' recommendations on calorie intakes and

U.S. Census Bureau data. From these figures, the agencies determined that the mean recommended calorie intake for the American population is about 2,350 calories a day. Based on public comment—and, in part, to make the number user-friendly—the number was rounded to 2,000 calories.

Also, the 2,000-calorie basis gives more appropriate dietary reference numbers for the group that often has the most difficulty obtaining adequate levels of nutrients—older women.

What do the % Daily Values mean?

These show how much of reference daily nutrient intakes a serving of food provides. For example, a food that lists 5 percent as the % Daily Value for fat contributes 5 percent (3 grams), of the maximum amount of fat a person on a 2,000-calorie diet could eat and still be within the Dietary Guidelines' recommendation of 30 percent or less of calories from fat (65 grams of fat or less). The percentage does not mean that the food is made up of 5 percent fat or that 5 percent of the calories come from fat.

How do you interpret "sugars" on the label?

Sugars are part of total carbohydrate and include sugars naturally present in the food (for example, lactose in milk and fructose in fruit), as well as those added to the food, such as table sugar, corn syrup, and dextrose. The label can claim "no sugar added" but still have naturally occurring sugar. An example is fruit juice.

Why do some labels lack nutrition information?

In addition to the possibility that the food may have been packaged before the August 1994 deadline, there are several other possible explanations. The Nutrition Labeling and Education Act of 1990—the law on which the food labeling regulations are based—specifically exempts some foods from nutrition labeling. These include:

- food produced by small businesses. FDA and USDA's definitions for a small business are based, in part, on the number of employees and amount of product produced.

- food in small packages that don't carry nutrient claims. Under FDA rules, a package of less than 12 square inches doesn't have to give nutrition information. However, it must provide an address or telephone number for consumers to get the required information. USDA exempts individually wrapped products weighing less than half an ounce.

- food served for immediate consumption, such as that served in restaurants, hospital cafeterias and airplanes, and that sold by food service vendors (for example, mall cookie counters, sidewalk vendors, and vending machines)

- ready-to-eat food that is not for immediate consumption but is prepared primarily on site (for example, bakery, deli and candy store items)

- medical foods—that is, those used to address the recognized nutritional requirements associated with particular diseases

- plain coffee and tea, some spices, and other foods that contain no significant amounts of any nutrients.

You also may find nutrition information missing on some odd-shaped packages. Only those that have received FDA's permission not to carry nutrition information because the shape makes it impractical are allowed this exemption. But these products must generally provide an address or telephone number for consumers to get the required information.

If you see a product without nutrition information that doesn't fit into these categories, it may be in violation of the law. Between Sept. 19 and Dec. 31, 1994—during the first six months of the law's implementation—FDA notified 625 food importers and 630 domestic companies that their food products were improperly labeled. The majority of them were missing nutrition information.

Consumers who believe a product is improperly labeled and in violation of the law may report this information to their local FDA office.

Label Accuracy

Can you trust the nutrition information on the label?

In most cases, yes, suggests an FDA study of 300 food products off store shelves. The study, conducted last fall—during the first six months of the labeling regulations' implementation—found that about

319

87 percent of eight or more nutrients measured were within regulatory limits.

For fat, 94 percent of the analyses showed that the amount listed on the label accurately reflected what was in the food. For calories, it was 93 percent.

FDA also found that products with new labels appeared to have a higher rate of conformance—88 percent of 1,680 new labels—than old labels—83 percent of 411 old labels.

"These results show that consumers can trust what it says on the new food label," said FDA Commissioner David A. Kessler, M.D.

by Paula Kurtzweil

Paula Kurtzweil is a member of FDA's public affairs staff.

Chapter 21

The New Food Label: Making It Easier to Shed Pounds

Sibyl Weiss of Van Nuys, Calif., is an avid food label reader—and for good reason.

Twenty-two years ago, the 59-year-old former nurse was obese; she carried more than 300 pounds on her 5-foot 5-inch frame. Today, she weighs in at under 150 pounds, a weight she says she's maintained for more than 20 years.

She credits her success to her participation in a self-help weight-control organization that uses group therapy, competition and recognition to help members lose and maintain their weight. As part of this program, Weiss says, she came to understand the importance of the food label in monitoring food intake.

"For so many years I didn't care what I poured into my body," she says. "Now I do."

Weiss has learned that label information can play an important role in weight management. That role is expected to take on even greater importance as the new food label makes its official debut this year.

Label Changes

In the past, diet-conscious consumers like Weiss couldn't always count on the food label to give complete nutrition information. The information was required only when a food contained added nutrients or when nutrition claims appeared on the label. In all other cases, the

DHHS Publication No. (FDA) 95-2287

nutrition information was voluntary. When it did appear, it was often hard to find and hard to read.

That's changing, though, as a result of the Nutrition Labeling and Education Act of 1990 and regulations from the Food and Drug Administration and the U.S. Department of Agriculture. Those regulations, most of which take effect this year, call for extensive food labeling changes designed to help ensure that there are a lot more success stories like Weiss'.

First, nutrition information in bigger, more readable type is now required for almost all packaged foods. The information also will be near many fresh ones, like fruits and vegetables. On packaged foods, it will usually appear on the side or back of the package under the heading "Nutrition Facts."

Second, the required nutrition information is more useful than before. A new column of information, the "% (percent) Daily Value," tells consumers at a glance how the food fits into a healthy diet.

Third, the information is more complete. The label now must include information about saturated fat, cholesterol, fiber, sugars, calories from fat, and other dietary components that are important to today's consumers. (See "'Nutrition Facts' to Help Consumers Eat Smart" in the May 1993 *FDA Consumer*.)

Fourth, serving sizes now more closely reflect the amount people actually eat.

Also, "light," "low-fat," "calorie-free," and other such claims must meet strict government definitions so when dieters see them, they can believe them. (See "A Little 'Lite' Reading" in the June 1993 *FDA Consumer*; this article is also reprinted in this section of *Diet and Nutrition Sourcebook*.)

"There's no doubt about it. There's going to be a lot of nutrition information on the label," says Camille Brewer, a registered dietitian and nutritionist in FDA's Office of Food Labeling. "And some of it is going to be particularly helpful to people trying to control their weight."

Focus on Fat

Contrary to popular belief, fat—not calorie—content is the most important information for dieters on the food label, Brewer says. The reason: Fat is the densest source of calories, with 9 calories per gram, while carbohydrate and protein each provide 4 calories per gram. (Alcohol, while not a nutrient, provides 7 calories per gram.) By limiting fat alone, consumers will likely lower their calories, as well, and thus their weight, Brewer said.

"In the past, dieters were told to focus entirely on calories, but the new trend really is for them to monitor and reduce grams of fat," Brewer says.

Calories can't be totally discounted. Brewer points out they serve as the basis for determining a person's recommended daily fat intake. Like the general population, dieters are usually advised to limit fat consumption to no more than 30 percent of their total day's calories. (Some health experts restrict it even more—to 20 percent or less, according to Brewer.) The 30 percent limit follows the Dietary Guidelines for Americans.

For example, most people who eat 2,000 calories a day should strive to limit their calories from fat to no more than 600 (2,000 x 0.30 = 600) or no more than 65 grams (g) fat (600 calories divided by 9 calories per gram fat = 67, rounded to 65).

The 2,000-calorie level happens to be the basis on which % Daily Values on the label are calculated. (For more information, see "'Daily Values' Encourage Healthy Diet" in the May 1993 FDA Consumer.) FDA and USDA chose 2,000 calories because, according to Ed Scarbrough, Ph.D., director of FDA's Office of Food Labeling, it is a "user-friendly" number that allows consumers to easily adjust Daily Value numbers to their own diet and calorie intakes.

The calorie level also provides more appropriate dietary reference numbers for one of the groups most often targeted for weight control— older women—he says.

Brewer acknowledges that not everyone needs 2,000 calories a day, especially people trying to lose weight. They often need to eat fewer calories to lose weight. But whatever their calorie intake, dieters still can use the % Daily Values to get a general idea of how high or low a food is in the major nutrients.

She advises people interested in losing weight to see a doctor, dietitian or nutritionist first. These professionals, she says, can help individuals determine appropriate calories and fat levels that will allow them to lose weight and still receive adequate nutrition.

Focus on Fiber

In addition to fat, Brewer suggests that dieters also check the label for a food's fiber content. Fiber can be an important aid in weight maintenance, she says, because eating enough of it can help make a person feel full and thus not eat as much.

FDA and USDA's reference amounts are set at 11.5 g fiber per 1,000 calories; thus, the Daily Value for fiber is 25 g. This Daily Value is based partly on the National Cancer Institute's recommendation that Americans eat 20 g to 30 g fiber a day. For most people, dieters included, a fiber intake of at least 25 g a day—100 percent of the Daily Value—is desirable.

Front Label Info

Dieters should begin their search for fat, fiber and calorie information on the front of the food package. This is where food manufacturers often place statements about the nutritional benefits of their products. Some of these, like "fat-free," "low-calorie" and "high-fiber," will be of particular interest to weight-watchers. (See "Dieters' Guide to Label Nutrient Claims.")

Brewer advises caution, however, when choosing foods that are labeled "fat-free" and "low-fat." Some of these foods, like "low-fat" cakes and cookies, still may be high in calories because of added sugars. So dieters should always check the Nutrition Facts panel to get complete information, she says.

% Daily Values

The column headed "% Daily Value" is the place to start under "Nutrition Facts." The numbers in this column can quickly tell if a food is high or low in the nutrients listed. For dieters, the % Daily Values for fat and fiber will be especially important to look at. If the % Daily Values are 5 or less, the food is considered low in that nutrient. So, the goal for dieters should be to select, as much as possible, foods that have a % Daily Value for fat of 5 or less and for fiber, 5 or more.

The overall goal should be to select foods that together add up to about 100% of the Daily Value for each nutrient.

"Dieters may occasionally select a higher fat item, such as a slice of pound cake that provides about 15 percent of the Daily Value for fat," FDA's Brewer says, "but they should monitor the other foods they eat that day and try not to go over 100 percent of the Daily Value for fat."

The idea, she says, is to give dieters some flexibility in making food choices, while enabling them to restrict their total daily fat intake and increase their total daily fiber intake.

Serving Size

Serving size information is important, too. It tells the amount of the food that will give the calories and nutrient levels listed. It is stated in both common household and metric measures.

Under the new regulations, serving sizes better approximate the actual amounts most people eat, although they are not necessarily the amounts recommended by various health groups. So, instead of being misleading, serving sizes offer a more useful measure for assessing a food's nutrient composition.

Also, the serving size must be about the same for like products—for example, different brands of potato chips—and for similar products within a category of foods—for example, potato chips, pretzels, and corn chips within the category of snack foods. This makes it easy to compare the nutritional qualities of related foods.

Here's an example: Ice cream and frozen yogurt are considered similar foods, so they have the same serving size—one half cup. A half cup of many brands of chocolate ice cream provides 7 g fat—11 percent of the Daily Value for fat. The same amount of frozen chocolate yogurt may yield 4 g fat, or 6 percent of the Daily Value for fat. If a person's goal is to reduce fat intake, the frozen yogurt would be the product to buy.

Other Nutrition Info

In addition to % Daily Values, information about a food's fat content is presented in two other ways on the Nutrition Facts panel—as calories from fat and as grams of fat.

"Calories from Fat" is listed below serving size information immediately following "total calories." Grams of fat are stated to the right of "Total Fat," which tops the list of nutrients. The grams of fat offers consumers the option of monitoring the number of grams of fat eaten. Both "calories from fat" and grams of fat can help consumers limit their fat intake to no more than 30 percent of their total day's calorie intake.

Here's how to use "calories from fat": At the end of the day, add up total calories and calories from fat eaten. Divide calories from fat by total calories. The answer gives the percentage of calories from fat eaten that day. For example, 450 calories from fat divided by 1,800 calories = 0.25 (25 percent), an amount within the recommended level of not more than 30 percent.

Consumers should refer to the % Daily Values for the other nutrients, as well, to determine how nutritious a food is overall. Whether the % Daily Values are for other nutrients most people should limit (for example, cholesterol and sodium) or eat more of (for example, total carbohydrate, vitamin A, and calcium), they can tell at a glance how the food compares nutritionally to others. With all this information, the new food label affords weight-conscious consumers an easier time of selecting a wide variety of foods that meets their dietary needs. That, in turn, can help them achieve and maintain their ideal weight.

Sibyl Weiss greets the changes enthusiastically: "There'll be a lot more information," she says. "I think that' s great."

Dieters' Guide to Label Nutrients Claims

Fat

Fat-free: less than 0.5 grams (g) fat per serving

Low-fat: 3 g or less per serving and, if the serving size is 30 g or less or 2 tablespoons or less, per 50 g of the food

Reduced or less fat: at least 25 percent less per serving than reference food

The following claims can be used to describe the fat content of meat, poultry, seafood, and game meats.

Lean: less than 10 g fat, 4.5 g or less saturated fat, and less than 95 milligrams cholesterol per serving and per 100 g

Extra lean: less than 5 g fat, less than 2 g saturated fat, and less than 95 mg cholesterol per serving and per 100 g

Calories

Calorie-free: fewer than 5 calories per serving

Low-calorie: 40 or fewer calories per serving and, if the serving size is 30 g or less or 2 tablespoons or less, per 50 g of the food

Reduced or fewer calories: at least 25 percent fewer calories per serving than the reference food

Calories and Fat

Light (two meanings):

* one-third fewer calories or half the fat of the reference food. (If the food derives 50 percent or more of its calories from fat, the reduction must be 50 percent of the fat.)

* a "low-calorie," "low-fat" food whose sodium content has been reduced by 50 percent of the reference food

("Light in sodium" means the food has 50 percent or less sodium than the reference food.)

Fiber

Foods making claims about increased fiber content also must meet the definition for "low-fat" or the amount of total fat per serving must appear next to the claim.

High-fiber: 5 g or more per serving

Good source of fiber: 2.5 g to 4.9 g per serving

More or added fiber: at least 2.5 g more per serving than the reference food

Sugar

Sugar-free: less than 0.5 g per serving

No added sugar, without added sugar, no sugar added:

* no sugar or ingredients containing sugars (for example, fruit juices, applesauce, or dried fruit) added during processing or packing

* no ingredients made with added sugars, such as jams, jellies, or concentrated fruit juice.

("Sugar-free" and "No added sugar" signal a reduction in calories from sugars only, not from fat, protein and other carbohydrates. If the total calories are not reduced, a statement will appear next to the "sugar-free" claim explaining that the food is "not low calorie" or "not for weight control." If the total calories are reduced, the claim must be accompanied by a "low-calorie" or "reduced-calorie" claim.)

Reduced sugar: at least 25 percent less sugar than the reference food

Consumers should check the Nutrition Facts to learn more about the food's calorie, fat, and other nutrient content.

Alternatives to High-fat Foods

If you find yourself constantly eating more than 100 percent of the Daily Value for fat each day, consider these low-fat and nonfat alternatives. For labeled items, check the % Daily Value for fat; try to select those foods that provide 5 percent or less per serving.

Instead of:	Eat:
fried foods	baked, broiled, steamed, microwaved, or roasted meat, fish, poultry, and vegetables
oils, salad dressings, sour cream, mayonnaise	reduced-calorie salad dressings and sour cream, low-fat or nonfat plain yogurt, mustard
whole milk	nonfat dry milk, skim or 1% milk
butter, margarine (as a spread)	jam, jelly, preserves, low-calorie apple butter
cake, pie, cookies, pastries	angel food cake, baked apple, fruit crisp, oatmeal cookies, ginger snaps, fresh or juice-pack fruit
snack crackers, chips	crisp breads, matzo, pretzels, rice cakes, melba toast, air-popped or microwaved popcorn

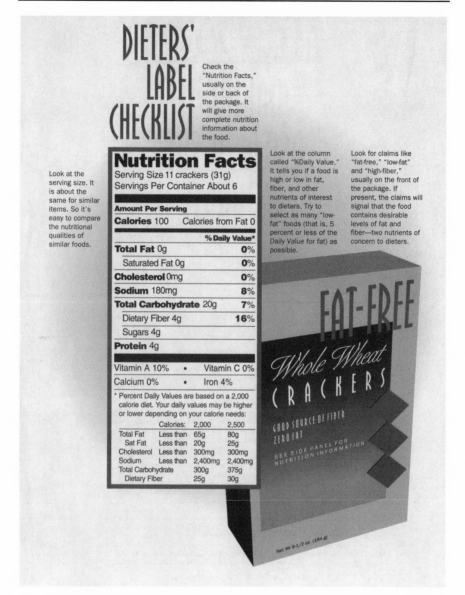

DIETERS' LABEL CHECKLIST

Check the "Nutrition Facts," usually on the side or back of the package. It will give more complete nutrition information about the food.

Look at the serving size. It is about the same for similar items. So it's easy to compare the nutritional qualities of similar foods.

Look at the column called "%Daily Value." It tells you if a food is high or low in fat, fiber, and other nutrients of interest to dieters. Try to select as many "low-fat" foods (that is, 5 percent or less of the Daily Value for fat) as possible.

Look for claims like "fat-free," "low-fat" and "high-fiber," usually on the front of the package. If present, the claims will signal that the food contains desirable levels of fat and fiber—two nutrients of concern to dieters.

Nutrition Facts

Serving Size 11 crackers (31g)
Servings Per Container About 6

Amount Per Serving

Calories 100   Calories from Fat 0

	% Daily Value*
Total Fat 0g	**0%**
Saturated Fat 0g	**0%**
Cholesterol 0mg	**0%**
Sodium 180mg	**8%**
Total Carbohydrate 20g	**7%**
Dietary Fiber 4g	**16%**
Sugars 4g	
Protein 4g	

Vitamin A 10%	•	Vitamin C 0%
Calcium 0%	•	Iron 4%

* Percent Daily Values are based on a 2,000 calorie diet. Your daily values may be higher or lower depending on your calorie needs:

	Calories:	2,000	2,500
Total Fat	Less than	65g	80g
Sat Fat	Less than	20g	25g
Cholesterol	Less than	300mg	300mg
Sodium	Less than	2,400mg	2,400mg
Total Carbohydrate		300g	375g
Dietary Fiber		25g	30g

FAT-FREE *Whole Wheat* CRACKERS

GOOD SOURCE OF FIBER
ZERO FAT

SEE SIDE PANEL FOR NUTRITION INFORMATION

Net Wt 6-1/2 oz. (184 g)

by Paula Kurtzweil

Paula Kurtzweil is a member of FDA's public affairs staff.

Chapter 22

The New Food Label: Scouting For Sodium And Other Nutrients Important to Blood Pressure

For years, consumers watching their sodium intake have had to plod through ingredient lists on many food labels like high school students through a Shakespearean play. They had to read a lot of unknown words and then do plenty of guessing.

Aiming to get some idea of a food's sodium content, consumers knowledgeable about sodium-restricted diets looked for names like sodium caseinate, monosodium glutamate, trisodium phosphate, sodium ascorbate, sodium bicarbonate, sodium stearoyl lactylate, and other sodium-containing ingredients, including salt (sodium chloride).

It wasn't easy, and it wasn't always accurate. Elizabeth Adams of Churchton, Md., can vouch for that. She started to limit her sodium intake 23 years ago. She recalled spending "a long time" in grocery stores reading ingredient lists and looking for nutrition information, which then was voluntary and, until recently, appeared on only about 60 percent of food labels.

"I got to the point where I didn't buy a food unless it had only one ingredient or carried nutrition information," she said. "I had no idea otherwise how much sodium the food had in it."

Resorting to such measures will no longer be necessary for the nearly 50 million Americans like Adams who suffer from hypertension (high blood pressure) and the many others who want to reduce their risk for it. The food label they depend on to help monitor their sodium intake—and thus control their blood pressure—now must state how much sodium a food contains per serving and how the food fits in with their daily diet.

DHHS Publication No. (FDA) 95-2284

Label Changes

These requirements are the result of the Nutrition Labeling and Education Act of 1990 and regulations from the Food and Drug Administration and the U.S. Department of Agriculture. Under these regulations, consumers are seeing:

- Nutrition information in bigger, more readable type on almost all packaged foods. It appears in the table headed "Nutrition Facts," which is usually on the side or back of the package. Nutrition information also will be available in stores near many fresh foods, like fruits and vegetables. (See "Nutrition Info Available for Raw Fruits, Vegetables, and Fish" in the January-February 1993 *FDA Consumer.*)

- "% (percent) Daily Values," which tell consumers at a glance the levels of important nutrients in a food and how those amounts fit into a daily diet.

- Serving sizes that closely reflect the amount people actually eat.

- Strictly defined nutrient-content claims, like "low-sodium," "salt-free," and "rich in potassium." This means that when consumers see such claims, they can believe them. (See "A Little 'Lite' Reading" in the June 1993 *FDA Consumer;* also reprinted in this section of the *Diet and Nutrition Sourcebook.*)

- Strict rules for using health claims, such as one that links low-sodium diets to a reduced risk of high blood pressure. (See "Starting This Month, Look for 'Legit' Health Claims on Foods" in the *FDA Consumer.*)

Sodium's Role

Some of the information—particularly that pertaining to sodium content—will be of special interest to people with blood pressure.

Sodium has long been a major dietary factor in reducing the risk of, and controlling, high blood pressure. (For more on hypertension, see "High Blood Pressure: Controlling the Silent Killer," in the December 1991 *FDA Consumer.*) This role was reiterated as recently as January 1993 in the fifth report of the Joint National Committee on Detection, Evaluation, and Treatment of High Blood Pressure. The committee noted that numerous studies have shown that reducing sodium intake can reduce blood pressure.

What is a reduced sodium intake? According to Camille Brewer, a registered dietitian and nutritionist in FDA's Office of Food Labeling, therapeutic sodium-restricted diets can range from below 1,000 milligrams (mg) to 3,000 mg a day.

"American adults, on average, eat too much sodium—between 4 to 6 grams (4,000 mg to 6,000 mg) daily," she said. "Most people would benefit from moderately reducing their sodium intakes."

Brewer advises people who are considering a sodium-restricted diet to consult a physician, dietitian or nutritionist first.

Under FDA's food labeling rules, the Daily Value for sodium is 2,400 mg. (Daily Values are a new label reference tool. See "'Daily Values' Encourage Healthy Diet" in the May 1993 *FDA Consumer*.) FDA established this value because it is consistent with recommendations and government reports that encourage reduced sodium intakes.

Salt and other sodium compounds used in food processing are the biggest contributors of sodium to most people's diets, Brewer pointed out. (One teaspoon of salt has about 2,000 mg of sodium.) These substances are used in food processing for preserving, flavoring and stabilizing other ingredients, she said.

"That's why the ingredient lists of canned, frozen, and other processed foods often contain the names of so many sodium compounds," she said.

Also, kosher beef, lamb and chicken have salt added.

Sodium also is present naturally in some foods, such as milk, cheese, meat, fish, and some vegetables.

Weight Reduction

Label information about fat, calories and fiber also will be important for people with high blood pressure who are overweight. These are the nutrients of most concern to those trying to lose weight or control it. (See "Making It Easier to Shed Pounds" in the July-August 1994 *FDA Consumer*; also reprinted in this section.)

Body weight, like sodium intake, often closely correlates with blood pressure: As weight goes up, blood pressure frequently does, too. If weight is reduced, blood pressure often goes down.

Other Nutrients

Hypertensives also may be interested in label information about potassium, calcium and magnesium. According to the Joint National Committee's report, evidence suggests that these nutrients may play a role in reducing the risk of high blood pressure. For this reason, nutrition experts often encourage people with hypertension to increase their intakes of these nutrients.

Information about a food's potassium and magnesium content is required on the Nutrition Facts panel only if the food contains added potassium or magnesium as a nutrient or if claims about those nutrients appear on the label. In all other cases, it is voluntary. When listed, potassium must appear below sodium on the Nutrition Facts panel, and magnesium must be shown in the list of vitamins and minerals.

The Daily Value for potassium is 3,500 mg. For magnesium, it's 400 mg.

Information about calcium is mandatory. It, too, appears in the list of vitamins and minerals. The Daily Value for calcium is 1 gram (g), or 1,000 mg.

% Daily Values

The place to begin is the "% Daily Value" column under Nutrition Facts. This column contains numbers that show whether a food is high or low in the nutrients listed. For people with high blood pressure, the % Daily Value for sodium is especially important.

If the % Daily Value for sodium is 5 or less, the food is considered low in that nutrient. So, the goal should be to select, as much as possible, foods that have a % Daily Value for sodium of 5 or less. The goal for the full day's diet should be to select foods that together add up to no more than 100 percent of the Daily Value for sodium.

People with high blood pressure also may want to check the % Daily Values for fat, fiber, calcium, and, if listed, potassium and magnesium. The goal for the full day's diet should be to select foods that together add up to no more than 100 percent of the Daily Value for fat and at least 100 percent for fiber and calcium.

Serving Size

Serving size information is important, too. It tells the amount of the food, stated in both common household and metric measures, to which all other numbers apply.

Under the new regulations, serving sizes are designed to reflect the actual amounts that most people eat, although they are not necessarily the amounts recommended by various health groups.

Also, the serving size must be about the same for like products—for example, different brands of potato chips—and for similar products within a category of foods—for example, potato chips, pretzels, and popcorn within the category "snacks." This makes it easier to compare the nutritional qualities of related foods.

Other Information

The Nutrition Facts panel also gives the amount in milligrams of a food's sodium content. This information can help consumers who monitor the milligrams of sodium they consume.

The % Daily Values for other nutrients are helpful, too, because they can help consumers determine how nutritious a food is overall. Whether the % Daily Values are for nutrients most people should limit—for example, saturated fat and cholesterol—or eat more of—for example, total carbohydrate, fiber, vitamin A, and calcium—the % Daily Values tell at a glance how the food compares nutritionally to others.

Food Label Claims

On some food packages, claims describing the food's nutritional benefits may appear. Often, they will show up on the front of the package where shoppers can readily see them.

Nutrient claims—like "sodium-free, "salt-free," and "very low sodium"—describe desirable levels of nutrients in the food. (See "Nutrient Claim Guide.")

Relative nutrient claims compare a product to the "regular" version of the food or to a similar food. For example, a "reduced-sodium" claim on the label of canned spaghetti sauce means the food has at least 25 percent less sodium than regular canned spaghetti sauce. A claim of "light in sodium" on canned spaghetti sauce means the sodium has been reduced by at least 50 percent.

Other claims simply show that a food is high or low in a nutrient, without any particular comparisons to other products. For example, "low-sodium" means the food has 140 mg or less per serving. "Very low sodium" means it has 35 mg or less per serving.

Also, health claims may be made about the relationship between a nutrient or food and a disease or health-related condition Only those health claims authorized by FDA may appear because they're the only ones supported by substantial scientific evidence.

The claim that diets low in sodium may reduce the risk of high blood pressure is an authorized claim. This claim can appear only on products that meet the definition of "low-sodium" and that provide 20 percent or less of the Daily Value for fat, saturated fat and cholesterol per serving. FDA incorporated this requirement so that low sodium foods would not be counterproductive by being high in other components that contribute to heart disease.

Whatever the source—health claims, nutrient claims, or the Nutrition Facts panel—consumers, especially those restricting their sodium intake, will find that the new food label puts an end to the guessing games they may have played before. Instead, they'll see that the label gives them more complete, accurate information to help them make more healthful food choices.

Nutrient Claim Guide

Sodium

Sodium-free: less than 5 milligrams (mg) per serving

Very low sodium: 35 mg or less per serving or, if the serving is 30 grams (g) less or 2 tablespoons or less, 35 mg or less per 50 g of the food

Low-sodium: 140 mg or less per serving or, if the serving is 30 g or less or 2 tablespoons or less, 140 mg or less per 50 g of the food

Light in sodium: at least 50 percent less sodium per serving than average reference amount for same food with no sodium reduction

Lightly salted: at least 50 percent less sodium per serving than reference amount (If the food is not "low in sodium," the statement "not a low-sodium food" must appear on the same panel as the "Nutrition Facts" panel.)

Reduced or less sodium: at least 25 percent less per serving than reference food
Salt (Sodium Chloride)

Salt-free: sodium-free (see above definition)

Unsalted, without added salt, no salt added:

- no salt added during processing, and

- the food it resembles and for which it substitutes is normally processed with salt

(If the food is not "sodium free," the statement "not a sodium-free food" or "for control of sodium in the diet" must appear on the same panel as the Nutrition Facts panel.)

Potassium

High-potassium: 700 mg or more per serving

Good source of potassium: 350 mg to 665 mg per serving

More or added potassium: at least 350 mg more per serving than reference food

Calcium

High-calcium: 200 mg or more per serving

Good source of calcium: 100 mg to 190 mg per serving

More or added calcium: at least 100 mg more per serving than reference food

(For weight-reduction claims, see "Making It Easier to Shed Pounds" in the August 1994 *FDA Consumer*.)

Alternatives to High-Sodium Foods

If you find yourself continually eating more than 100 percent of the Daily Value for sodium each day, consider these lower sodium alternatives. For labeled items, check the % Daily Value for sodium; try to select foods that provide 5 percent or less per serving.

Instead of:	Eat:
smoked, cured, salted, and canned meat, fish and poultry	unsalted fresh or frozen beef, lamb, pork, fish, and poultry
regular hard and processed cheese, regular peanut butter	low-sodium cheese, low-sodium peanut butter
crackers with salted tops	unsalted crackers
regular canned and dehydrated soups, broths and bouillons	low-sodium canned soups, broths and bouillons
regular canned vegetables	fresh and frozen vegetables and low-sodium canned vegetables
salted snack foods	unsalted tortilla chips, pretzels, potato chips, and popcorn

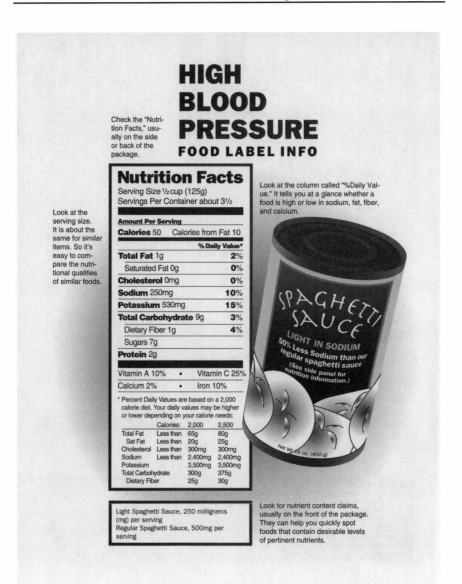

by *Paula Kurtzweil*

Paula Kurtzweil is a member of FDA 's public affairs staff

Chapter 23

The New Food Label: Better Information for Special Diets

The right diet is important for everyone, but for Tony Robinson of Orlando, Fla., it truly is his lifeblood.

Robinson has end-stage renal disease. Three times a week, he goes to a local medical center, where a dialysis machine does what his kidneys no longer can: purify his blood.

Between treatments, he's careful about what he eats because some nutrients can cause harmful—sometimes deadly—levels of substances to build up in his blood. He eats a diet low in protein, sodium and potassium to keep those dangerous substances minimal, and high in calories to maintain his weight.

Until recently, he and his wife, who does most of the cooking, kept mainly to foods listed in a brochure of "foods to eat" and "foods to avoid" for people with end-stage renal disease. But now they're using the new food label as another source of information.

"The new label adds to what we already know," Robinson said. "And mandatory nutrition labeling gives us the information we need to choose from a wider range of food products."

Label Benefits

Under the Nutrition Labeling and Education Act of 1990 and regulations from the Food and Drug Administration and the U.S. Department of Agriculture, virtually all food labels must now give information about a food's nutritional content.

DHHS Publication No. (FDA) 95-2291

That wasn't always the case. Until 1994, nutrition information was voluntary. Manufacturers had to provide it only when a food contained added nutrients or when nutrition claims appeared on the label. Nearly 40 percent of products didn't carry nutrition information.

"Just to have the information on the label is a big plus for consumers on therapeutic diets," said Camille Brewer, a registered dietitian and nutritionist in FDA's Office of Food Labeling.

Another group the regulations help is people with food sensitivities. Every product with two or more ingredients must now list the ingredients on the label. That includes standardized foods, such as peanut butter, and some baked goods. These foods previously were exempt from ingredient labeling because at one time, most Americans were familiar with the recipes since they were foods routinely prepared at home.

Also, the source of some ingredients (for example, hydrolyzed soy protein) must now be identified.

Get the Nutrition Facts

Consumers looking for nutrition information about a food should first look at "Nutrition Facts," usually on the side or back of the package.

For many people on special diets, the amount of the nutrient in grams or milligrams is most important because their diets are based on a set amount of one or more nutrients a day specific to their needs— for example, 60 grams (g) of protein, 2,000 milligrams (mg) of sodium a day. Special dieters can find the amount by weight of nutrients listed in the top part of the Nutrition Facts panel.

Some important points about the Nutrition Facts panel: The values listed for total carbohydrate include all carbohydrates, including dietary fiber and sugars listed below it.

The sugars include naturally present sugars, such as lactose in milk and fructose in fruits, as well as those added to the food, such as table sugar, corn syrup, and dextrose. The label can claim "no sugar added" but still have naturally occurring sugar. An example is fruit juice.

Also, potassium may be listed voluntarily with the nutrients listed on the top part of the panel, just below sodium. Its % Daily Value is based on a recommended intake of 3,500 mg a day.

Other vitamins and minerals may be listed on the Nutrition Facts panel, along with vitamins A and C, iron, and calcium.

Amounts of vitamins and minerals are only presented as percentages of the Daily Value.

Calorie information appears at the top of the Nutrition Facts panel, following serving size information. This information is important for those needing to increase or decrease their calories.

Serving Size

The serving size information gives the amount of food to which all the other numbers on the Nutrition Facts panel apply.

Now serving sizes are more uniform among similar products and are designed to reflect the amounts people actually eat. Also, serving sizes must be about the same for the same types of products—for example, different brands of frozen yogurt—and for similar products within a food category—for example, ice cream, ice milk, and sherbet within the category frozen dairy-type desserts.

Having more uniform serving sizes makes it easier to compare the nutritional values of related foods.

People who follow special diets should be aware that the serving size on the label may not be the same as that recommended for their specific needs. For example, the label serving size for cooked fish is 3 ounces (84 g). A person following a 60 gram protein diet may be allowed only 1 ounce (28 g) of fish at a meal. So, in this case, the nutrient values would have to be divided by 3 to determine the nutritional content of the 1-ounce portion eaten.

Ingredients

The ingredient list is a source of information especially useful for people with food sensitivities. (See Ingredient Labeling: What's in a Food?" in the April 1993 FDA Consumer.) Some new requirements that provide more information in the list are:

- Listing protein hydrolysates by source—instead of "hydrolyzed vegetable protein," the list must state the type of vegetable (for example, "hydrolyzed corn protein").

- Stating FDA food-certified color additives by name—for example, "FD&C Blue No. 1" and "FD&C Yellow No. 6." Before, they could be listed simply as "colorings."

- Declaring caseinate as a milk derivative in foods that claim to be non-dairy, such as coffee whiteners.

343

On some labels, the ingredient list may state the source of sweeteners, too, although this is voluntary. For example, instead of "dextrose" or "dextrose monohydrate," the ingredient may be listed as "corn sugar monohydrate."

Nutrient Claims

Elsewhere on the label, consumers may find claims about the food's nutrient content. Often, these claims appear on the front of the package, where shoppers can readily see them. These claims signal that the food contains desirable levels of certain nutrients.

Some claims, such as "low-sodium" "high in calcium," or "good source of fiber," describe nutrient levels. (See "A Little 'Lite' Reading," in the June 1993 *FDA Consumer*; also reprinted in this section of the *Diet and Nutrition Sourcebook*.) Some, but not all, highlight foods containing beneficial amounts of nutrients for some people with special dietary needs. The same claim may warn other consumers, for whom the nutrient is detrimental, to avoid the product. For example, a product claiming to be an "excellent source of potassium" is not a wise buy for a person following a low-potassium diet. (See "Nutrient Claims Guide for Individual Foods.")

Health Claims

Health claims describe a relationship between a nutrient or food and a disease or health-related condition. FDA has authorized eight such claims; they are the only ones that can be used in a label. The claims may show a link between:

- calcium and a lower risk of osteoporosis

- fat and a greater risk of cancer

- saturated fat and cholesterol and a greater risk of coronary heart disease

- fiber-containing grain products, fruits and vegetables and a reduced risk of cancer

- fruits, vegetables and grain products that contain fiber and a reduced risk of coronary heart disease

- sodium and a greater risk of high blood pressure

- fruits and vegetables and a reduced risk of cancer

- folic acid and a decreased risk of neural tube defect-affected pregnancy.

Nutrient and health claims can be used only under certain circumstances, such as when the food contains appropriate levels of the stated nutrients.

The intent of the new food label is not just to ensure that label information is truthful but to provide more complete and useful nutrition and ingredient information for consumers' use. People with special dietary needs will likely find the labeling changes a welcome bonus.

Nutrient Claims Guide For Individual Foods

Fiber

High-fiber: 5 grams (g) or more per serving

Good source of fiber: at least 2.5 g per serving

More or added fiber: at least 2.5 g more per serving than the reference food. (Label will say 10 percent more of the Daily Value for fiber.)

Protein

High-protein: 10 g or more of high-quality protein per serving

Good source of protein: at least 5 g of high-quality protein per serving

More protein: at least 5 g more of high quality protein per serving than reference food (Label will say 10 percent more of the Daily Value for protein.)

Calcium

High-calcium: 200 milligrams (mg) or more per serving

Good source of calcium: at least 100 mg per serving

More calcium: at least 100 mg more than reference food. (Label will say 10 percent more of the Daily Value for calcium.)

Vitamin D

High in vitamin D: 80 International Units (IU) or more per serving

Good source of vitamin D: at least 40 IU per serving

More or fortified with vitamin D: at least 40 IU more than reference food. (Label will say 10 percent more of the Daily Value for vitamin D.)

Special Diets

Label information can help individuals select foods appropriate for their special dietary needs, determined by a physician, registered dietitian, or nutritionist. Some medical conditions that require special attention to diet are:

Kidney Disease

For many people whose kidneys have failed or are failing, protein, potassium and sodium are restricted. The nutrient phosphorus also may be restricted.

People undergoing dialysis may be encouraged to eat 20 to 25 grams (g) of fiber daily because fluid restrictions, lack of exercise, and some kidney medications can cause constipation. The Daily Value for fiber, which is based on a 2,000-calorie diet, is 25g.

Daily Values are reference numbers based on recommended dietary intakes to help consumers use label information to plan a healthy diet. (See "'Daily Values' Encourage Healthy Diet" in the May 1993 *FDA Consumer*.)

Liver Disorders

People with hepatitis, cirrhosis and other liver diseases often need a high-calorie, low-protein diet to help rejuvenate the damaged liver and maintain adequate nutrition. They also may need to increase their intake of vitamins—particularly folic acid, vitamin B_{12}, and thiamin—and minerals.

Food Sensitivities

According to the Food Allergy Network (a national nonprofit organization), the most common food allergens are milk, eggs, wheat, peanuts and other nuts, and soy. The treatment: Avoiding the food or foods containing them.

Celiac Disease

This is a genetic disorder in which the body cannot tolerate gliadin, the protein component of the gluten in wheat, barley, rye, and oats. So, people with celiac disease must avoid all products containing these grains—even foods that may contain only small amounts of the protein such as vinegar, bouillon, and alcohol-containing flavorings. The intolerance leads to malabsorption—not only of the offending food but virtually all nutrients.

Cancer

Because weight loss is common during cancer treatment, many cancer patients need to increase their calories and protein intake.

In the case of bowel obstruction—either from surgery, radiation or the tumor—cancer patients may need to eat less fiber. But, they may need more if they become constipated.

To help reduce their risk of developing cancer again, following treatment, patients may want to choose foods and nutrients whose role in reducing cancer risk has been borne out by significant scientific evidence. (See "Look for 'Legit' Health Claims on Foods" in the May 1993 *FDA Consumer.*)

Bowel Disease

Increased fiber is often recommended for people with chronic constipation, irritable bowel syndrome, and diverticulosis. Low-fiber diets may be called for during flare-ups of these and other bowel diseases, such as Crohn's disease and ulcerative colitis.

Osteoporosis

In osteoporosis, bone mass decreases, causing bones to become brittle and easily broken, especially in later life. A low-calcium intake throughout life is thought to be a major risk factor. The Daily Value for calcium, based on calcium needs for all ages, is 1,000 milligrams. Vitamin D also is important because it aids calcium absorption. The Daily Value for vitamin D is 400 International Units.

by Paula Kurtzweil

Paula Kurtzweil is a member of FDA's public affairs staff

Chapter 24

The New Food Label: Coping With Diabetes

Pat Coyle, of Rockville, Md., is a 67 year-old woman with diabetes, vitamin B_{12}-deficiency anemia, and osteoporosis. So she has to pay attention to her diet. But ask her what she likes most about the new food label, and you won't hear much about serving sizes, names of nutrients, and % Daily Values. Instead, you'll get rave reviews about the print size and background color.

The nutrition information on the new label is in bigger type, and FDA requires that it appear on a white or other neutral contrasting background, when practical.

Those are benefits for Coyle because she has diabetic retinopathy, an eye condition that can lead to blindness. She already has had two surgeries to correct poor eyesight. Before the surgeries, she had trouble reading food labels.

"I needed a magnifying glass to read [the nutrition information]," she recalls, referring to the small type and shaded backgrounds on the old labels. "I'm looking forward to not having to read the teeny tiny print."

For people with diabetes, easily readable labeling information is vital because diet is important in managing diabetes.

Other Label Benefits

New food labeling regulations that went into effect May 1994 now require labels on most packaged foods to provide nutrition informa-

---

DHHS Publication No. (FDA) 95-2289

tion. That previously was voluntary and appeared on only about 60 percent of such foods.

Also, nutrition information for fresh fruits and vegetables and raw meat and fish may appear at the point of purchase. (See "Nutrition Info Available for Raw Fruits, Vegetables, Fish" in the January-February 1993 *FDA Consumer.*)

The nutrition information is now more complete. Labels continue to provide information about calories, fat, carbohydrate, sodium, protein, iron, calcium, and vitamins A and C. But now they also contain additional information about saturated fat and cholesterol. These two nutrients are important to people with diabetes because diabetes increases the risk of heart disease, and heart disease is also linked to high intakes of saturated fat and cholesterol.

Diet for Diabetes

How beneficial the new label will be for people with diabetes depends on the type of meal plan they follow. Today, diabetes experts no longer recommend a single diet for all people with diabetes. Instead, they advocate dietary regimes that are flexible and take into account a person's lifestyle and particular health needs.

The American Diabetes Association (ADA) described some common options in a 1994 position paper. A first step, for example, is to encourage people with diabetes to follow the government's Dietary Guidelines for Americans and Food Guide Pyramid.

According to Phyllis Barrier, a registered dietitian and director of council affairs for ADA, this step alone may be enough to maintain normal blood glucose, or sugar, levels. Maintaining these levels helps reduce the risks of retinopathy and other diabetes-related complications, such as kidney and heart disease.

Other people use the Exchange Lists for Meal Planning, she said. This system, established by the American Dietetic and American Diabetes associations, separates foods into six categories based on their nutritional makeup. People following this plan choose a set amount of servings from each category daily, depending on their nutritional needs.

A more sophisticated method of meal planning is "carbohydrate counting" in which grams of carbohydrate consumed are monitored and adjusted daily according to blood glucose levels. Some people count protein and fat grams, too. These two nutrients also can affect blood sugar levels, although to a lesser extent.

Whatever method used, ADA recommends these general dietary guidelines for people with diabetes:

- Limit fat to 30 percent or less of daily calories.

- Limit saturated fat to 10 percent or less of daily calories.

- Limit protein to 10 to 20 percent of daily calories. For those with initial signs of diabetes-induced kidney disease, restrict protein to 10 percent of daily calories.

- Limit cholesterol to 300 milligrams or less daily.

- Consume about 20 to 35 grams of fiber daily.

Most of these guidelines are a good idea for the general population, as well.

Those who are overweight also may moderately restrict calories. ADA recommends a calorie reduction of 250 to 500 calories less than normally eaten per day. That should result in a weight loss of about 0.2 to 0.5 kilograms (one-half to 1 pound) a week, ADA's Barrier said. The calorie restriction, along with increased exercise, should help an overweight person achieve a weight loss of 5 to 10 kilograms (11 to 22 pounds) in about six months to one year. The weight loss, although moderate, can help improve diabetes control.

Carbohydrate intake can vary, but, contrary to popular belief, the type of carbohydrate is not a factor. As ADA points out in its position paper, people with diabetes have for years been told to avoid "simple" sugars, such as table sugar and those found in sugary snacks, because they were thought to elevate blood glucose more quickly and more severely than other carbohydrates.

"There is, however, very little scientific evidence that supports this assumption," ADA wrote in its position paper. The organization recommended that the focus be on total carbohydrate—not source of carbohydrate. If sugar and sugar-containing foods are eaten, the amounts must be figured into the daily allotment of carbohydrate.

Get the Nutrition Facts

Considering these factors, how should people with diabetes go about using the new food label?

They can begin with the Nutrition Facts panel, usually on the side or back of the package. A column headed % Daily Values shows whether a food is high or low in many of the nutrients listed.

353

People with diabetes should check the % Daily Values for fat, saturated fat, and cholesterol. As a rule of thumb, if the number is 5 or less, the food may be considered low in that nutrient.

The goal for most people with diabetes is to pick foods that have low % Daily Values for fat, saturated fat, and cholesterol and high % Daily Values for fiber. Other label nutrition information can help people with diabetes see if and how a food fits into their meal plan.

Serving Sizes

The serving size information gives the amount of food to which all other numbers on the Nutrition Facts panel apply.

Serving sizes now are more uniform among similar products and reflect the amounts people actually eat. For example, the reference amount for a serving of snack crackers is 30 g. Thus, the serving size for soda crackers is 10 crackers and for Goldfish Tiny Crackers, 55, because these are the amounts that come closest to 30g.

The similarity makes it easier to compare the nutritional qualities of related foods.

People who use the Exchange Lists should be aware that the serving size on the label may not be the same as that in the Exchange Lists. For example, the label serving size for orange juice is 8 fluid ounces (240 milliliters). In the exchange lists, the serving size is 4 ounces (one-half cup) or 120 mL. So, a person who drinks one cup of orange juice has used two fruit exchanges.

Calorie and Other Information

The Nutrition Facts panel also gives total calories and calories from fat per serving of food. This is helpful for people who count calories and monitor their daily percentage of calories from fat.

Here's how to use calories from fat information: At the end of the day, add up total calories and then calories from fat eaten. Divide calories from fat by total calories. The answer gives the percentage of calories from fat eaten that day. For example, 450 calories from fat divided by 1,800 total calories = 0.25 (25 percent), an amount within the recommended level of not more than 30 percent calories from fat.

The label also gives grams of total carbohydrate, protein and fat, which can be used for carbohydrate counting.

The values listed for total carbohydrate include all carbohydrate, including dietary fiber and sugars listed below it. Not singled out is complex carbohydrates, such as starches.

The sugars include naturally present sugars, such as lactose in milk and fructose in fruits, and those added to the food, such as table sugar, corn syrup, and dextrose.

The listing of grams of protein also is helpful for those restricting their protein intake, either to reduce their risk of kidney disease or to manage the kidney disease they have developed.

Front Label Info

Elsewhere on the label, consumers may find claims about the food's nutritional benefits. Often, they appear on the front of the package, where shoppers can readily see them. These claims signal that the food contains desirable levels of certain nutrients.

Some claims, such as "low-fat," "no saturated fat," and "high-fiber," describe nutrient levels. (See "A Little 'Lite' Reading," in the June 1993 *FDA Consumer;* this article is also reprinted in this section of the *Diet and Nutrition Sourcebook.*) Some of these are particularly interesting to people with diabetes because they highlight foods containing nutrients at beneficial levels. (See "Nutrient Claims Guide.")

Other claims, called health claims, show a relationship between a nutrient or food and a disease or health condition. FDA has authorized eight such claims; they are the only ones about which there is significant scientific agreement. (See "Starting This Month: Look for 'Legit' Health Claims on Foods" in the May 1993 *FDA Consumer.*)

Two that relate to heart disease are of particular interest to people with diabetes:

• A diet low in saturated fat and cholesterol may help reduce the risk of coronary heart disease.

• A diet rich in fruits, vegetables and grain products that contain fiber, particularly soluble fiber, and are low in saturated fat and cholesterol may help reduce the risk of coronary heart disease.

Both claims also must state that heart disease depends on many factors.

Nutrient and health claims can be used only under certain circumstances, such as when the food contains appropriate levels of the stated nutrients. So now, when consumers see the claims, they can believe them.

The intent, though, is not just to ensure the label information is truthful, but also to enable the consumer to use it to choose healthier foods. For people with diabetes, that's especially important because of the increased risk of other chronic diseases. Pat Coyle is one person with diabetes who realizes this.

"I'm looking forward to greater health because I won't have any excuses," she says. "The information . . . is right there." And, she adds, "I especially like the large print."

Nutrient Claims Guide For Individual Foods

Fat

Fat-free: less than 0.5 grams (g) fat per serving

Low-fat: 3 g or less per serving and, if the serving size is 30 g or less or 2 tablespoons or less, per 50 g of the food

Reduced or less fat: at least 25 percent less per serving than reference food

Saturated Fat

Saturated fat free: less than 0.5 g and less than 0.5 g of trans fatty acids per serving

Low saturated fat: 1 g or less per serving and not more than 15 percent of calories from saturated fatty acids

Reduced or less saturated fat: at least 25 percent less per serving than reference food

Cholesterol

Cholesterol-free: less than 2 milligrams (mg) and 2 g or less of saturated fat per serving

Low-cholesterol: 20 mg or less and 2 g or less of saturated fat per serving and, if the serving is 30 g or less or 2 tablespoons or less, per 50 g of the food

Reduced or less cholesterol: at least 25 percent less than reference food and 2 g or less of saturated fat per serving

The following claims can be used to describe meat, poultry, seafood, and game meats:

Lean: less than 10 g fat, 4.5 g or less saturated fat, and less than 95 mg cholesterol per serving and per 100 g

Extra lean: less than 5 g fat, less than 2 g saturated fat, and less than 95 mg cholesterol per serving and per 100 g

Healthy

- "low fat," "low saturated fat," with 60 mg or less cholesterol per serving (or, if raw meat, poultry and fish, "extra lean")

- at least 10 percent of Daily Value for one or more of vitamins A and C, iron, calcium, protein, and fiber per serving

- 480 mg or less sodium per serving, and, if the serving is 30 g or less or 2 tablespoons or less, per 50 g of the food. (After Jan. 1, 1998, maximum sodium levels drop to 360 mg.)

Calories

Calorie-free: fewer than 5 calories per serving

Low-calorie: 40 or fewer calories per serving and, if the serving size is 30 g or less or 2 tablespoons or less, per 50 g of the food

Reduced or fewer calories: at least 25 percent fewer calories per serving than the reference food

Light (two meanings)

- one-third fewer calories or half the fat of the reference food—if the food derives 50 percent or more of its calories from fat, the reduction must be 50 percent of the fat

- a "low-calorie," "low-fat" food whose sodium content has been reduced by 50 percent from the reference food ("Light in sodium" means the food has 50 percent or less sodium than the reference food and may be used on foods that are not "low-calorie" and "low-fat.")

357

Fiber

High-fiber: 5 g or more per serving

Good source of fiber: 2.5 g to 4.9 g per serving

More or added fiber: at least 2.5 g more per serving than the reference food. (Label will say 10 percent more of the Daily Value for fiber.)

Foods making claims about increased fiber content also must meet the definition for "low-fat" or the amount of total fat per serving must appear next to the claim.

Sugar

Sugar-free: less than 0.5 g per serving

No added sugar, without added sugar, no sugar added:

- no sugar or ingredients that functionally substitute for sugar (for example, fruit juices) added during processing or packing

- no ingredients made with added sugars, such as jams, jellies, or concentrated fruit juice

("Sugar-free" and "No added sugar" signal a reduction in calories from sugars only, not from fat, protein and other carbohydrates. If the total calories are not reduced or the food is not "low-calorie," a statement will appear next to the "sugar-free" claim explaining that the food is "not low-calorie," "not reduced calorie," or "not for weight control." If the total calories are reduced, the claim must be accompanied by a "low-calorie" or "reduced-calorie" claim.)

Reduced sugar: at least 25 percent less sugar than the reference food

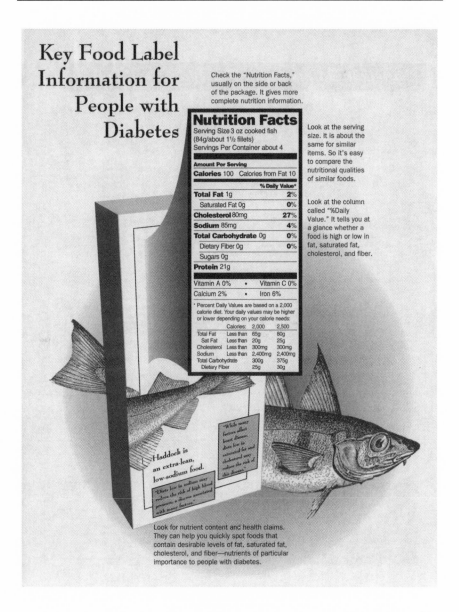

Key Food Label Information for People with Diabetes

Check the "Nutrition Facts," usually on the side or back of the package. It gives more complete nutrition information.

Nutrition Facts
Serving Size 3 oz cooked fish (84g/about 1½ fillets)
Servings Per Container about 4

Amount Per Serving
Calories 100 Calories from Fat 10

	% Daily Value*
Total Fat 1g	2%
Saturated Fat 0g	0%
Cholesterol 80mg	27%
Sodium 85mg	4%
Total Carbohydrate 0g	0%
Dietary Fiber 0g	0%
Sugars 0g	
Protein 21g	

Vitamin A 0%	•	Vitamin C 0%
Calcium 2%	•	Iron 6%

* Percent Daily Values are based on a 2,000 calorie diet. Your daily values may be higher or lower depending on your calorie needs:

	Calories:	2,000	2,500
Total Fat	Less than	65g	80g
Sat Fat	Less than	20g	25g
Cholesterol	Less than	300mg	300mg
Sodium	Less than	2,400mg	2,400mg
Total Carbohydrate		300g	375g
Dietary Fiber		25g	30g

Look at the serving size. It is about the same for similar items. So it's easy to compare the nutritional qualities of similar foods.

Look at the column called "%Daily Value." It tells you at a glance whether a food is high or low in fat, saturated fat, cholesterol, and fiber.

Haddock is an extra-lean, low-sodium food.

Diets low in sodium may reduce the risk of high blood pressure, a disease associated with many factors.

While many factors affect heart disease, diets low in saturated fat and cholesterol may reduce the risk of this disease.

Look for nutrient content and health claims. They can help you quickly spot foods that contain desirable levels of fat, saturated fat, cholesterol, and fiber—nutrients of particular importance to people with diabetes.

by Paula Kurtzweil

Paula Kurtzweil is a member of FDA 's public affairs staff.

Chapter 25

Labeling Rules for Young Children's Food

How much fat should we eat to stay healthy? For adults, the answer is clear: The Dietary Guidelines for Americans tell us to restrict fat to no more than 30 percent of our total calorie intake.

But for infants and toddlers, the answer is less straightforward; the Dietary Guidelines don't apply to children under 2. In fact, health experts advise against restricting fat in young children's diets because they need the calories and nutrients fat provides to grow and develop properly.

For this reason, FDA and the U.S. Department of Agriculture's Food Safety and Inspection Service have established special rules to govern the labeling of foods for children under 4. (USDA regulates labeling of meat and poultry products. FDA oversees labeling of all other foods.)

Just as for other foods, the regulations require labels for foods for young children to include information about nutrients important to health—for example, fat, sodium, carbohydrate, protein, vitamins, and minerals. This is to help parents choose foods that contain the appropriate kinds and amounts of nutrients their children need.

But the new regulations forbid labels for foods for children under 2 to carry certain nutrition information because the presence of the information may lead parents to wrongly assume that certain nutrients should be restricted in young children's diets, when, in fact, they should not.

DHHS Publication No. (FDA) 95-2292

In addition, the labels for foods for children under 4 cannot show how the amounts of some nutrients correspond to Daily Values—recommended daily intakes. The reason is because Daily Values for some nutrients, such as fat, fiber and sodium, have not been established for children under 4. This is because current dietary recommendations do not specify appropriate levels for young children. FDA has set Daily Values only for vitamins, minerals and protein for this age group because the National Academy of Sciences has established appropriate levels of these nutrients for this age group in the Recommended Dietary Allowances. FDA incorporated those recommendations in the Daily Values. (See " 'Daily Values' Encourage Healthy Diet" in the May 1993 *FDA Consumer.*)

Up-to-Date Label

These labeling requirements stem from the Nutrition Labeling and Education Act of 1990, which, among other things, requires labels of most foods—including those for children under 4—to carry nutrition information.

The children's nutrition labeling rules apply to most foods whose labels suggest that the food is intended for infants and toddlers. This includes infant cereals, infant strained meats, vegetables and fruits, "junior" foods, teething biscuits, and infant and "junior" juices. The regulations do not apply to infant formula, which has special nutrition labeling requirements.

Many foods for infants and toddlers have carried some nutrition information since at least the 1970s, when voluntary nutrition labeling went into effect. But now, for many such foods, the information is required and more pertinent to today's health concerns. (See "Good Reading for Good Eating" in the May 1993 *FDA Consumer.*)

Importance of Fat

Concerns about excessive fat and cholesterol intake for most of the population don't apply to children under 2, however. Fat is one of six nutrient categories essential for proper growth and development. (The others are protein, carbohydrate, water, vitamins, and minerals.) At no other age does fat play such an important role as in infancy and early childhood, a period of rapid growth and development. Dietary fat serves as:

- a source of energy (infants and toddlers have the highest energy needs per kilogram of weight of any age group)

- a carrier for the fat-soluble vitamins A, D, E, and K and as an aid in their absorption in the intestine

- the only source of linoleic acid, an essential fatty acid.

Fat also gives taste, consistency, stability, and palatability to foods and converts to body fat, which is necessary to hold organs in place, absorb shock, and insulate the body from temperature changes.

Some parents fail to realize fat's importance for young children. According to a Gerber Products Co.'s telephone survey of 1,076 adults, nearly one in five respondents said they reduce the amount of fat in their baby's diet.

Yet, according to Virginia Wilkening, a registered dietitian and consumer safety officer in FDA's Office of Food Labeling, case reports have shown that limiting fat intakes in very young children can cause them to "fail to thrive."

"Babies need fat and cholesterol in their diets for proper growth and development," Wilkening said. "Parents should be aware of this and avoid reducing fat in their young children's diets."

Restrictions

For foods for children under 2, the amount of saturated fat, polyunsaturated fat, monounsaturated fat, cholesterol, calories from fat, and calories from saturated fat in the food cannot be listed on the label.

Labels of foods for children under 2 also cannot carry most of the claims about a food's nutritional content—such as "low-fat" and "low-cholesterol"—that labels of other foods can. (See "A Little 'Lite' Reading in the June 1993 *FDA Consumer;* this article is also reprinted in this section of the *Diet and Nutrition Sourcebook.*) And, they cannot carry the eight FDA-approved health claims about the relationship between a nutrient or food and a health problem—for example, dietary fat and cancer—that other labels can. (See "Starting This Month, Look for 'Legit' Health Claims on Foods" in the May 1993 *FDA Consumer.*)

Allowed Facts

What information is allowed? The following is a list of dietary components about which information is allowed on the Nutrition Facts panel on the labels of foods for children under 2. Information usually appears on the side or back of the package and is mandatory for underlined components.

- <u>total calories</u>

- <u>total fat</u>

- <u>sodium</u>

- potassium

- <u>total carbohydrate</u>

- <u>dietary fiber</u>

- soluble fiber

- insoluble fiber

- <u>sugars</u>

- sugar alcohol

- <u>protein</u>

- <u>vitamin A</u>

- <u>vitamin C</u>

- <u>calcium</u>

- <u>iron</u>

- other essential vitamins and minerals.

(Information about them is mandatory only when they are added to enrich or fortify a food, or when a claim is made about them on the label.)

Labels for foods for children 2 to 4 also must give the amount of cholesterol and saturated fat per serving. They can voluntarily provide the calories from fat and calories from saturated fat, and the amount of polyunsaturated and monounsaturated fat per serving.

The % Daily Values for protein and vitamins and minerals present in significant amounts must be listed. This helps parents see how a serving of food fits into their child's total daily diet. The amount of other nutrients is given in grams or milligrams.

Serving Size

The serving size, under "Nutrition Facts," is the basis on which manufacturers declare the nutrient amounts and % Daily Values on the label. It is the amount of food customarily eaten at one time—not necessarily the amount recommended by dietary guidelines.

The serving size is based on FDA- and USDA-established lists of "Reference Amounts Customarily Consumed Per Eating Occasion." FDA has established 11 groups of foods specially intended for children under 4. USDA has four such groups.

The serving size must be stated in both common household units and metric measures—for example, for dry instant cereal, "1/4 Cup (15 g)."

These standardized serving sizes make it easier to compare the nutritional quality of similar foods.

Nutrient and Health Claims

FDA and USDA's regulations also extend to label claims.

Among the few allowed in children's nutrition labeling are claims that describe the percentage of vitamins or minerals in the food as they apply to the Daily Values for children under 2—for example, "provides 50 percent of the Daily Value for vitamin C." This type of claim also is allowed in the labeling of dietary supplements for children under 2.

Also allowed for foods for children under 2 are the claims "unsweetened" and "unsalted." FDA believes that for foods for this age group, these claims refer to taste and not nutrition.

Two claims—"no sugar added" and "sugar free"—are approved only for use on dietary supplements for children under 2 because they often contain added sugar.

If presented with sound evidence, however, FDA will consider allowing other nutrient content claims, as well as health claims, in the labeling of foods for children under 2.

365

These and other rules are intended to help consumers select the best foods for children. The absence of some information allowed in labeling for other foods can help them do that.

As long as the products meet the definitions of the terms, the claims "sugar free" and "no sugar added" are allowed on the labels of dietary supplements for children under 2. But those claims, and many others that are allowed elsewhere, can't be used on regular foods for children of that age.

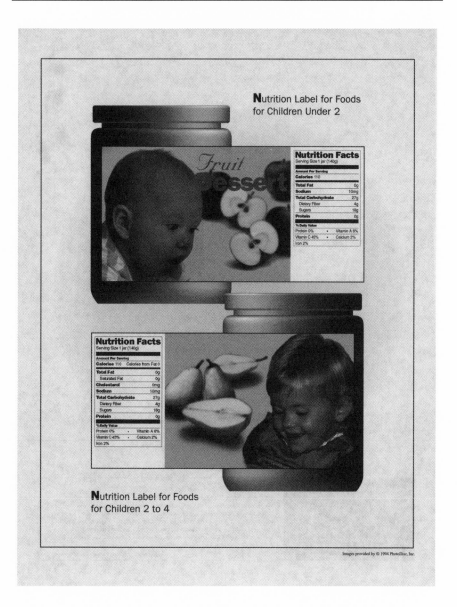

Nutrition Label for Foods for Children Under 2

Nutrition Label for Foods for Children 2 to 4

Images provided by © 1994 PhotoDisc, Inc.

by Paula Kurtzweil

Chapter 26

A Little 'Lite' Reading

"Low fat." "No cholesterol." "High in oat bran." "Light." And don't forget "lite."

Until now, many of these claims have been nothing more than advertising hype. The public has been misled with products like the "light" vegetable oil that was just light in color and the "lite" cheesecake that was just light in texture.

But with the publication of new food labeling regulations in January 1993, the Food and Drug Administration and the U.S. Department of Agriculture's Food Safety and Inspection Service (FSIS) address the problem of misleading nutrition claims and help reestablish the credibility of the food label. The regulations spell out which nutrient content claims are allowed and under what circumstances they can be used.

There are 11 core terms:

- free
- low
- lean
- extra lean
- high
- good source
- reduced

FDA Consumer / June 1993

- less
- light
- fewer
- more

Let Freedom Ring

The new regulations allow manufacturers the option to use the following synonyms for the term "free":

- without
- trivial source of
- negligible source of
- dietarily insignificant source of
- no
- zero

Whatever term the manufacturer chooses, the product must either be absolutely free of the nutrient in question or, if the nutrient is in the food, the amount must be dietetically trivial or physiologically insignificant.

For example, zero fat cannot be required because it is impossible to measure below a certain amount. So, the regulation will allow a fat-free claim on foods with less than 0.5 grams (g) of fat per serving, an amount that is physiologically insignificant even if a person eats several servings.

Foods that don't contain a certain nutrient naturally must be labeled to indicate that all foods of that type meet the claim. For example, a fat-free claim on applesauce would have to read "applesauce, a fat-free food."

"Free" also can be used in reference to saturated fat, cholesterol, sodium, sugars, and calories.

The Lowdown

A food meets the definition for "low" if a person can eat a large amount of the food without exceeding the Daily Value for the nutrient.

The synonyms allowed for 'low" are:

- little

- few

- contains a small amount of

- low source of

"Low" claims can be made in reference to total fat, saturated fat, cholesterol, sodium, and calories.

A claim of "very low" can be made only about sodium.

Lean, Mean Eating Machine

"Lean" and "extra lean" can be used to describe the fat content of meat, poultry, seafood, and game meats. (FSIS regulates meat and poultry products; FDA oversees seafood and game meats.)

"Lean" means the food has less than 10 g of fat, less than 4 g of saturated fat, and less than 95 milligrams (mg) of cholesterol per serving and per 100 g. An example of a serving is 55 g (2 oz.) for fish, shellfish or game meat. Some "lean" foods are Spanish mackerel, bluefin tuna, and domesticated rabbit.

"Extra lean" means the food has less than 5 g of fat, less than 2 g of saturated fat, and less than 95 mg of cholesterol per serving and per 100 g. Examples of "extra lean" foods are haddock, swordfish, clams, and deer.

Percent Fat Free

FDA and FSIS believe that this claim implies, and consumers expect, that products bearing "percent fat free" claims contain relatively small amounts of fat and are useful in maintaining a low-fat diet. Therefore, products with these claims must meet the definitions for low fat.

371

In addition, the claim must accurately reflect the amount of fat present in 100 g of the food. For example, if a food contains 2.5 g of fat per 50 g, the claim must be "95 percent fat free."

Take the High Road

"High" and "good source" focus on nutrients for which higher levels are desirable. To qualify for the "high" claim, the food must contain 20 percent or more of the Daily Value for that nutrient in a serving. Approved synonyms for high are "rich in" or "excellent source."

"Good source" means a serving contains 10 to 19 percent of the Daily Value for the nutrient.

Comparison Claims

Manufacturers who want to compare a nutritionally altered product with the regular product may make a relative claim—that is, "reduced," "less," "fewer, "more," or "light." The regular products, or reference foods, may be either an individual food or a group of foods representative of the type of food—for example, an average of three market leaders.

Restrictions on these claims and the reference foods include:

- A relative claim must include the percent difference and the identity of the reference food.

- "Reduced," "less" and "light" claims can't be made on products whose nutrient level in the reference food already meets the requirement for a "low" claim.

- Reference foods for "light" and "reduced" claims must be similar to the product bearing the claim—for example, reduced fat potato chips compared with regular potato chips.

- Reference foods for "less" and, in the case of calories, "fewer" may use dissimilar products within a product category—for example, pretzels with 25 percent less fat than potato chips.

At the other end of the spectrum, a serving of a food carrying a "more" claim (or claims of fortified, enriched or added) must have at least 10 percent more of the Daily Value for a particular nutrient (that is, dietary fiber, potassium, protein, or an essential vitamin or mineral) than the reference food that it resembles

Let There Be Light/Lite

"Light" or "lite" can mean one of two things:

First, that a nutritionally altered product contains one-third fewer calories or half the fat of the reference food. If the food derives 50 percent or more of its calories from fat, the reduction must be 50 percent of the fat.

Second, that the sodium content of a low-calorie, low-fat food has been reduced by 50 percent.

The term "light in sodium" is allowed if the food has at least 50 percent less sodium than a reference food. If the food still does not meet the definition for "low sodium," the label must include the disclaimer "not a low-sodium food."

"Light" will be allowed to describe color or texture, provided qualifying information is included. However, names that have a long history of use, such as "light brown sugar," can still be used without qualifying information.

Meals and Main Dishes

Any product represented as or in a form commonly understood to be breakfast, lunch or dinner is subject to the special rules for meat products. Examples include frozen dinners, some pizzas, and shelf-stable items.

Under FDA rules, a main dish must weigh at least 6 ounces and contain at least two different foods from at least two of four specified food groups. (While FDA endorses the five food groups recommended in current dietary guidelines, the agency believes treating fruits and vegetables as separate groups in this situation would allow the inappropriate classification of a fruit and a vegetable product as a main dish.)

FDA requires a "meal" to weigh at least 10 ounces and have at least three different foods from at least two of the four specified food groups.

USDA defines a meal-type product as one weighing between 6 and 12 ounces per serving and containing ingredients from two or more of four specified food groups.

Claims that a meal or main dish is "free" of a nutrient, such as sodium or cholesterol, must meet the same requirements as those for individual foods

"Low" claims can be made if the main dish or meal has:

- 120 calories or less per 100 g

- 14.0 mg sodium or less per 100 g

- 3 g fat or less and no more than 30 percent of calories from fat per 100 g

- 1 g saturated fat or less and no more than 10 percent calories from saturated fat per 100 g or

- 20 mg cholesterol or less per 100 g and no more than 2 g of saturated fat per 100 g.

Implied Claims

"Made with oat bran" and "no tropical oils" are examples of statements that may be implied nutrient content claims. Such claims are prohibited when they wrongfully imply that a food contains or does not contain a meaningful level of a nutrient. They are allowed if the food's nutrient content meets the definition for appropriate nutrient content descriptors that are implied by the claim.

For example, FDA considers statements about some types of oil as an ingredient, such as "made with canola oil" or "contains corn oil," to imply that the oil in the product is low in saturated fat. Therefore, to carry that claim, a food would have to meet the definition of "low saturated fat."

The statement "made only with vegetable oil" implies that because vegetable oil is used instead of animal fat, the oil component contributes no cholesterol and is low in saturated fat. In this case, the claim could be used only if the food meets the definition of "cholesterol free" and "low saturated fat."

And the statement "contains no oil" implies that the product contains no fat and thus is fat free. Such a claim on a product that contained another source of fat, such as animal fat, would be misleading. Therefore, this statement would be allowed only if the food is truly fat free.

Claims that imply a product contains a particular amount of fiber, such as "high in oat bran," can be made only if the food actually meets the definition for "high" fiber or "good source" of fiber, whichever is appropriate.

Statements that don't fall under the rules for nutrient content implied claims and therefore are still allowed are:

- those that help consumers avoid certain foods because of religious beliefs or dietary practices—for example, a "milk-free" claim

- those about nonnutritive ingredients, such as "no preservatives" or "no artificial colors"

- those about ingredients that provide added value, such as "contains real fruit"

- statements of identity, such as "Colombian coffee" and "100 percent corn oil"

Fresh

Although not mandated by the Nutrition Labeling and Education Act of 1990, as regulations for the other nutrient content claims are, FDA has issued a regulation for the term "fresh." Under this regulation, "fresh" can be used only on a food that is raw, has never been frozen or heated, and contains no preservatives. (Irradiation at low levels is allowed.) "Fresh frozen," "frozen fresh," and "freshly frozen" can be used for foods that are quickly frozen while still fresh. Blanching (brief scalding before freezing to prevent nutrient break down) is allowed.

Other uses of the term "fresh," such as in "fresh milk" or "freshly baked bread, are not affected.

Healthy

Along with the final rule on nutrient content claims published last January, FDA and FSIS published proposed rules that would allow manufacturers to make a "healthy" claim on the label. Under FDA's proposal, "healthy" could be used if the food is low in fat and saturated fats and a serving does not contain more than 480 mg of sodium or more than 60 mg of cholesterol. USDA's proposal would allow the term if the food meets the definition for "lean" and contains no more than 480 mg of sodium per serving.

Special Situations

"Standards of identity" define a food's composition and specify the ingredients it must contain. The government originally developed these standards to protect consumers from economic deception.

But some standards of identity require high amounts of nutrients that many consumers would like to avoid. For example, the standard for sour cream requires that the food contain 18 percent fat and the standard for mozzarella cheese requires it to be 45 percent fat. Before the new regulations, "reduced-fat" sour cream or mozzarella cheese were required to have their own standards of identity or be called "imitation" or "substitute," names that consumers may perceive as negative.

The new regulations allow manufacturers to reduce the fat content of such products and call them "low fat" or "light," as appropriate, as long as the food is still nutritionally equivalent to the regular version. For example, sour cream can be called "light" as long as its fat content is reduced to 9 percent and it has vitamin A added to replace the amount lost when the fat was removed. If the company decides not to add the vitamin A, it must call the product "imitation light sour cream."

FDA is not allowing nutrient content claims on foods for infants and children under 2, unless explicit permission has been given.

FDA allows manufacturers to use the terms "unsweetened" and "unsalted" on these foods because these claims are considered to be about taste rather than nutrient content. However, current dietary guidelines do not call for limiting salt or sugar in the diets of children under 2. Therefore, FDA will not allow phrases that imply low or reduced amounts of sodium and calories, such as "no salt added" and "no sugar added," on these types of foods.

Getting Specific

Here are examples of the meaning of some descriptive words for specific nutrients.

Sugar

Sugar free: less than O.5 grams (g) per serving

No added sugar, Without added sugar, No sugar added:

- No sugars added during processing or packing, including ingredients that contain sugars (for example, fruit juices, applesauce, or dried fruit).

- Processing does not increase the sugar content above the amount naturally present in the ingredients. (A functionally insignificant increase in sugars is acceptable from processes used for purposes other than increasing sugar content.)

- The food that it resembles and for which it substitutes normally contains added sugars.

- If the food doesn't meet the requirements for a low- or reduced-calorie food, the product bears a statement that the food is not low calorie or calorie-reduced and directs consumers' attention to the nutrition panel for further information on sugars and caloric content

Reduced sugar: at least 25 percent less sugar per serving than reference food

Calories

Calorie free: fewer than 5 calories per serving

Low calorie: 40 calories or less per serving and if the serving is 30 g or less or 2 tablespoons or less, per 50 g of the food

Reduced or Fewer calories: at least 25 percent fewer calories per serving than reference food

Fat

Fat free: less than 0.5 g of fat per serving

Saturated fat free: less than 0.5 g per serving and the level of trans fatty acids does not exceed 1 percent of total fat

Low fat: 3 g or less per serving, and if the serving is 30 g or less or 2 tablespoons or less, per 50 g of the food

Low saturated fat: 1 g or less per serving and not more than 15 percent of calories from saturated fatty acids

Reduced or Less fat: at least 25 percent less per serving than reference food

Reduced or Less saturated fat: at least 25 percent less per serving than reference food

Cholesterol

Cholesterol free: less than 2 milligrams (mg) of cholesterol and 2 g or less of saturated fat per serving

Low cholesterol: 20 mg or less and 2 g or less of saturated fat per serving and, if the serving is 30 g or less or 2 tablespoons or less, per 50 g of the food

Reduced or Less cholesterol: at least 25 percent less and 2 g or less of saturated fat per serving than reference food

Sodium

Sodium free: less than 5 mg per serving

Low sodium: 140 mg or less per serving and, if the serving is 30 g or less or 2 tablespoons or less, per 50 g of the food

Very low sodium: 35 mg or less per serving and, if the serving is 30 g or less or 2 tablespoons or less, per 50 g of the food

Reduced or Less sodium: at least 25 percent less per serving than reference food

Fiber

High fiber: 5 g or more per serving. (Foods making high-fiber claims must meet the definition for low fat, or the level of total fat must appear next to the high-fiber claim)

Good source of fiber: 2.5 g to 4.9 g per serving

More or Added fiber: at least 2.5 g more per serving than reference food

A serving of a food carrying a "more" claim (or claims of fortified, enriched or added) must have at least 10 percent more of the Daily Value for a particular nutrient (that is, dietary fiber, potassium, protein, or an essential vitamin or mineral) than the reference food that it resembles.

by Dori Stehlin

Dori Stehlin is a member of FDA's public affairs staff

Part Five

Recent Developments in Nutritional Research

Chapter 27

Bioavailability: How the Nutrients in Food Become Available to Our Bodies

Bioavailability is the degree to which food nutrients are available for absorption and utilization in the body. It is a critical issue for many nutritional concerns.

Why Do We Care About Measuring Bioavailability?

The role of bioavailability is important in establishing nutrient requirements and using those requirements in food labeling. The amount of a nutrient in a food that the body can actually use may vary depending on age and physiologic condition, such as pregnancy. Nutrient availability is also important in testing and marketing infant foods, nutritional supplements, and enteral formulas (for patients who can't digest solid foods).

An understanding of bioavailability is also important because consumers continually change their dietary patterns for reasons of health, economics, or personal preference, and knowledge of nutrient bioavailability may influence their choices. Furthermore, as the range of food products from which consumers may choose constantly increases (especially with production of new and unconventional convenience foods), the food processing industry has a critical interest in the effects of food processing and preparation on the bioavailability of nutrients.

Excerpt from *Nutrition: Eating for Good Health*, U.S. Department of Agriculture, Agriculture Information Bulletin 685

Demographic changes also expand food choices, so that determining the nutrient availability and adequacy in ethnic foods is of greater concern. The use of vitamin and mineral supplements by as many as 50 percent of Americans suggests a need for accurate data on the availability of nutrients in these supplements. Finally, nutrient-drug interactions may alter nutrient bioavailability and thus affect nutritional status in individuals who are taking certain drugs.

Analyzing and Measuring Bioavailability

Bioavailability refers to the amount of a nutrient in a food that the body may ultimately use to perform specific physiological functions.

Several factors influence the bioavailability of a nutrient. These include:

- Digestion,

- Absorption,

- Distribution of the nutrient by the circulating blood, and

- Entry of the nutrient into the specific body tissues and fluids in which it may be physiologically effective.

Each of the steps involved in the process that makes nutrients bioavailable can be affected by a variety of factors in the food itself, and also by the nutritional status of the individual. It is particularly difficult to assess bioavailability when the nutrients are present in many different forms in foods and tissues.

As complicated as it appears to be, the assessment of nutrient bioavailability still remains critical to our understanding of how humans utilize essential nutrients from consumed foods and to our appreciation of how foods satisfy our nutritional requirements.

Researchers have found new analytic techniques that permit more accurate identification and measurement of nutrients in foods and tissues, and they have creatively applied these techniques to improve our understanding of observed variations in the bioavailability of a nutrient from different foods.

Individual Nutrients and Food Factors That Affect Bioavailability

A variety of components in foods may reduce or enhance the bioavailability of the nutrients. Some components may form complexes with a nutrient and prevent its digestion or absorption or even degrade the nutrient, as is the case with foods that contain an enzyme that breaks down the B vitamin, thiamin. Protein inhibitors that often reduce nutrient bioavailability are generally destroyed by cooking. Other complexes can increase solubility and, thus, enhance absorption. Recent developments in the availability of selected nutrients are summarized below:

Calcium

Efforts to understand the metabolic and dietary factors that lead to osteoporosis, or the loss of skeletal mass with aging, emphasize the importance of calcium bioavailability. Calcium in foods exists mainly as complexes with other factors (phytates, oxalates, fiber, lactate, fatty acids) from which the calcium must be released to be absorbed.

Plant constituents of the diet, in particular, may reduce calcium bioavailability so that people who do not use dairy products are less likely to obtain adequate amounts of calcium. Oxalates, present in some foods, normally bind with calcium in the gut, and the body excretes both of them together, thus limiting calcium absorption and availability. Researchers are using plants intrinsically labeled with tracer forms of calcium to evaluate the effects of plant food constituents on calcium bioavailability. Calcium supplements are also being evaluated by these techniques to determine their availability to humans.

Recent research has shown that the bioavailability of calcium from calcium carbonate, a widely used supplement, is similar to that from milk. It has also been shown that vitamin B_6 deficiency may reduce calcium availability.

Iron

Iron deficiency is widespread in the United States and is a major cause of anemia in susceptible populations, especially in those whose demand for iron is high, such as growing children or pregnant women. Many factors, including dietary components (phytates, tannins, phosphates, and high calcium intake), exercise, menstruation, and maturity may increase or reduce iron availability. Iron absorption and utilization increase as iron stores are depleted, but inhibiting factors in such foods and beverages as soybeans and tea can impair iron absorption. Conversely, including meat or foods containing vitamin C in a meal enhances iron absorption. It is not known how meat achieves this effect, but recent research suggests that some factors in meat form a complex with iron to increase its absorption. Meat also increases gastric acid secretion, which may increase iron availability and absorption.

The optimal criterion for measuring the bioavailability of iron is not clear. The most commonly used response criterion is hemoglobin concentration in blood. The most recent research suggests that regeneration of red-blood-cell hemoglobin (an oxygen-transporting protein) can be used to measure iron bioavailability, thereby providing an easily obtained index of iron availability. Protocols are being developed to predict the bioavailability of iron in humans based on animal models. Recent research also shows that interactions of other minerals, such as zinc and calcium, with iron may reduce iron bioavailability. Copper deficiency, cooked meat, and raw vegetables are thought to enhance iron absorption.

Copper

Copper deficiency can result in anemia, bone disease, and diminished immune competence. Excessive intake of copper can lead to toxic effects, especially vascular problems such as low blood pressure and high blood-cholesterol levels. The bioavailability of copper is affected by a variety of factors. Among those which decrease bioavailability are sub-optimal levels of acid in the gastrointestinal tract; the boiling of foods, which may leach away copper; and the consumption of uncooked protein foods. Copper bioavailability may also be reduced by interaction with other minerals such as iron, zinc, lead, cadmium, and selenium.

Lead

Intake of lead has become a major public health concern. Lead toxicity is most widespread in children, in whom it may lead to impaired mental development. In poorly nourished populations, it commonly results in anemia by interfering with the availability of essential nutrients, such as iron and copper. Recent research indicates that increasing meat intake reduces lead absorption from drinking water or other sources of ingested lead. Additional copper intake is more effective than either iron or zinc in reducing lead absorption, although intake of all three minerals seems to protect against lead toxicity.

Vitamin B_{12}

Vitamin B_{12} deficiency rarely occurs from inadequate dietary intake but can become a problem for the elderly, leading to serious hematologic, neurologic, or gastrointestinal consequences. With age, the stomach secretes less of a protein necessary for the absorption of B_{12}. Research indicates that pectin and other soluble dietary fibers can interfere with absorption of vitamin B_{12} from foods, as well as with reuse of the vitamin made available from secretions into the intestine. Inadequate knowledge of the actions of such fibers in the digestive tract, along with dietary recommendations for increased fruit and fiber intake, indicates a need for additional research.

Folic acid (folate)

Studies implicating folic acid in birth defects from impaired development of the spinal column and brain suggest that the recommended dietary allowances need to be reexamined as more accurate data on folate bioavailability and utilization are obtained. This will be especially critical for pregnant women. The bioavailability of folate in a typical U.S. diet is about 50 percent. An examination of folate-depleted rats indicates that folate bioavailability varies from about 70 to 100 percent depending on the food source.

Vitamin B_6

Vitamin B_6 occurs in several forms in foods and is necessary for normal lipid and amino acid metabolism, red-blood-cell function, hormone production, and immune competence. The forms present in plant sources may include a complex with a glucose molecule, which appears to reduce the bioavailability of other forms of vitamin B_6 present in foods. The vitamin B_6 present in foods from animal sources exhibits very high availability—as much as 100 percent in tuna—while availability in foods from plant sources is low, 20 to 40 percent, due in part to the presence of the complex. Vegetarians are thus at particular risk for low vitamin B_6 intake. Vitamin B_6 status also appears to decline with age for reasons that may include reduced absorption. Research on the bioavailability of vitamin B_6 is emphasizing the effects of the glucose complex in foods.

Improving Our Food Choices

Knowledge of nutrient bioavailability is key to our understanding of the role of nutrients in maintaining human health. Improved knowledge of nutrient bioavailability can help in providing definitive, quantitative dietary guidance, and it can help us translate what we know into optimal and desirable eating patterns and food choices.

David S. Wilson
Assistant Professor,
Department of Nutrition,
University of Nevada, Reno,
and
Andrew J. Clifford
Professor,
Department of Nutrition,
University of California, Davis

Chapter 28

Energy Metabolism

What Is Energy Metabolism?

Energy can be defined as the capacity for doing work. Metabolism is the sum of processes by which the body handles a particular substance. When scientists study energy metabolism, therefore, they are studying the processes that handle energy in the body.

What Is a Calorie?

The energy value of foods or beverages is expressed in terms of the kilocalorie. If a food is burned and the heat produced is measured, the quantity of heat produced expressed in kilocalories represents the gross energy value of the food. The gross energy value of food does not represent the energy available to the body (fig. 1). No food is completely utilized, since some of the energy is excreted in urine and feces. When corrections are made to account for this loss of excreted energy, the corrected energy value of foods is designated "metabolizable" energy. Energy values listed in food tables represent metabolizable energy. Although it is common to call the energy value of food "calories," it is more accurate to use the term "kilocalories."

Excerpt from *Nutrition: Eating for Good Health*, U.S. Department of Agriculture, Agriculture Information Bulletin 685

Is a Calorie Really a Calorie?

The energy content of foods varies depending primarily on the amount of protein, fat, and carbohydrate contained in the specific food. The amounts of metabolizable energy in a gram of protein, fat, and carbohydrate are 4.0, 9.0, and 4.0 kilocalories, respectively. Although these nutrients are metabolized differently within the body, a kilocalorie from carbohydrate is the same as a kilocalorie from fat or protein.

What Is Energy Balance, or How Can I Maintain a Stable Body Weight?

Fig. 1 is a diagram detailing energy balance in humans. After adjusting energy intake (from food and beverages) for energy excreted in human wastes, one can determine the calories absorbed by the body—or metabolizable energy. In order for a person to maintain a stable body weight, metabolizable energy must be equally balanced with energy expenditure—that is, the calories expended to perform physical and metabolic work.

When metabolizable energy is greater than energy expenditure, the excess energy is stored in the body as protein, carbohydrate, or largely as fat. If energy expenditure is greater than metabolizable energy, then energy is mobilized from body energy stores. In fact, this storage and mobilization of energy is an ongoing cycle. During the day we store energy as either glycogen or fat; during sleep we mobilize energy to meet the metabolic work needs of the body. When a person is in energy balance, this daily rhythm is such that weight varies by only 2-3 pounds around a particular weight. However, when a person is in positive energy balance, then energy is being stored and weight increases. In order to lose weight, therefore, it is necessary to decrease energy intake below energy expenditure or to increase energy expenditure beyond energy intake.

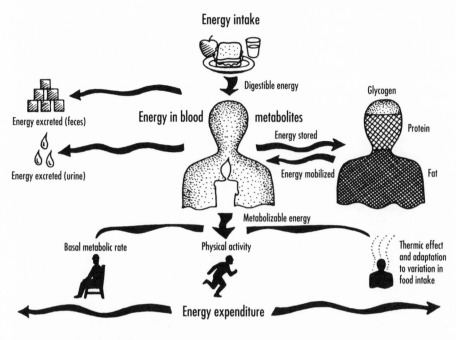

Figure 1: *Principles of energy expenditure*

What Is Basal Metabolic Rate?

The amount of energy expended by a fasting person completely at rest (but awake) prior to getting out of bed for the day is defined as basal metabolic rate or BMR. The relationship between BMR and total energy expenditure is depicted in fig. 2. For a sedentary person, BMR accounts for about 60-70 percent of daily energy expenditure; the remaining 30-40 percent is from physical activity and from body heat produced after a meal. Physical activity is responsible for as much as 50-60 percent of total energy expenditure in people who include frequent aerobic exercise into their lifestyle.

How Is Energy Expenditure Measured?

In the research or hospital setting, energy expenditure is determined by examining inhaled and exhaled air and measuring the person's oxygen consumption and carbon dioxide production. The ratio between oxygen consumption and carbon dioxide production is called the respiratory quotient or RQ. Daily energy expenditure in kilocalories is calculated from an equation that accounts for the number of units of oxygen and carbon dioxide exchanged by a person under specific conditions. This technique for measuring energy expenditure is called indirect calorimetry because it measures heat production (calories) indirectly from respiratory gas exchange.

In the United States, a number of laboratories have built room-sized indirect calorimeters. Volunteers stay in the room for a total of 24 hours. During this time they are served meals and snacks, and they have access to a TV, VCR, telephone, desk, chair, bed/couch, and toilet facilities. While this technique accurately determines energy expenditure, the physical activity of the volunteers is typically lower than their normal daily physical activity because they are confined to the room calorimeter.

Scientists have recently turned to a technique called doubly labeled water ($^2H_2^{18}O$) to estimate the energy expenditure of free-living human volunteers. This technique requires volunteers to consume small amounts of water that contain the nonradioactive isotopes of hydrogen and oxygen—deuterium (2H) and oxygen-18. Each volunteer's rate of excretion of deuterium and oxygen-18 is measured in daily spot urine samples for 14 days to estimate carbon dioxide production and oxygen consumption. From these two determinations, energy expenditure can be determined in individuals who have been free to go about their daily activity. This technique has successfully estimated individual energy expenditure and is currently being used in many laboratories around the country.

How Is Energy Stored in the Body?

Like a combustion engine, the body utilizes fuel (food and drink) for energy and combusts the fuel to give energy, water, and carbon dioxide. In a car excess fuel (gasoline) is stored in the gasoline tank; in humans, excess fuel is stored in the body. When energy intake exceeds energy requirements, the energy is stored within the body as glycogen and fat.

Glycogen is the storage form of carbohydrate in the body. Both liver and muscle are capable of synthesizing glycogen and breaking it down when energy is needed for muscle and liver function or other purposes. Since glycogen is a large molecule, it cannot be stored within the muscle or liver in great quantities. Energy is stored in the body primarily as fat.

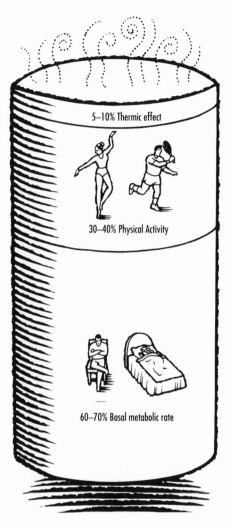

Figure 2: *Components of energy expenditure for a sedentary person*

5–10% Thermic effect

30–40% Physical Activity

60–70% Basal metabolic rate

When fat is stored, it is stored in adipose tissue by two processes: hypertrophy and hyperplasia. The primary form of storage during early childhood is hyperplasia, an increase in the number of adipose tissue cells. During puberty and adulthood, adipose tissue cells change in size with weight loss or weight gain. If weight is gained, they increase in size by hypertrophy, the process of enlarging adipose cells to accommodate additional fat. If weight is lost, then the fat is mobilized from the adipose tissue cells and the cells decrease in size.

In early childhood, energy is stored and mobilized to facilitate growth and development. Therefore it is important that the overall energy balance be positive. That is, more energy must be taken in than expended in the child's daily activity to provide energy for growth. Children increase in weight until the end of adolescence, when they reach their adult weight.

The goal for adults is to maintain this healthy adult weight and not increase it. In order to maintain weight, adults must be in energy balance; that is, their energy intake must be closely matched with energy expenditure. When energy intake exceeds energy expenditure, a person is said to be in positive energy balance and gains weight.

Within the scientific community there is currently much discussion as to the exact definition of the term "ideal body weight." The USDA-Health and Human Services 1990 Dietary Guidelines are one of many sources that suggest healthy body weights. (See Part I, Chapter 1.)

393

Am I an "Apple" or a "Pear"?

During the last 10 years, researchers in Europe and America have gathered data in large populations of men and women to demonstrate the importance of the location of fat on a person's body. They found that the risk for disease (cardiovascular disease, hypertension, and diabetes) and premature death increases in obese populations that have greater deposits of fat around their abdomen (or waist) than around their hips. This distribution of fat is typical of obese males and is named "android" or "apple." Women typically have more fat deposited around the hips and buttocks than around the abdomen. This distribution pattern is named "gynoid" or "pear."

To determine whether you are an "apple" or a "pear," you must first know your waist-to hip ratio (WHR). This ratio is determined by dividing the waist circumference measurement by the hip circumference measurement. Men having a WHR greater than 1.0 and women having a WHR greater than 0.85 are consider "apples." Conversely, men having a WHR less than 1.0 and women having a WHR less than 0.85 are consider "pears." In people who are significantly overweight or

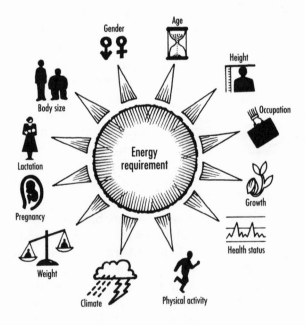

Figure 3: Factors affecting energy requirements

obese, fat distribution has great significance. "Apples" have increased risk for cardiovascular disease, hypertension, and diabetes.

Most of this research has been conducted in Europeans or in Americans of European descent, and it is not certain at this time if these generalizations hold true for African-Americans, Hispanic-Americans, Asian-Americans, or Native Americans. One ARS study found that African-American women have greater amounts of fat on their upper bodies than European-American women. Further research is being conducted in ARS and other laboratories to see if these generalizations concerning disease risk are applicable to the whole American population.

Recent research studies have found that within the abdominal region, location of fat can be predictive of disease and premature death. Fat located just below the skin is called subcutaneous fat, while fat surrounding vital organs is called visceral fat. While most people with a high WHR have larger deposits of visceral fat than those with a low WHR, some people with high WHR have their fat located more subcutaneously. In epidemiological studies, large deposits of visceral fat in the abdominal region (near the waist) have been associated with greater risk for disease and premature death.

Can I Change My WHR or Fat Deposit Pattern?

In ARS and other research studies, magnetic resonance imaging (MRI) has been used to determine the location of fat within the abdominal region and also to monitor fat loss during a weight-reducing regimen. When a person loses weight, fat is lost from all over the body. However, the largest amount of adipose tissue will be lost from the regions of the body having the largest adipose tissue deposits at the beginning. This means that if one has large fat deposits on the buttocks and hips, these regions will lose the most fat. At the end of a weight-losing regimen, these regions of fat may still be large, but the amount of fat will be reduced. While it may be difficult to change the body's fat patterning or WHR with weight loss, some studies report small changes. The benefit of weight loss for the person with large amounts of visceral fat is the decrease in visceral fat and therefore a presumed decrease in risk for disease and premature death.

How Can I Assess My Body Composition?

While there are many sophisticated methods of determining one's body composition in the laboratory, the familiar "pinch-an-inch" test (pinching fat tissue between the thumb and forefinger) is probably the easiest way to determine the presence of fat deposits on one's body. While it may seem imprecise, it has some merit.

Is It True That the More Weight One Loses, the Harder It Is To Continue Losing Weight?

Research studies at ARS have not supported the common belief that it becomes harder to lose weight the longer one diets. In fact the decrease in energy expenditure or metabolic rate seen in dieting individuals can be explained by the decrease in energy intake and the decrease in lean tissue that is obligatory with weight loss. Perhaps the single most important predictor of one's energy requirement is physical activity, such as walking, running, swimming, cycling. Frequently this type of physical activity decreases during a weight-loss regimen.

What Determines a Person's Energy Requirement?

The amount of energy a person requires to maintain energy balance is called the energy requirement. As shown in fig. 3, many factors influence one's energy requirement. Energy metabolism can be affected by any or all of these factors, making the study of energy requirements very complex.

Joan M. Conway
Research Chemist,
Energy and Protein Nutrition Laboratory,
Beltsville Human Nutrition Research Center,
Agricultural Research Service, USDA,
Beltsville, MD

Chapter 29

Nutrition, Brain Function, and Behavior

It is widely accepted that a well-balanced diet and good nutrition are necessary to ensure normal growth, prevent disease, and maintain physical performance. Despite much speculation and some important early findings about general malnutrition, relatively little is known about how specific nutrients affect the brain and other organ systems in relation to mental activities, emotional states, and behavior in healthy individuals. With few exceptions (for example, vitamin B_{12} and iron), the behavioral consequences of deficiency are not presently considered as criteria when establishing recommended dietary allowances. However, the involvement of a broader range of disciplines and recent methodological advances have led to the reemergence of studies on brain function and behavior in relation to nutrition. This area of research represents a unique approach to assessing the functional consequences of altered nutrition.

This chapter focuses on this nutrition research; describes current methods of assessing nutrition, brain function, and behavior; highlights several interesting findings; and discusses future challenges.

Why Study Brain Function and Behavior?

Among the public, there is a strong and persistent belief that what we eat affects our mental and emotional states and, in general, our ability to perform day-to-day activities and to meet life's demands. It

Excerpt from *Nutrition: Eating for Good Health*, U.S. Department of Agriculture, Agriculture Information Bulletin 685

seems we all have theories, or at least suspicions, about the functional importance of this or that food or specific nutrient. In fact, some of us alter our diets and take supplements and freely advise others to do likewise, with the firm belief that such changes will improve the way we feel and our ability to perform.

This belief often creates a psychological environment amenable to food faddism and uncritical acceptance of claims made by self-styled "nutritionists." Today's "smart" foods, promoted as a way to increase "brain power" and enhance memory, are a recent example. Scientific evidence to support most of these claims of the beneficial effects of specific nutrients or diets is at best conflicting and, more typically, simply lacking. The study of nutrition, brain function, and behavior responds to public interest and will, with time, produce the experimental data needed to assess the legitimacy of health claims and provide reliable criteria useful for evaluating nutritional status and making recommendations for dietary intakes.

The consumption of nutrients (biologically active chemicals), in the form of foods or supplements, affects body chemistry which, in turn, affects brain chemistry and function. Neural impulses are largely the result of sodium and potassium exchange, but numerous other minerals, carbohydrates, amino acids, proteins, and vitamins affect cell membrane permeability, neurotransmitter metabolism, and the glial cells that provide structural and nutritional support to neurons.

The delicate chemical balance of the brain is somewhat protected by the blood-brain barrier, which restricts entry of certain chemicals to the brain via the blood. Nevertheless, the brain is highly susceptible to changes in body chemistry resulting from nutrient intake and deficiency.

The brain receives, stores, and integrates sensory information and initiates and controls motor responses. These functions correspond to mental activities and form the basis for behavior. Thus, theoretically, there is a direct connection between nutrition, brain function, and behavior. Furthermore, behavior may be unique as a criterion for establishing nutritional adequacy, in that it represents the functional integration of all biological systems, including homeostatic and other compensatory mechanisms that determine the practical importance of a nutritional deficit or excess.

Who Studies Brain Function and Behavior?

In the United States, studies on nutrition and brain function are conducted at private laboratories and hospitals, academic institutions, and government research laboratories. Government-supported research in this area is concentrated in the Department of Defense (DOD), USDA, and the National Institutes of Health (NIH). DOD nutrition programs focus on enhancing performance during combat and in other stressful environments, while NIH nutrition programs focus on the brain and behavior related to disease states and drugs used in treating disease. Only USDA addresses the relationships among nutrition, brain function, and behavior in the population as a whole.

One of the six principal objectives stated in USDA's 1992-98 Agricultural Research Service (ARS) Program Plan is to "develop the means for promoting optimal human health and well-being through improved nutrition" and to "define adequate and safe ranges of intake for nutrients." To meet this objective, the plan explicitly recognizes the need to acquire "information about the effects of foods and nutritional adequacy on behavior and performance."

Within ARS, the Grand Forks Human Nutrition Research Center, in North Dakota, has been a leader in studying the effects of nutrition on brain function and behavior in both humans and animals for more than a decade. The human nutrition research centers located in San Francisco, CA, Boston, MA, Beltsville, MD, and Houston, TX, have also conducted studies in this area.

The need for broad institutional support is clear because this research is truly multidisciplinary, drawing heavily from the fields of biochemistry, physiology, neuroscience, psychology, and medicine, and, less frequently, from epidemiology, sociology, and anthropology. Technological and analytical advances have further involved the fields of biotechnology, computer science, and multivariate statistics. Coordinating and integrating the activities of scientists from these diverse fields is a significant challenge and key to successful research on nutrition, brain function, and behavior.

Important Issues To Consider

Several considerations are common to most studies of nutrition, including those on brain function and behavior. Inadequate dietary intakes result in deficiency states that occur by degree, ranging from suboptimal to marginal to severe. By definition, a severe clinical deficiency in any essential nutrient is going to have profound effects, particularly during periods of early development. However, cases of marginal or subclinical deficiencies are far more common (at least in the United States) and thus probably merit greater attention by researchers and a larger share of experimental resources.

Optimal intakes for all nutrients are difficult to determine and have not yet been established. This issue of optimal intakes is particularly important to the study of brain function and behavior, and interest arises in part from the increasing emphasis of medical and allied professionals on promoting health rather than treating illness and in part from the belief that brain function and behavior within the normal range can and should be improved.

The choice of an animal or human model is important. Animal studies permit greater control over genetic and environmental variation, assessment of effects over an entire life span and even across generations, and extensive analysis of brain chemistry and anatomy. They can also be useful in assessing brain physiology, mental processes, and some emotional responses, such as anxiety. However, there are often significant differences between humans and animals in nutrient metabolism; human brain function and cognition are considerably more complex, and the behavioral repertoire of humans, including speech, greatly exceeds that found in animals. Thus, the ability to generalize findings from animal studies to humans is limited and many aspects of function simply cannot be studied in animals.

Even within a healthy population, nutritional effects on brain function and behavior must be studied separately in numerous distinct groups. These groups may be defined by characteristics such as age, sex, body composition, exercise, stress, and dietary choices including consumption of vegetarian and other restricted diets, caffeine, and alcohol. The overwhelming majority of existing studies on nutrition, brain function, and behavior were conducted on children.

The diet contains both nutrients and non-nutrients. Examples of the latter are preservatives, artificial sweeteners, and substances like caffeine and alcohol. Studies that assess the effects of excessive amounts of either nutrients or non-nutrients may be considered toxicological rather than nutritional in nature. When nutrient intakes are manipulated by supplementation, amounts can be at either physiologic (appropriate to the body's normal functioning) or pharmacologic amounts. Although pharmacologic or therapeutic amounts may be required for a brief period to remedy a severe deficiency, they are in excess of amounts that can be reasonably acquired from the typical diet.

Highlights From Human Studies

Studies of severe protein-calorie malnutrition in children have a long history and are by far the most common of any nutritional studies. They have reliably found that malnourished children have abnormal EEG's, reduced activity levels, and impaired attention. A variety of other behavioral consequences have been frequently, but not consistently, reported, including impaired or delayed mental (particularly verbal) and motor development, impaired intersensory integration, reduced academic performance, increased crying in infancy, hyperactivity, apathy, withdrawal, and impaired social skills. With rare exceptions, however, these studies were correlational in design such that brain and behavioral effects were confounded by an impaired interaction of the child with his or her social and physical environment.

An ongoing series of experimental studies has repeatedly shown that eating a high-carbohydrate, low-protein meal on an empty stomach increases the relative availability of the amino acid tryptophan, and promotes synthesis of the neurotransmitter serotonin. Under these conditions, several behavioral effects have been consistently observed: impaired attention and slowed reaction times, increased fatigue and sleepiness, and reduced pain sensitivity.

Severe deficiencies in several B vitamins have profound effects for brain function and behavior, including abnormal EEG's, impaired memory, anxiety, confusion, irritability, and depression. Subclinical deficiencies in thiamin (B1), riboflavin (B2), niacin (B3), pyridoxine (B6), cobalamin (B12), and folic acid are also commonly found in elderly and psychiatric populations. However, experimental studies have not been done to determine the involvement of individual vitamins in memory processes or in thought and affective (emotional) disorders. Experimental pyridoxine and vitamin E deficiencies produce abnormal brain electrical activity in humans and animals, and vitamin C supplementation in rather large doses (1-2 grams per day) seems to influence brain activity, although in varying ways.

The relationship of iron to brain function and behavior has received considerable attention, particularly in children. Iron deficiency reliably results in impaired attention and learning, hyperactivity, and apathy, which are consistent with findings of reduced dopamine (a brain neurotransmitter) in iron-deficient animals. In several studies with young adults, iron intake and status were related to EEG and EP responses and to performance on tasks assessing short-term memory; the findings indicate that low levels of iron result in reduced alertness and impaired memory.

401

Supplementation and correlational studies have found increased brain and behavioral excitability with low zinc intakes and status. Subclinical experimental magnesium depletion was also found to increase brain electrical activity. Nutritional copper deficiency reduces brain excitability, consistent with reported reductions in several neurotransmitters in copper-deficient animals. Behaviorally, calcium supplementation has been related to relief of pain during menstruation.

Boron, a mineral not yet recognized as essential for humans, has shown effects on brain electrical activity and cognitive performance in several studies with older adults. When compared with higher boron intakes, EEG changes noted with low boron intake were in the direction of those found with other forms of malnutrition. Low boron intake also increased reaction times on attention, perception, memory, and motor tasks.

Future Research

The complexity of research on nutrition, brain function, and behavior is evident, but so too is its potential to generate knowledge that has broad practical application and benefits. Future studies will no doubt identify new relationships and better characterize existing ones, while attempting to discover underlying mechanisms. Although the focus of early studies was on the effects of general malnutrition in children, future studies will more likely focus on specific nutrients and their effects on brain function and behavior in adults. Experimental (in contrast with correlational) studies offer the best hope of distinguishing nutritional from nonnutritional effects on these critical aspects of function.

It is also highly probable that future research will attempt to identify nutrient intakes that will result in optimal performance (psychonutrition). To be sure, one challenge for researchers in this area will be to present findings in a manner that tempers the public's tendency to uncritically embrace new findings before they are replicated and refined and to overgeneralize highly specific findings obtained under the controlled conditions of the laboratory.

James G. Penland
Research Psychologist,
Grand Forks Human Nutrition Research Center,
Agricultural Research Service, USDA,
Grand Forks, ND

Chapter 30

Nutrition and a Robust Immune System

Introduction

Nature has provided scientists with early opportunities to learn about the effect of nutrition on the immune system. Low-nutrient soils have caused mineral deficiencies in some populations of livestock and humans. By studying these populations, scientists discovered the importance of selenium to the immune system. Famines, natural disasters, severe poverty, and wartime have likewise provided us with many of our early learning opportunities about the relationships among nutrition, immune functions, and health. Many essential micronutrients (vitamins and minerals), such as copper and zinc, were once believed to be unessential to the human diet but are now known to be important for normal immune function.

Thorough examination of the effects of nutrient deficiencies, combined with clinical observations and detailed investigations, is helping us understand the relationship between nutrition and immune function. This chapter briefly highlights the effects of nutrient deficiencies and overnutrition on a competent immune system and mentions some current research.

Excerpt from *Nutrition: Eating for Good Health*, U.S. Department of Agriculture, Agricultural Information Bulletin 685

Nutrient Deficiencies

Generalized malnutrition, historically referred to as protein-energy malnutrition (PEM), often coexists with deficiencies of one or more micronutrients. PEM is one of the earliest forms of malnutrition to have attracted the interest of the medical community. The association between severe PEM and atrophy of the thymus gland (primary lymphoid tissue) was described nearly 150 years ago, even before it was realized that the thymus is a principal body organ of the immune system. Beginning as early as 1911, several investigators documented that thymus atrophy results from malnutrition due to food scarcity or from illness associated with cachexia (severe weight loss due to diseases such as cancer). Malnutrition also commonly causes atrophy of the tonsils (secondary lymphoid tissue).

During the first half of this century, an association between severe PEM and increased infections was described. But it was not until the 1960's, when the important role of the thymus as a primary source of cells (T-lymphocytes) of the immune system became known, that the relationships among nutrition, immunity, and health were established. During the past 20 years, it has become clear that PEM in children and adults reduces the number and function of T-helper immune lymphocytes, which promote an active immune-protective response against infectious and other diseases, such as cancer.

Healthy subjects who are fed balanced meals, but in restricted amounts, show suppressed immunity similar to that of children and hospital patients with PEM. ARS and U.S. Army researchers have found that young, healthy men consuming less energy in the form of food and drink than is required during heavy work and exercise show decreased immune function. In contrast to unhealthy subjects, such individuals show rapid correction of their immune functions when they receive enough calories to balance their energy demands.

The role of micronutrients in the immune system has been studied in individuals suffering from micronutrient deficiencies, such as hospitalized patients receiving liquid diets that lacked an unknown essential micronutrient, children living in regions deficient in select micronutrients, livestock grazing on mineral-deficient grassland, and research animals. Through such studies, the essential role of several minerals (iron, zinc, copper, magnesium, and selenium) and several vitamins (vitamin A, vitamin C, B-group vitamins, and vitamin E) has been demonstrated for normal immune functions. The mechanisms of their functions on the immune system and the safe range of intake are not fully understood. As with many nutrients, micronutrients interact with each other in maximizing their role in immune function.

High-Fat Diets

Consuming too much fat can have a suppressive effect on the immune system. The lifestyle of many people of the industrialized world leads to diets that are high in fat.

From animal and human studies, it is known that both the concentration and type of dietary fats play a crucial role in the function of the immune system. Diets high in fat cause reduced resistance to infectious diseases in animals and suppressed cellular immune function in both animals and humans. At high concentration, polyunsaturated fats that are low in vitamin E appear to be more immunosuppressive than saturated fats.

The immunosuppressive effects of high-fat diets can be lessened by eating foods containing antioxidants (certain vitamins and minerals) that neutralize these effects. Foods that have a stabilizing effect on the immune system include those containing vitamin E (oils, shortening, margarine, fruits, and green leafy vegetables), vitamin C (fruits and vegetables), beta-carotene (brightly colored fruits and vegetables), selenium (meats, cereals, dairy products, fruits, and vegetables), copper (liver, nuts, and whole-grain cereals) and manganese (nuts, whole-grain cereals, dried legumes, and tea).

Current and Needed Work

Early studies on nutrition and the immune system involved severe nutritional deficiencies. Since more sophisticated laboratory techniques are now available, ARS researchers are now able to compile information to establish the effects of moderate nutritional alteration on the immune system. Although our understanding of the role of nutrition in the immune system is increasing, considerably more work is needed before we can use the information to improve health.

Work describing maturation of the immune system in breast-fed and bottle-fed infants is needed. Most milk formulas for infants in the Western World are now considered to meet the conventional nutritional requirements of newborn infants. Despite this, investigation of the effects of breast- and bottle-feeding on select immune functions has shown that breast-feeding has contrasting effects on the development of immunity. In the early neonatal period, up to 6 weeks of age, there are enhanced immune responses in the breast-fed infants. But by 3 months of age, many of the immune responses are higher in formula-fed infants. These results suggest that, during the first 6 weeks, breast-fed infants are receiving enhanced immune protection from breast milk, while formula-fed infants must produce this immunity themselves. Developing immunity is not usually a problem for formula-fed infants in societies where the public health standards are high.

Many studies have documented the frequent occurrence of nutritional deficiencies in the elderly. Observations show that these deficiencies are associated with undernutrition due to reduced calorie intake; overall reduced intake; and lower blood levels of iron, zinc, vitamin C, B vitamins, and vitamin E. Socioeconomic deprivation, physical disability, isolation, dental problems, and increased nutrient needs due to underlying disease are common causes of nutritional problems in the elderly. Although it is logical to try to correct nutritional deficiencies in the elderly in order to improve their immune responses and reduce the risk of infectious disease and other age-related disorders, the desirability of taking megadose supplements of vitamins and minerals is questionable.

During the 150 years since a relationship between severe undernutrition and atrophy of the thymus gland was first described, our understanding of the role of nutrients on the immune system has increased tremendously. ARS researchers are now reaching the point where more can be learned about the effects of marginal changes in nutrition on immune protection against diseases. During this time, it is comforting to know that the body has tremendous capabilities for efficiently using nutrients, even in unbalanced amounts, and maximizing responsiveness of the immune system.

Tim R. Kramer
Research Biologist,
Beltsville Human Nutrition Research Center, ARS, USDA
Beltsville, MD

Chapter 31

Recent Advances in Maternal and Infant Nutrition

Milk fat provides infants with the essential fatty acids important for the growth of their neurological tissue and cell membranes. It also provides about 50 percent of their energy needs. Scientists need to understand how dietary fat is used to produce human milk, so food recommendations can be formulated for breastfeeding mothers.

Maternal Nutrition and Lactation

Most of the dietary fatty acids consumed by lactating women are (1) converted to energy through oxidation, (2) secreted into milk, or (3) stored in maternal adipose tissues. The Children's Nutrition Research Center has studied what happens to dietary fats in lactating, well-nourished women who consume either a low-fat diet or a high-fat diet. The diets were randomly assigned to 16 women who were nursing their infants. Figure 1 shows how dietary fat was used for energy, secreted into milk, or stored as fat.

The results of the study indicate that women on the low-fat diet had a lower concentration of fat in their milk but produced greater amounts of milk. Thus, their daily secretion of milk fat did not change, but their total carbohydrate production increased. The study also indicates that women with more body fat are better able to store dietary lipids and consequently may have difficulty losing weight.

Excerpt from *Nutrition: Eating for Good Health*, U.S. Department of Agriculture, Agriculture Information Bulletin 685

In contrast, Otomi Indian women living in rural Mexico who consume a low-fat diet and have low body fat may produce milk that has a low fat content. Lactation was studied in these women because their infants were growing poorly. The Otomi women consume a low-fat, corn-predominant diet. Although their milk production rates were actually 15-20 percent higher than rates reported for well-nourished women, the concentrations of fat and energy in their milk were lower and may have contributed to the poor growth of their infants.

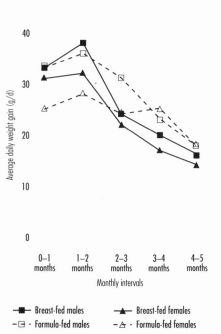

Infant Nutrition

Composition of weight gain in breast-fed and formula-fed infants

Growth standards for infants from the National Center for Health Statistics (NCHS), Washington, DC, were derived primarily from formula-fed infants studied 20-50 years ago (fig. 2). Efforts are now under way to revise growth standards for infants. In a study at the Children's Nutrition Research Center, the growth of breast-fed and formula-fed infants was monitored for 9 months. Investigators found that formula-fed infants gained more weight after 3 months than breast-fed infants of the same age.

Until recently, most nutrition studies in infants relied on measurements of weight and length to estimate growth and body composition. Today, however, scientists have new techniques, such as total body electrical conductivity, to measure lean and fat body mass. Surprisingly, initial studies suggest that breastfed infants may have more body fat than formula-fed infants. Other methods make it possible to measure how infants use the nutrients in the food they eat. Using indirect calorimetry and the doubly labeled water ($^{2}H_{2}^{18}O$) method, investigators have shown that breast-fed infants not only consume fewer calories than formula-fed babies but also expend fewer calories.

Besides differences in how breast-fed and formula-fed infants use calories, there are important differences in their biochemical makeup.

408

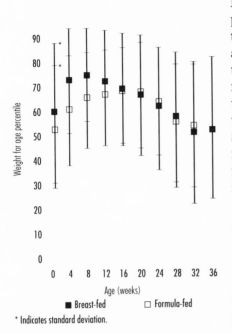

* Indicates standard deviation.

Growth of breast-fed and formula fed infants measured by growth standards of the National Center for Health Statistics (Courtesy of J.E. Stuff)

Breast-fed infants have higher plasma cholesterol concentrations than formula-fed infants, presumably because of the higher cholesterol content of human milk than formula. The synthesis of cholesterol in breastfed infants is one-third that of formula-fed infants. Scientists are now trying to determine how cholesterol intake in infancy affects cholesterol levels in adulthood.

Nutrition of the Preterm Infant

The survival rate of preterm infants has increased dramatically in the last several years; at least 90 percent of infants born prematurely survive. Scientists are studying differences in the composition of human and cow's milk to determine the levels of nutrients most suitable for preterm infants. Feeding human milk to preterm infants appears to be advantageous, because (1) the fat content of human milk is more appropriate than that of cow's milk for infant brain development, and (2) the levels of immunoglobulins in human milk may increase an infant's ability to defend against infection. Human milk, however, is "designed" by nature for full-term infants, whose bones are more fully developed, so investigators at the Children's Nutrition Research Center are studying how much additional calcium and phosphorus must be added to human milk to ensure healthy bone growth in preterm infants.

Studying Postnatal Growth and Development

Some infant nutrition questions must be studied in animals, such as the infant pig, to avoid the possibility of harming human subjects.

Scientists at the Children's Nutrition Research Center are studying genetically lean and obese piglets to learn how fat and cholesterol are used in early life. They have found that cholesterol levels in genetically obese piglets continue to rise when their diets contain cholesterol, suggesting that these piglets may not be able to shut down cholesterol synthesis when cholesterol is provided in the diet. Studies have also shown that piglets with low levels of plasma cholesterol grow more slowly than piglets with higher levels. Because infant formula has very little cholesterol compared with human milk, both findings are important in designing human infant formulas, whether for full-term or preterm infants.

Rats are also studied to learn more about human infants. Because they are particularly immature at birth, rats are relevant to studies of preterm infants. Investigators have found that before 10 days of age, the weight gain of rat pups consists almost entirely of protein, with very little increase in body fat. This phenomenon can also be seen in preterm infants. From the studies in rats, scientists have learned that adequate nutrition immediately after birth is very important to ensure normal maturation.

Continuing Research

Nutrient utilization in lactating females and their offspring is being investigated through noninvasive techniques and animal models. We have yet to fully understand how maternal diet and nutritional status affect milk composition and how dietary manipulation of infant weight gain, body composition, and serum cholesterol affects health later in life. Studies to ensure that preterm infants get adequate nutrition will enable normal growth and development and promote optimal cognitive and immune functions. Both short- and long-term effects of infant nutrition on the developing organism are important in defining the nutritional requirements of infants.

Nancy F. Butte
Associate Professor,
USDA-ARS Children's Nutrition Research Center,
Department of Pediatrics,
Baylor College of Medicine,
Houston, TX

Chapter 32

Recent Advances in Nutrition: From Adolescence to Adulthood

Diet recommendations for adolescents cannot be improved until scientists have more information about nutrient intakes, body compositions, and energy expenditures for adolescents.

Basic Nutritional Requirements of Adolescents

Most recommendations have relied on body measurements to index growth. To date, nutrient requirements for growth during adolescence have been estimated from studies of fetuses or adults. Because tissue composition during growth differs among different age groups, it is not appropriate to measure growth in teenagers using techniques that were developed to measure growth in adults and fetuses. In addition, most studies have been done on Caucasians; very few have been conducted on individuals of other ethnic groups. Data in the literature suggest that there are differences among ethnic groups in growth rate, metabolic rate, body composition, and onset of fertility.

To assess the nutritional needs of teenagers (including obese or pregnant teens), scientists must collect data on nutrient intakes, body composition, and energy expenditure from healthy adolescents who represent different ethnic groups.

Adolescence is the transition period between childhood and adulthood. The growth spurt that occurs during adolescence includes rapid bone growth, increased muscle mass, and increased body fat. The

Excerpt from *Nutrition: Eating for Good Health*, U.S. Department of Agriculture, Agriculture Information Bulletin 685

411

growth and development of adolescents reflect their genetic background and their dietary history during infancy and childhood. The food choices made by adolescents affect not only their growth and development during puberty but also their reproductive capacity and susceptibility to degenerative diseases when they become adults.

Nutritional Problems of Adolescents

Obesity

Because of the high fat content of the American diet, obesity affects 10 to 35 percent of adolescents. Researchers have shown that infant weight correlates strongly with adult weight and that children who are overweight before puberty have a 75 percent chance of becoming obese adults. It has also been shown that those who are overweight after puberty have a 95 percent chance of becoming obese adults. It is not surprising, therefore, that data from the Second National Health and Nutrition Examination Survey (1976-80) indicated that approximately 34 million American adults (25.7 percent) are overweight.

Although fat deposition during puberty is essential for teenage girls in preparation for reproduction and lactation, the incidence of obesity in the United States is unfortunately high, especially in adult women. Obesity is associated with increased risk of diabetes, high blood pressure, heart disease, gallbladder disease, colon cancer, postmenopausal breast cancer, and menstrual irregularities. Unless obese women eat a prudent diet during pregnancy, they have a great risk of complications.

Pregnangy and Osteoporosis

The National Center for Health Statistics recently documented the sharpest rise in teenage pregnancies in 15 years; the annual incidence in the United States is now 1 in 10. The effects of pregnancy during adolescence on long-term health status are not completely understood. A female adolescent generally attains 99 percent of her mother's bone size and 80 to 95 percent of her mother's bone mass and bone density by 14 years of age. The growth spurt and onset of fertility that occur during puberty impose substantial nutrient demands on female adolescents.

The consequences of these changes during puberty depend on individual nutritional status, level of sexual maturity, and genetic background. An increasing health problem in the United States is posed by pregnant and lactating teenaged girls, who must accommodate the additional nutrient demands of reproduction. These girls are at high risk of nutrient deficiencies, such as calcium deficiency, and thus have a higher risk of developing osteoporosis later in life. There are many nutrition questions to be answered about pregnancy during adolescence

Cholesterol and Atherosclerosis

Cholesterol is an essential component of cell membranes and is required for cell growth, replication, and maintenance. Plasma cholesterol concentrations are known to be higher in breast-fed infants than in formula-fed infants, perhaps because human milk has a higher cholesterol content than formula. Although cholesterol causes atherosclerosis in humans, animal studies have shown that a diet high in cholesterol early in life may protect against diets high in cholesterol later in life. The protective mechanism, however, has not been documented in humans.

Nutrition Research at the Children's Nutrition Research Center

The Children's Nutrition Research Center (CNRC) has developed numerous noninvasive techniques to measure lean body mass, fat mass, bone mineral content and density, basal metabolic rate, and total energy expenditure. Several studies are in progress at the CNRC to assess the nutrient requirements of adolescents.

In one cross-sectional study, nutrient intakes, cardiorespiratory fitness, body composition, energy expenditure, plasma lipid profile, and plasma iron status are being measured in 200 healthy female adolescents between 10 and 16 years of age. Equal numbers of adolescents representing four ethnic groups (white, black, Hispanic, and Asian) are being studied. Nutrient intakes for a 3-day period are being analyzed from food records. Cardiorespiratory fitness is being evaluated by determining the maximal heart rate and maximum oxygen utilization while the subject is walking and running on a motorized treadmill. Body density is being measured by weighing the subject in and out of the water. Because fat is less dense than water, lower body density reflects higher body fat. Lean body mass is being estimated in a total body electrical conductivity (TOBEC) machine. The TOBEC machine has been approved for use on infants, children, and adults by the Food and Drug Administration. Total body bone mineral content and density are being measured by a technique called dual-energy x-ray absorptiometry. The subject lies in a supine position during the whole-body scan, which takes approximately 15 minutes.

The energy required for daily activities, including sleep, is being measured while the subject is inside a whole-body indirect calorimeter for 24 hours. The whole-body calorimeter is similar in size to a small bedroom and has a bed, table, chair, television, VCR, stereo system, exercise bicycle, telephone, and toilet facilities. The subject also eats breakfast, lunch, and dinner in the calorimeter. The 24-hour energy expenditure measured reflects the caloric needs of the subject while being confined in the chamber. Activities inside the calorimeter, however, are limited. Because the subject is being monitored constantly inside the chamber, behavior and activity patterns are not typical. The whole-body calorimeter provides important information on basic energy needs but does not provide an accurate estimate of the caloric needs of the subject in a free-living environment.

The energy needs of free-living subjects are being estimated using the doubly labeled water method. After a baseline saliva sample is collected, each subject drinks a known amount of water containing the stable isotopes deuterium and oxygen-18. The energy expenditures of the free-living subjects are calculated from the rates of disappearance of these isotopes in subsequent saliva samples. A blood sample is collected from each subject after the subjects have fasted overnight. Each sample is tested for plasma total cholesterol, triglyceride, high-density and low-density lipoprotein cholesterol, apolipoproteins A-1 and B, total iron, and ferritin. The relationships of nutrient intake, body composition, caloric needs, cardiorespiratory fitness, plasma lipid profile, and iron status to each other and to sexual maturity and race are being evaluated.

Another study underway at the CNRC will establish a body composition database for both men and women. Results from this study will define the relationships between nutrient intake and body composition of healthy children from infancy through adolescence for different ethnic groups. The data will also establish acceptable upper and lower limits within which to evaluate children who are ill. Approximately 1,000 healthy children under 18 years of age from 3 ethnic groups (white, black, and Hispanic) are being studied in the Metabolic Research Unit and Body Composition Laboratory at the CNRC.

Two studies at CNRC are designed to define the nutrient needs of pregnant and lactating teenagers. One longitudinal study will estimate the nutrient intakes, changes in body composition, and changes in energy expenditure of 20 healthy pregnant teenagers under 17 years of age. These teenagers are being studied four times between 8 and 40 weeks of gestation and immediately after delivery. The other study will measure the dietary intakes, milk production, and changes in body composition and growth in lactating adolescents. Preliminary results indicate that body weight, lean body mass, and body fat in lactating adolescents are maintained during the first 3 months after giving birth. This conservation of body mass may occur at the expense of milk production in the adolescent mother.

To test the hypothesis that early neonatal ingestion of large quantities of cholesterol protects the infant from high-cholesterol diets later in life, the CNRC is planning to study the effects of dietary cholesterol on in vivo cholesterol synthesis. The studies will be conducted in 4-month-old infants: 12 exclusively breastfed, 12 formula-fed, and 12 formula-fed with added cholesterol. Later, all infants will be fed a formula with low cholesterol levels. The same procedure will be repeated at 11 months of age. The infants will then be fed a diet high in cholesterol, and the effects of the diet on the cholesterol levels in the infants will be evaluated.

The United States is confronted with phenomenal economic costs from obesity, adolescent pregnancy, poor birth outcomes, and cardiovascular heart diseases related to atherosclerosis. The data collected in the CNRC studies will provide important information for the formulation of food recommendations for healthy teenagers as well as obese and pregnant teenagers. We hope these recommendations, besides helping to provide adequate education, will also help reduce nutrition-related health costs in our society.

William W. Wong
Associate Professor,
USDA-ARS Children's Nutrition Research Center,
Department of Pediatrics,
Baylor College of Medicine,
Houston, TX

Part Six

Nutrition in Public Health

Chapter 33

Feeding America's Future: USDA's Child Nutrition Programs

Only children who eat well can learn well. And only children who learn well can build the future.

USDA's food assistance programs recognize the inseparable links among health, nutrition, and educational success; therefore, a number of programs are specifically for children. The continuum of care begins with the Special Supplemental Food Program for Women, Infants, and Children (WIC), which serves the Nation's youngest children who are at nutritional risk. Other child nutrition programs pick up from there.

The Child Nutrition Programs administered by USDA's Food and Nutrition Service (FNS) are designed to give children access to a more nutritious diet, to improve their eating habits through nutrition education, and to encourage the consumption of foods produced by American farmers. Many of these programs benefit the Nation's most needy children.

Long-Term Commitment

As early as 1853, the need for child feeding programs was recognized in the United States. Initial efforts to provide school food services were sporadic yet persistent, and they culminated in the establishment of the National School Lunch Program in 1946.

Excerpt from *Nutrition: Eating and Good Health*, U.S. Department of Agriculture, Agriculture Information Bulletin 685

Over the years, as the National School Lunch Program grew in public and nonprofit private schools and institutions, program operations became more sophisticated, and the relationships among nutrition, health, and educational success became more pronounced. In addition, several other school feeding programs were established to fill in gaps in the nutritional needs of school-age children.

The School Breakfast Program was established to offer a nutritious breakfast in schools. The Special Milk Program for Children was designed to encourage the consumption of milk by children in schools. The Summer Food Service Program (SFSP) was created to provide a food service program during the summer months when school was not in session.

While the nutritional needs of school-age children were being addressed, those of preschool children were not. The Child and Adult Care Food Program (CACFP) was developed to address the nutritional needs of children in child care centers and family day care homes. The WIC Program was also created, to focus on the nutritional needs of pregnant women, infants, and young children at home.

Over the years, each of these programs has undergone changes to accommodate new research in nutritional health and education trends, while maintaining a commitment to providing nutritional food to keep children healthy enough to learn.

The National School Lunch Program

At the turn of the century, a penny lunch program was started in Philadelphia. A program in rural Wisconsin schools provided lunches for children prepared in the homes of women and heated in pint jars set in a bucket of hot water on top of a stove.

The Depression of the 1930's spurred the growth of school feeding programs. Widespread unemployment meant less money for food. At the same time that the market for farm products declined and surpluses grew, many children were going hungry.

In 1935, new legislation authorized USDA to buy price-depressing surplus foods. Needy families and school lunch programs provided outlets for those commodities. In a separate action, under the Works Progress Administration, the preparation and serving of school lunches became a source of employment.

The expansion in school feeding programs seen in the 1930's slowed in the 1940's. World War II resulted in the growth of defense industries which provided work for many. The huge requirements for food to support the armed services resulted in fewer commodities being available to school lunch programs. The threat to school feeding programs activated a number of groups concerned with such issues as children's health, the disposal of surplus agricultural commodities, the effects of consolidating rural schools in the South, jobs, and the fact that many men rejected for military service had health problems related to nutritional deficiencies.

In 1946, these concerns converged when Congress enacted the National School Lunch Act, "as a measure of national security, to safe guard the health and well-being of the Nation's children, and to encourage the domestic consumption of nutritious agricultural commodities and other food."

The National School Lunch Program (NSLP) makes free or low-cost lunches available to about 25 million children each school day in approximately 93,000 schools throughout the Nation. More than half these children get their meals free or at a reduced price. The program is available to 98 percent of public school children, and to 90 percent of all school children.

Participating schools receive cash assistance and donated foods from USDA, which serve to lower the cost of the meal to the paying child. Schools are provided with more than 60 different kinds of food including meat, fruits and vegetables, fruit juices, vegetable shortening, peanut products, vegetable oil, and grain products such as flour.

In return, participating schools must serve lunches which meet the minimum meal pattern requirements, and they must offer those lunches free or at a reduced price to needy children. The lunch pattern specifies the minimum amount of five food items a school must offer to receive Federal reimbursement: meat or meat alternate, bread or bread alternate, milk, and two fruits and/or vegetables. Efforts are being made to serve more nutritious, healthful foods. Schools have been provided new recipes which emphasize reductions in sugar, fat, and salt, and many improvements have been made in the foods provided by USDA.

The School Breakfast Program

The School Breakfast Program (SBP) makes low-cost breakfasts available to more than 5 million children in nearly 55,000 schools and institutions each school day. It is not as widely offered as the school lunch program and is more likely to operate in schools where economic need is greater.

As in NSLP, participating schools receive cash assistance to lower the cost of the breakfast to the paying child. In addition, the schools have access to the donated foods made available under the NSLP.

Participating schools must serve breakfasts which meet the minimum meal pattern requirements, and they must offer breakfast free or at a reduced price to needy children. The breakfast pattern specifies the minimum amounts of four food items a school must offer in order to receive Federal reimbursement: a serving of fluid milk, a serving of fruit or vegetable or both, and two servings of bread/bread alternate or meat/meat alternate or one serving of each.

Grants from USDA over the last 4 years have encouraged schools to start breakfast programs. More than 6,000 schools and a million children have been added to the program since the startup grants were first issued in 1989.

The Special Milk Program for Children

Expansion of the school lunch and breakfast programs, which include milk, has led to a reduction in the School Milk Program (SMP) since its peak in the late 1960's. Participation is now limited to schools, summer camps, and child care institutions that have no federally supported meal program, or to prekindergarten or kindergarten children who attend half-day sessions and have no access to meal programs provided by the schools. Low-income children may, at local option, qualify to receive their milk free.

The SMP encourages the consumption of fluid milk by children in over 10,000 schools and institutions which do not participate in any federally assisted meal service program.

Schools and institutions may choose from among pasteurized fluid types of unflavored or flavored whole milk, lowfat milk, skim milk, and cultured buttermilk. All contain vitamins A and D at levels specified by the Food and Drug Administration.

The Summer Food Service Program

The Summer Food Service Program (SFSP) funds meals and snacks for children in needy areas—where at least half the children come from families with incomes below 185 percent of the Federal poverty level—when schools are not in session during the summer. More than 1.9 million children participate in the SFSP.

The meal service can be sponsored by public or private nonprofit school food authorities, residential camps, colleges operating the National Youth Sports Program, units of State and local government, and private nonprofit organizations that meet specific criteria.

In areas where schools operate year-round, the SFSP may be available at times other than summer. The Ninth Street School in Los Angeles, for example, offers SFSP at other times of the year. Of the 555 children attending the school during the 1991-92 school year, virtually all participated in the lunch program, and three-quarters of the children participated in the breakfast program. Most of the children ate free meals.

Until recently, the school operated on the standard, single-track school year. Children were offered breakfast and lunch during the summer months through the SFSP. When the school switched to a year-round system, the children who were out of classes, or "off track," were left without a meal program. To remedy this, a local organization worked with the school district to develop an "off track" meal program which provided children who were on break with two meals each school day through the SFSP, even if "summer break" occurred in November or March.

The Child and Adult Care Food Program

The CACFP is the fastest growing of FNS' food assistance programs, with 1.9 million children and nearly 30,000 adults served in 1992.

The CACFP provides funds and USDA-donated foods year-round to help provide meals to children up to age 12 in day care centers, family day care homes, and afterschool care programs. It also provides support for meals served to impaired and elderly adults in nonresidential care centers.

All participating institutions must serve meals which meet the meal pattern requirements specified in program regulations. Centers and family day care homes may be approved to receive assistance for up to three meals per person per day, at least one of which must be a morning or afternoon snack. In addition, centers may be approved to receive assistance for three meals and one snack or two meals and two snacks for children maintained in care for 8 hours or more per day.

Stanley C. Garnett Director,
Child Nutrition Division,
Food and Nutrition Service, USDA
Alexandria, VA

Chapter 34

Food and Nutrition Service Programs Serving Special Populations

Approximately 1 in every 10 Americans benefits from the Food Stamp Program, USDA's largest food assistance program. However, USDA also offers other, less widely known food programs that serve special populations. These include the Special Supplemental Food Program for Women, Infants, and Children (WIC); the WIC Farmers' Market Nutrition Program (FMNP); and the Food Distribution Program on Indian Reservations (FDPIR), all administered by USDA's Food and Nutrition Service. The Administration on Aging in the U.S. Department of Health and Human Services oversees the Nutrition Program for the Elderly (NPE) with financial and commodity support from USDA.

Special Supplemental Food Program for Women, Infants, and Children

WlC's goal is to improve the health of pregnant, breastfeeding, and nonbreastfeeding postpartum women; infants; and children under 5 years old, by providing supplemental foods, nutrition education, and access to health services. Eligibility is determined by income (185 percent of Federal poverty income guidelines or below, or participation in the Aid to Families with Dependent Children, Food Stamp, or Medicaid Programs). Applicants must also be at nutritional risk as determined by a health professional.

Excerpt from *Nutrition: Eating and Good Health*, U.S. Department of Agriculture, Agriculture Information Bulletin 685

Each month, more than 5 million participants receive vouchers that can be redeemed at retail food stores for specific foods that research has shown are rich sources of the nutrients frequently lacking in the diet of low-income mothers and children.

The program nurtures new mothers who breastfeed, so that they can stay healthy and successfully nurse their babies. Infants and children receive foods that will help them grow and prepare them to learn in school. WIC also provides nutrition education, which helps participants to form good eating habits, and refers them to other local health and social services.

A recent study showed that women who participated in the WIC program during their pregnancies had lower Medicaid costs for themselves and their babies than did women who did not participate. Each dollar spent in prenatal WIC benefits was found to be more than offset by reduced Medicaid costs for both mother and baby after birth. For every WIC dollar invested in pregnant women, between $1.77 and $3.13 in Medicaid costs is saved for newborns and their mothers. For newborns only, the savings range from $2.84 to $3.90.

WIC works, but it does not work alone. WIC is a "gateway" program. Many people enter the social service system through WIC. During their first visit to the WIC clinic, they learn about other programs designed to meet their needs, such as the Food Stamp Program, the Aid to Families with Dependent Children Program, and the Medicaid Program. At all levels, WIC staff work closely with other agencies that provide complementary services to participants, including prenatal care, infant and childhood immunization, and alcohol and drug abuse counseling. Through the WIC Program, USDA has also assumed a leading role in the promotion of breastfeeding, which is generally the best way to nourish infants.

A Case Study

Maria Foster of Springfield, VA, was having a difficult pregnancy. When her weight fell to 85 pounds, she entered the hospital. She was soon discharged, 5 pounds heavier. But weight was not all she had gained. Rebecca King, a nutritionist at the hospital, counseled Foster on nutrition and immediately enrolled her in WIC, which allowed her to stretch her limited earnings as domestic helper to include many of the foods she needed during her pregnancy. The monthly food package for pregnant and breastfeeding women includes milk, cheese, eggs, cereals, and peanut butter, dry beans, or peas.

King continued to advise her on nutrition during her pregnancy, specifically on the importance of WIC foods in her diet. Instead of the small, sickly infant she originally feared she might have, Foster gave birth to healthy 7-pound, 7-ounce Cindy Vanessa. Foster followed King's advice and breastfed her baby. While she breastfed, she continued to participate in WIC, and thus to receive the high-protein foods she required for nursing.

WIC Farmers' Market Nutrition Program

In some areas, WIC recipients can participate in USDA's newest food assistance program, the WIC Farmers' Market Nutrition Program (FMNP). The program began in 1992 and provides WIC participants with coupons that can be used to buy fresh fruits and vegetables at authorized farmers' markets.

WIC participants receive $10-20 a year in FMNP coupons, in addition to their regular WIC food benefits. They can use the coupons to buy produce from farmers who have been authorized by the State to accept them. The State agency also provides nutrition education to encourage FMNP recipients to improve their diets by adding fresh fruits and vegetables and to advise them in preparing the foods they buy with FMNP coupons.

The FMNP is now authorized in certain areas of 11 States: Connecticut, Iowa, Maryland, Massachusetts, Michigan, New York, North Carolina, Pennsylvania, Texas, Vermont, and Washington. New State agencies will be added as funds become available. States that choose to operate the FMNP must contribute at least 30 percent of the total cost of the program.

Food Distribution Program on Indian Reservations

The Food Distribution Program on Indian Reservations (FDPIR) provides an alternative to the Food Stamp Program (FSP) for low-income Native Americans. In 1974, Congress mandated operation of the FSP in all counties nationwide. At that time, many Native Americans expressed a preference for continuation of the Needy Family Commodity Distribution Program, through which they had traditionally received food assistance. They indicated that the remote location of most reservations makes it difficult to participate in the FSP.

Food stamp offices, as well as grocery stores where Food Stamps can be transacted, are often located far from where Native Americans live. Furthermore, the few, smaller stores characteristically found in such remote rural areas tend to have higher prices, thus reducing the purchasing power of Food Stamps. In response to these concerns, Congress established the FDPIR as an alternative to Food Stamps in 1977. Eligible households cannot participate simultaneously in both programs, but may switch from one to the other on a monthly basis. The program is administered by States and Indian tribal organizations.

A Case Study

In 1991, USDA and the Wind River Indian Reservation in Wyoming added a new nutrition education initiative to the FDPIR menu. USDA's Expanded Food and Nutrition Education Program (EFNEP), administered by the Extension Service, provided a 3-week basic nutrition training course at the University of Wyoming for two aides hired from the reservation. The aided returned to the reservation to conduct cooking demonstrations, hold nutrition workshops, and counsel individual families in their homes.

Through home counseling, nutrition aide Val Whiteman taught Josephine Lynch, of the Arapaho Tribe, to deal successfully with a serious health condition. Lynch was overweight and required insulin injections to control her diabetes. Whiteman helped her to improve her diet, and she lost 57 pounds. Her eyesight also stabilized. Through proper nutrition, Lynch also ended the need for injections. Her doctor could prescribe oral medication instead, and he considered her diabetes to be under control. Other Indian tribal organizations are adapting successful efforts like the Wind River initiative to their own tribal environments.

Nutrition Program for the Elderly

Established by the Older Americans Act of 1965, the Nutrition Program for the Elderly (NPE) provides prepared meals to persons at least 60 years old and their spouses regardless of age. Eligibility is based solely on age; a means test is not required. USDA provides per-meal support in the form of commodities or cash for meals that average one-third of the Recommended Daily Allowance of nutrients.

Projects must serve at least one meal a day for 5 or more days each week, except in rural areas, where States can approve less frequent meal service.

NPE offers congregate meals served in recreation centers or other facilities and "Meals on Wheels" delivered directly to the homebound elderly. Many older Americans are not able or inclined to cook for themselves, and they may live in relative isolation. Congregate feeding addresses both of these tendencies by providing nutritious meals in a social setting. Meals on Wheels responds to the needs of the frail and homebound elderly, who might otherwise have no alternative but an extended-care residential facility.

Philip K. Cohen
Chief, Program Administration Branch,
Food Distribution Division,
Food and Nutrition Service, USDA,
Alexandria, VA

Chapter 35

Gleaning

In an age when thousands of Americans go without food every day, it is distressing to note that up to 20 percent of the American harvest each year is left to rot. It is hard to imagine that thousands of cans and packages of edible food in canneries, packing houses, food markets, and restaurants are routinely cast aside. Yet, research has found this to be the case.

Why the waste? Often produce may not meet market standards due to shape, size, or quantity. Other times, produce may not be harvested due to a lack of farm labor. Overproduction, dented cans, broken boxes, and expired marketing dates are more reasons why perfectly edible food is disposed of. The challenge is how to retrieve this discarded, yet edible, food and distribute it to the needy. The answer is known as "gleaning."

"Gleaning" is an organized activity in which hundreds of people collect unused and discarded food and provide it to those in need. Through gleaning, needy individuals, including low-income and unemployed persons, can receive agricultural products from farmers, processors, or retailers without charge. There are many groups, such as food banks and other charities involved with feeding the poor, that organize volunteer gleaning programs. During recent years, some USDA agencies have become key players in the gleaning effort

Section 1774 of the Food, Agriculture, Conservation, and Trade Act of 1990 includes a Gleaning Clearinghouse provision. This authorizes

---

Excerpt from *Nutrition: Eating for Good Health*, U.S. Department of Agriculture, Agriculture Information Bulletin 685

431

the Secretary of Agriculture to provide information and technical assistance to public and nonprofit groups that want to participate in gleaning projects. The Cooperative Extension System (CES), through its national educational network, is providing information to interested groups and individuals on ways to conduct gleaning programs. Extension has served as a resource on the Executive Council of Feeding Sites—bringing food providers and the "hunger and poverty network," the public, and other groups together. Extension field faculty also provide information to farmers and growers on gleaning legislation and to producers and processors about the needs of the poor.

Active State Programs

A 1992 CES survey of State gleaning efforts showed that 23 States had some form of gleaning program. The wide range of State gleaning activities includes setting up soup kitchens to preserve excess food, helping to train Master Food Preservers, and providing technical assistance on food preservation. CES staff members also serve as liaison with the State Department of Agriculture.

In Georgia, excess, prepared, and perishable foods are being collected from food service donors and distributed to feeding sites. Extension then contacts the recipients, encouraging them to sign up for a program of their interest, such as the Expanded Food and Nutrition Education Program (EFNEP).

Professionals at Oregon State University's Agriculture Experiment Station take a different approach to gleaning. They arrange for teams from the Gleaning Network, Inc., a three-county effort in Oregon, to glean the garden at the Experiment Station in Medford, OR, as well as the Master Gardener areas. For years, it has been a cooperative effort boasting positive results.

"All of our gleaning team members fall within USDA poverty guidelines," said Carol McLaughlin, program coordinator of the Gleaning Network, Inc. "They keep the gleanings they collect. Any excess is given to our organization, which then distributes it to team adoptees."

The adoptees, McLaughlin explains, are individuals who are at least 55 years old, or disabled, and who fall within the poverty guidelines. Teams are organized according to neighborhoods in Klamath, Jackson, and Josephine counties, and may consist of as few as 5 or as many as 48 households. To prepare for gleaning at the Agriculture Experiment Station and Master Gardener areas, team members must participate in a 2-day Gleaning Network training program in which they are taught how to collect produce without damaging crops.

"We usually glean between 10 and 15 times a year at the Experiment Station and Master Gardener areas. This year we collected tomatoes, onions, squash, green peppers, two varieties of corn, and three varieties of green beans." said McLaughlin.

The concept of "harvesting after the harvest" is popular in other States as well. Washington State University Cooperative Extension personnel developed a project to specially train individuals to harvest produce left in fields and orchards. A distributor from the local area emergency food banks comes directly to the fields to collect the harvest. The food banks then immediately distribute the surplus produce to homeless people or others in need of food.

Steven Garrett is the supervisor, Expanded Food and Nutrition Education Program in Pierce County, Washington State University Cooperative Extension Service. Local EFNEP personnel and volunteers do the gleaning.

"In 1992, EFNEP personnel and volunteers gleaned 160,000 pounds of leftover fruits and vegetables," reports Garrett. "We had 96 volunteers giving a total of 4,600 hours. Seventy-five percent of the food collected went to the Emergency Food Network in Pierce County, which distributed it to local food banks. The other 25 percent went to the volunteer gleaners."

Training the Gleaners

Garrett recalled that prior to 1990 local farmers had been somewhat reluctant to allow gleaners on their property for fear of potential crop and property damage. In the spring of 1990, David Ottey, executive director of the Emergency Food Network, and Margaret Movius, who was then the EFNEP supervisor in the Pierce County Cooperative Extension Office, decided to train volunteers—recruited from the county's EFNEP program—in the proper way to harvest crops. They also contacted area farmers to assure them that, because of the training, their farm property wouldn't be damaged by the volunteer gleaners. As a result of this effort, more local farmers and Tacoma-area home gardeners were willing to invite gleaners onto their properties. Besides collecting fresh fruit and vegetables for themselves and for other needy individuals, the EFNEP volunteer gleaners also have the option of taking classes in food preservation, which are conducted by an Extension volunteer food advisor.

Throughout the Nation, more and more farmers, farmers' markets, producers, retailers, institutions, restaurants, and backyard gardeners are contributing to gleaning programs, as this humanitarian effort continues to become more popular. Brochures, fliers, toll-free hotlines, and promotional videos are just some of the means by which county Extension offices are getting the word out on gleaning.

Nancy Leidenfrost
National Program Leader,
and
Rita Rogers
Public Affairs Specialist,
Extension Service, USDA,
Washington, DC

Chapter 36

Helping Low-Income Americans With USDA Commodities

Every day, thousands of low-income people have a nutritious meal prepared with USDA commodity foods. Sometimes these meals are prepared at home; other times the meals are served at schools, soup kitchens for the homeless, day care centers, summer camps, senior centers, hospitals, nursing homes, and half-way houses for battered women or recovering substance abusers. In dollar terms (about $1 billion annually), the USDA commodity programs are small compared to other domestic food assistance efforts such as the Food Stamp or National School Lunch Programs. However, their reach is great.

A Depression Program

Through its commodity programs, the USDA has been providing food to people and help to farmers since the Great Depression of the 1930's. It was then that the Federal Government began to buy surplus crops from farmers to stabilize agricultural markets and guarantee producers a fair return for their labors in the face of eroding consumer purchasing power and dislocations in foreign trade. Although the emphasis then was on the removal of surpluses from the market, by 1938 USDA was distributing $54 million dollars worth of food annually to local public assistance agencies that gave it to the poor.

Schools also received surplus commodities to help them provide nutritious meals for millions of students who were unable to pay for

Excerpt from *Nutrition: Eating for Good Health*, U.S. Department of Agriculture, Agriculture Information Bulletin 685

their school lunches. This marrying of interests between helping the American farmer and providing for the food needs of low-income people has continued to varying degrees throughout the history of the commodity programs.

The Delicate Balance

Today, USDA provides regular commodity support to a wide variety of low-income people through eight different programs:

- The Child Nutrition Programs

- The Nutrition Program for the Elderly

- The Commodity Supplemental Food Program

- The Charitable Institution Program

- The Program for Summer Camps

- The Food Distribution Program on Indian Reservations

- The Emergency Food Assistance Program

- The Soup Kitchen/Food Bank Program

Commodity assistance is also available to victims of natural disasters.

Sometimes these commodities are surplus foods and their purchase plays an important role in stabilizing agricultural markets. This is true for some of the commodities that are provided to the Child Nutrition Programs and the Emergency Food Assistance Program (TEFAP), and all of the commodities donated to the Charitable Institution Program. For other programs—such as the Commodity Supplemental Food Program, the Food Distribution Program on Indian Reservations, and the Soup Kitchen/Food Bank Program—funds appropriated by Congress are intended to purchase commodities specifically tailored to the needs of recipients. In these instances, surplus removal gives way to other considerations such as the particular nutritional needs of program participants.

Surplus food is not lower in quality or less appealing than other food. Over the years, USDA has donated millions of pounds of meat, poultry, fish, fruits, vegetables, grain, and dairy products when they were in surplus. Purchase specifications require high quality standards; all commodities are processed using on-site USDA inspection to assure that purchase specifications are met.

The administrative agency, the Food and Nutrition Service (FNS), also pays attention to the Dietary Guidelines for Americans when selecting commodity foods. Over the last decade, purchase specifications have been changed: commodity canned fruits are now packed only in light syrup or natural juice, the fat content of canned and frozen meat has been significantly lowered, tuna is packed in water, and peanuts are unsalted. Commodity foods—surplus or otherwise—are under constant review to ensure that they meet current nutrition standards.

Since the passage of the Commodity Distribution Reform Act of 1987, FNS has collected annual preference information from all of its commodity program operators. This allows FNS to determine whether the foods it provides will be consumed once they are distributed.

Working Together

The commodity programs represent a successful melding of the interests of American agriculture and the people who need assistance in obtaining a nutritionally adequate diet. However, other important partners in this effort include State and local governments, a variety of nonprofit institutions, and thousands of volunteers.

Commodity foods are served to senior citizens in many different settings—including senior centers, churches, and Meals-on-Wheels programs—through the Nutrition Program for the Elderly. Low-income Native Americans receive commodities as an alternative to the Food Stamp Program on 223 reservations throughout the country. In FY 1992, approximately 2.1 billion meals were served through the Charitable Institution Program by more than 14,000 nonprofit institutions— such as hospitals, food pantries, nursing homes, and shelters for the homeless—using surplus commodities. Over the years, USDA has provided foods such as rice, pasta, peanut butter, dairy products, flour, fish, vegetables, and fruits to these institutions.

Low-income children also receive the benefit of as many as 90 different commodity foods through the National School Lunch Program, the Child and Adult Care Program, and the Summer Food Service Program. In school year 1992-93, FNS gave school meal providers 14 cents worth of commodities for every meal served in the National School Lunch Program.

These efforts require State agencies to develop and maintain systems for warehousing and distributing commodities to local distributing organizations. State governments play a critical role in the operation of the commodity programs. Several of the programs are also heavily dependent on the efforts of local nonprofit organizations and volunteers.

All over the country, volunteer groups provide community-based services to low-income adults and children. And foods donated by USDA and private sources help them meet basic needs. Once those needs for shelter and food are met, people can turn their attention to other things that will help them become self-reliant and productive. A study of groups providing meals to the homeless, completed in 1989, found that "the higher proportion of USDA commodity foods that a provider gets, the more calories, protein, and carbohydrates are present in meals served, and the more food groups are present in the meals."

Case Studies

In Duluth MN, the Damiano Center not only provides food, shelter, and clothing, but also offers the homeless an opportunity, through its Handy Hands job program, to earn some much needed money at a community day labor program. If workers prove reliable, Handy Hands helps with references that can lead to full-time employment. "Damiano Center is based on the belief that the best hope for eliminating hunger is in actively working with people, enabling them to provide food for themselves," says Jim Dwyer, who coordinates the Emergency Food Assistance program (TEFAP) at the center. "Once their basic food needs are met, we try to create opportunities for low income people to learn to be more self-reliant."

In Boston, more than 120 volunteer groups donate or help with meals at the Pine Street Inn for the homeless. In addition to providing food and shelter, Pine Street has an onsite clinic and provides clothing, a work rehabilitation program, permanent housing services, and a special program for women who have been chronic substance abusers and their children. This special program for women works in tandem with USDA's Supplemental Food Program for Women, Infants, and Children (WIC).

At Baltimore's Bayard Street recreation center, police officers volunteer to cook meals and help the children learn social skills and positive values.

The Emergency Food Assistance Program

The Emergency Food Assistance Program (TEFAP) joins agricultural surpluses, USDA support for the food needs of low-income people, and the efforts of volunteer groups. TEFAP began in December 1981 as a special distribution of cheese to reduce large dairy surpluses at a time of high unemployment. Subsequently, other surplus commodities—such as flour, butter, nonfat dry milk, rice, honey, and cornmeal—were added to the distributions. Volunteer groups and local governments in all States provided the people needed to give out these foods every month to low-income households who needed supplemental food assistance. At TEFAP's peak in 1987, community action agencies, food pantries, churches, senior centers, and welfare offices distributed $850 million in commodities.

Today, these large surpluses do not exist. TEFAP continues because in 1989 Congress passed the Hunger Prevention Act, which provided USDA with $120 million a year for the purchase of nutritious foods to augment those that remained in surplus. In addition, the Hunger Prevention Act created a new commodity program, the Soup Kitchen/Food Bank Program. In 1992, USDA purchased $32 million in commodities primarily for those organizations that serve meals to the homeless. When States find that they cannot use all of the commodities allocated to them to meet the needs of the homeless, they can give them to food banks for distribution to other low-income clients.

The funds appropriated by Congress allow USDA to purchase a wider variety of foods for both TEFAP and the Soup Kitchen/Food Bank Program. Canned meat, peanut butter, juice, fruit, vegetables, and rice are among the commodities available. Without the surpluses of overproduction, the program is smaller now than it has been. Now it is much more common for the 17,000 local distribution sites across the country to integrate USDA foods with those obtained from private sources. In some States, food banks are now the primary source of USDA foods. In these situations, needy households can go to a food pantry or other local nonprofit organization whenever they have an emergency need for food, rather than having to wait for the scheduled TEFAP distribution.

The Commodity Supplemental Food Program

The Commodity Supplemental Food Program (CSFP) operates at 47 sites in 20 States and one Indian Tribal Organization. It provides specially tailored commodity foods to supplement the diets of low-income pregnant, postpartum, and breastfeeding women and their children up to age 6. In some sites, the program also serves elderly persons. The goals of CSFP are similar to those of the Special Supplemental Food Program for Women, Infants, and Children (WIC), but it provides food rather than a voucher for the purchase of food. Clients cannot participate in both programs during the same month.

CSFP started in 1968 as the predecessor to WIC, and it served approximately 342,539 participants last year. The food packages are tailored to meet the needs of women and children. The packages include such items as juice, infant cereal, infant formula, nonfat dry milk, fruits, vegetables, and canned meat. Like many other USDA commodity programs, it is heavily dependent at the local level on the efforts of nonprofit organizations and volunteers.

Sites in Denver, Des Moines, and Detroit use a supermarket concept to provide efficient and educational service to their clients. At these sites, clients are provided with a shopping list of eligible foods and are then responsible for selecting from commodity foods those items and quantities that match family ages and numbers. Nutrition education, including food preparation demonstrations, is available to help CSFP clients make food choices.

In Des Moines, a well-baby clinic that offers immunizations, lead-poisoning screening, and iron-level blood tests is also housed on the premises. Denver has begun an innovative "Food for Thought" program through which children can get children's books provided by private donations.

Since it began its CSFP operation in Detroit, Focus: Hope, which was originally formed as a civil rights organization, has been able to garner support from private and public sources to offer high technology job training to inner city residents. 'The USDA food assistance available through CSFP has made it possible for us to realize our mission of eradicating racism, poverty, and injustice through practical and intelligent action," says Eleanor Josaitis, co-founder of Focus: Hope. 'There's a lot more left to be done, but our partnership with USDA is so vital to the basic well-being of the 85,000 women, babies, and elderly citizens we serve each month. A stable source of good food allows people to start addressing other life issues that can lead to self-reliance and a brighter future for their children."

Alberta C. Frost
Director, Supplemental Food Programs Division,
and former Director, Food Distribution Division,
Food and Nutrition Service, USDA,
Alexandria, VA

Chapter 37

A Sturdy Safety Net—Food Stamps

May 29, 1961, marks the beginning of today's Food Stamp Program. On that day, Mr. and Mrs. Alderson Muncy of Paynesville, WV, bought a can of pork and beans at Henderson's Supermarket. They were the first in the Nation to be issued modern Food Stamps and to use them to purchase food for their family. McDowell County, WV, was one of eight sites beginning "pilot programs" for Food Stamps in 1961. The pilots were intended to discover whether this method of helping poor families to buy food would work.

Mr. and Mrs. Muncy had no idea what they were inaugurating. No one could have predicted just how successful the program would become. In 1992, 25 million persons, on average, received Food Stamps each month. Approximately 1 in 10 Americans received some assistance from Food Stamps, making the program one of the most enduring and effective safety nets for Americans in economic distress.

How It Works

Food coupons, or stamps, are used to supplement the food buying power of eligible low-income households. The program is administered nationally by USDA's Food and Nutrition Service (FNS) and locally by State welfare agencies.

Available under the same rules and restrictions in every State and all counties in the United States, the Food Stamp Program is recog-

Excerpt from *Nutrition: Eating for Good Health*, U.S. Department of Agriculture, Agriculture Information Bulletin 685

nized as a potential source of help by most Americans. Grocers throughout the Nation understand the program, appreciate the additional purchasing power it has given their poorer customers, and regularly deposit redeemed Food Stamps in their local banks. The Federal Government, through the USDA Food and Nutrition Service, makes these deposits good. Most important, recipients of Food Stamps realize that this system allows them great freedom in choosing those foods they believe are most useful to their families and in choosing where they wish to shop.

Farmers and food processors benefit because their products can be purchased by people who otherwise might not be able to buy enough food. Studies show that Food Stamps substantially increase the nutrients in home food supplies, including such important problem nutrients as calcium, vitamin C, and iron.

The program is flexible and convenient. Unlike the direct distribution of canned goods and other foods to individuals in distress, which often occurs after disasters, the Food Stamp Program requires no special warehouses, inventories, or trucks to distribute food. As long as there are participating grocery stores with food stocks, recipients can redeem their stamps. When economic times are tough, the program expands to provide help to all those who are eligible. When times are better, and the unemployed gain jobs, the program shrinks accordingly.

Using uniform rules, local welfare office workers examine each applicant's income, assets, and family characteristics to make sure that only those in need receive stamps. Persons who are found to be guilty of fraud are made to repay their benefits, and disqualified from further participation. Grocery store owners who sell ineligible items (such as liquor, tobacco, cosmetics, and other nonfood items) for Food Stamps also lose the privilege of participating in the program.

Grocers or individuals who traffic in Food Stamps, buying them from poor persons at a fraction of their face value and redeeming them through a bank, face prosecution, possible imprisonment, and permanent disqualification from the program. States that become lax in administering the program, granting undeserved benefits to applicants, wind up owing the Federal Government sizable amounts of money; a quality control system finds errors.

Eligibility

To get Food Stamps, someone in the household fills out an application form at the nearest welfare office. Once this is done, an interview with an eligibility worker takes place. At the interview, the applicant provides documents verifying such factors as income, assets, employment status, and age of each member of the household. Benefits are geared to household size, a household being those persons who regularly prepare and eat food together.

The key eligibility factors are assets and income; tests are in place to assure that households with high income and large amounts of assets do not qualify for the Food Stamp Program. Some assets are not counted, such as a home and lot. Some vehicles are not counted as assets, such as those used to produce income most of the time. For other vehicles, the fair market value is determined, and everything above $4,500 counts toward the limit on assets.

Special deductions from gross monthly income may be applied. There is a deduction that encourages people to work or keep working by counting only part of their earnings as income. This deduction results in a smaller reduction in their benefits than they otherwise would get because of their increased income. There are other deductions for dependent care, excess medical expenses for the elderly and disabled, and excess shelter costs.

Once the eligibility worker has verified that the applicant household has less than the allowed $2,000 in countable resources (it is $3,000 for households with at least one person 60 or older), and has net income within the specified limits, the applicant may be certified to receive Food Stamps. The net monthly income limits and maximum Food Stamp allotments for each family size are as follows:

Household size	Net monthly income limits*	Maximum Food Stamp allotments*
1	$568	$111
2	766	203
3	965	292
4	1,163	370
5	1,361	440
6	1,560	528
7	1,758	584
8	1,956	667
Each additional person	+199	+83

*For the 48 contiguous States and the District of Columbia. There are different income limits and maximum allotment amounts for Alaska, Hawaii, Guam, and the Virgin Islands. These amounts are in effect through September 1993.

Delivery of Food Stamps

The eligibility worker determines the appropriate amount of Food Stamps which will be issued. Beginning with the date of application, the State has no more than 30 days to deliver benefits. (Where the household is very needy, benefits must be made available within 5 days.)

Some States issue eligible households Authorization to Participate cards, which are exchanged for the appropriate amount of Food Stamps. Other States mail the Food Stamps to the household. Still other States use a photo identification system in issuing Food Stamps. Once they are received, the Stamps may be used by the household at any authorized retailer whenever it is convenient.

Spending Food Stamps

Retail food stores must apply to the Food and Nutrition Service in order to be allowed to receive Food Stamps. When a store is authorized, it is given identifying signs and decals to post and any program participant may spend Food Stamps there. Special care is taken by the Food and Nutrition Service to make certain that enough retailers are authorized in low-income areas, so that poor people will have access to food. There are currently about 210,000 authorized stores.

The Food Stamp customer may use stamps only for food and for plants and seeds to grow food for the household. Food Stamps cannot be used to buy:

- alcoholic beverages

- tobacco or cigarettes

- household supplies, soaps, and paper products

- medicines or vitamins

- any other nonfood items

- food that will be eaten in the store

- hot foods that are ready to eat, such as barbecued chicken

- pet foods

Sales tax cannot be charged on eligible items purchased with Food Stamps. Any ineligible items purchased by the Food Stamp customer must be paid for in cash. These provisions help ensure that poor households receive enough nutritious food.

Food Stamps are issued in booklets of $1, $5, and $10 coupons. The grocer can give cash change only up to 99 cents. Change in even dollar amounts is given in Food Stamps.

Changes in Eligibility

Each Food Stamp household is periodically re-examined to make sure it is still eligible. In addition, Food Stamp households are required to report changes in their circumstances (such as a new job and income or more household members) which might affect their benefits. Benefits may be adjusted upward or downward appropriately.

Food Stamp recipients have rights and responsibilities, which are carefully explained when they are certified. People who break Food Stamp rules may be disqualified from the program, fined, imprisoned, or all three. If a person is disqualified, the first time is for 6 months; the second time is for a year; and the third time is permanent.

Households may continue to receive food stamps as long as they remain eligible. Children in these families are automatically eligible for free school lunch and breakfast.

The Average Food Stamp Household

A summer 1991 study of Food Stamp households showed that slightly more than half the recipients were children. The average food stamp household size was 2.6 persons with an average monthly gross income of $472 and an average monthly net income of $261; half the households had gross monthly incomes of less than $500. Almost 77 percent of all households had no countable assets and another 18 percent had countable assets of $500 or less. Those food stamp recipients who were able to work were working or otherwise meeting the work requirement—for example, by being in training or receiving education.

Food Stamps, then, go to the neediest Americans in those households with little or no income. And the Food Stamp Program does serve as a safety net: half of all recipients are on the program for 6 months or less.

Using Food Stamps for Good Nutrition

Low-income shoppers face tough decisions when spending their Food Stamps. More than most Americans, they need to get the maximum nutrition at the lowest cost for their stamps and the money with which they supplement them. Many are astute shoppers, buying generic brands and using discount coupons. Others are not as knowledgeable.

The Food and Nutrition Service makes publications available for distribution to Food Stamp recipients with information about shopping for low-cost nutrition. These publications discuss using food labels to make smart choices, the economy of preparing food rather than buying convenience foods, meal planning, cooking for one or two persons, and building a better diet. In addition, many major food chains distribute free publications with shopping advice.

If a particular nutrition problem exists in a State, that State can add a special nutrition education component to its annual Food Stamp operating plan. Federal funds are available to pay half the expenses of these components, and States are encouraged to take advantage of this opportunity to better serve Food Stamp recipients.

Access to Food Stamps

The increase in Food Stamp program participation during recent years clearly shows that the program responds to changes in the economy and in the circumstances of individual households, enabling those who need Food Stamps to get them. State and local governments have exerted tremendous effort to ensure that people in need receive the benefits to which they are entitled. In many cases, they have done so in the face of reduced State and local budgets.

Some numbers illustrate the ease with which the program absorbs the newly eligible: Average monthly participation in the Food Stamp Program increased from 18.8 million in 1989 to 25.8 million in 1992—an increase of 7 million persons and 37 percent in 3 years.

Aside from active and compassionate administrators, several program features make access easier. These include:

- Applicants must be given an application and allowed to file it the first day they contact a Food Stamp office. If the applicant cannot come to the office, the application must be mailed.

446

- States can combine the application process for the Food Stamp Program with that for other assistance programs. This saves the applicant the time and inconvenience of completing two or more applications, possibly at different locations.

- In cases where the applicant is homebound, handicapped, or otherwise unable to visit the office, an authorized representative may be appointed to represent the household in certification interviews or to get and use Food Stamps.

- If the household can't come to the food stamp office and can't appoint an authorized representative, interviews can be conducted by telephone, or an eligibility worker can be sent to the home. Face-to-face interviews can be waived for households where all members are 65 or older or are mentally or physically handicapped.

- Households in which all members receive Supplemental Security Income (SSI) can be certified through Social Security Offices, saving the household a trip to the Food Stamp office.

Electronic Benefits Transfer

One of the problems caused by growth in the Food Stamp Program is the difficulty of handling so many Food Stamps. Currently, about 4 billion new food stamps are distributed each year. This means that a special currency (hard to counterfeit) must be produced, stored in safe quarters, and transported by armored car to locations all over the United States where it can be stored and prepared for distribution in the correct amounts to eligible participants. Food Stamps must be available at the State and local levels when they are needed by recipients, so the process of moving stamps around is a big job.

Once the Food Stamps have been spent in grocery stores, each store must count and bundle its Food Stamps (usually each day) for redemption at a bank. The bank must also count and handle the Food Stamps as it prepares them to be submitted to the Federal Reserve Bank, which, in turn, pays the local bank. Finally, the Food Stamps must be sent to a central location for accounting and destruction. This process is costly and time-consuming.

With so many Food Stamps in circulation, there are greater opportunities for the unscrupulous to undermine the Food Stamp Program by fraud. A crooked retailer can lure Food Stamp recipients into giving up $100 worth of food purchasing power by offering, say, $50 in cash for the stamps. This sort of wrongdoing not only undermines the nutritional purpose of Food Stamps but also results in an illegal gain by the retailer, who deposits the stamps in a bank account. It is difficult to prevent such fraud and abuse from occurring when there are so many stamps and so many recipients.

One way to counter these problems is the electronic benefit transfer (EBT) system. EBT makes food assistance funds available to the household in a special account which can be used only by the household in approved grocery stores to purchase food.

The Food Stamp office enters the household's benefit amount in the special account each month. When the recipient buys food at the grocery store, all eligible Food Stamp items are totaled by the grocer. A plastic card (like a credit card) is passed through a reader by the recipient. Next, the recipient verifies the purchase by entering a private personal identification number into a keyboard at the checkout stand.

Both the amount of purchase and the identification number are electronically sent to the central accounts and the purchase is deducted from the account. Only the total amount available in the account can be spent for food. Only a recipient with a correctly coded card and the right personal identification number can have access to that particular account. Each time the recipient makes a purchase, a receipt is provided showing the amount purchased and the remaining balance. No money or Food Stamps are involved. Each month the Food Stamp office replenishes the benefit dollars available in the account if the household is still eligible.

Currently, there are five EBT demonstration projects, located in Reading, PA; Ramsey County (St. Paul), MN; Bernalillo County (Albuquerque), NM; Linn County (Cedar Rapids), IA; and Maryland, which operates a State-wide system. A sixth EBT project is underway in Dayton, OH, where the off-line approach is being tested. In an off-line system, benefit information is stored in a computer chip in the card itself and purchases are deducted directly from the card at the supermarket terminal.

Early experience suggests there may be a number of advantages to EBT:

- No Food Stamps are involved, and accounting for benefits can easily be accomplished.

- Problems of transportation and storage are eliminated.

- Retailers like the elimination of Food Stamp handling and the ease and speed of settlement with the bank.

- Banks are pleased that EBT eliminates their coupon issuance role and reduces their costs for handling and redeeming benefits.

- Recipients find EBT easier to use and less time-consuming than food stamps. They particularly like using the card; unlike Food Stamps, it does not overtly identify them to other store customers as food stamp recipients.

Reporting on a June 2, 1993 "town hall meeting" held by Vice President Gore in St. Paul MN, the Washington Post noted:

"Mary Jass, 35, moved here from California three years ago. She still receives welfare assistance, but without an affront to her dignity, she said.

"'We happened to live in a more affluent city and most of the people in the grocery store were not me. And I would get out my Food Stamp coupons and, kind of trembling, tear them out. I wanted to get this done with, and then they had to stamp every one of them. And it was very embarrassing and I didn't like it at all and I ended up going to other stores where I wouldn't be known. Coming to Minnesota it is entirely different. No one knows, it seems, that I'm even on welfare. They think it's a credit card.'"

Welfare Reform

Many Food Stamp households receive other public assistance as well. For these families, surviving on welfare means dealing with several different Government offices and program requirements, a confusing and time-consuming task. FNS is actively working with other Government programs, such as Aid to Families with Dependent Children (AFDC), Medicaid, and the Department of Housing and Urban Development (HUD), to find ways to simplify these programs for the recipients. Concepts such as "one-stop shopping" and using the same or similar eligibility requirements for different programs are being tested.

A major stumbling block is the fact that each public assistance program is authorized by a different law, often by different committees in Congress. This makes change a slow process, but each time

Congress reviews a program, changes are proposed to make it conform to the others. They are debated and often accepted.

It is now widely recognized that Government assistance may be a necessity for some recipients, not a preferred way of life. Greater attention and effort are being devoted to breaking the chains of public dependency for those who are able to do so. Work requirements for the able-bodied are part of the Food Stamp Program, as they are for several other programs.

Incentives for persons on welfare to gain the education, skills, and experience they need for successful self-support through employment are being built into programs. A number of States are experimenting with ways to more effectively integrate welfare recipients into the mainstream of American life, and we may learn from these experiments which paths to follow in the years ahead.

Richard G. Woods
Assistant to the Deputy Administrator,
and
Carol S. Stobaugh
Food Program Specialist,
Food Stamp Program,
Food and Nutrition Service, USDA,
Alexandria, VA

Appendix A

Advice on Purchasing Foods

Section 1

How to Buy Cheese

Because it is such a well-liked food, cheese is a favorite among cooks and food lovers. With the wide variety of flavors, colors, and consistencies to choose from, cheeses are suitable for any meal of the day, from appetizers to desserts and snacks.

Points to Consider

Wholesomeness. . .nutritive value. . .quality. . .informative labeling...and use are some of the points to consider when purchasing cheese.

Wholesomeness

Before grading or inspection of a cheese product is provided, the processing plant must meet the U.S. Department of Agriculture's specifications for quality and sanitation. A USDA dairy inspector checks the plant, incoming raw products, and processing and packaging techniques.

Nutritive Value

Cheese, like many other milk products, provides protein, vitamins, minerals, fat, saturated fat, and cholesterol. While cheese is one of

Agricultural Marketing Service Home and Garden Bulletin No. 256

the best sources of calcium, it may also be high in sodium and saturated fat. A 1 1/2-ounce serving of natural cheese supplies the same amount of calcium as 1 cup of milk or yogurt, as well as 12 to 14 grams total fat, 9 grams saturated fatty acids, 44 milligrams cholesterol, and 173 calories. For sodium, while 1 cup of milk contains 120 milligrams, 1 1/2 ounces of natural cheese could contain from 110 to 450 milligrams, while 2 ounces of process cheese could contain 800 milligrams. Use the Nutrition Facts panel on each individual product label to learn about the nutrient content of that food and how it fits into an overall daily diet.

Choose a diet low in fat, saturated fat, and cholesterol to help reduce the risk of getting certain diseases and to help maintain a healthy weight. The Dietary Guidelines for Americans suggest choosing a diet containing 30 percent or less of calories from fat and less than 10 percent of calories from saturated fatty acids. Also, some health authorities suggest that dietary cholesterol be limited to an average of 300 milligrams or less per day.

The Food Guide Pyramid (see Chapter 2) suggests 2 to 3 servings each day of food from the milk, yogurt, and cheese group. Count as a serving 1 1/2 ounces of natural cheese or 2 ounces of process cheese.

Tips: Fat-free, "part skim," or lowfat cheeses are available. When you choose a higher fat cheese, balance your fat intake by choosing other foods that are low in fat.

Quality Assurance

USDA's Agricultural Marketing Service has established U.S. grade standards for four varieties of cheese: Cheddar, Colby, Monterey and Swiss. The cheese industry uses the grade standards to identify levels of quality, to have a basis for establishing prices at wholesale, and to provide consumers with the qualities they want. Generally, these grades do not appear on consumer packages, but the U.S. Grade shield may appear on some consumer packages of Cheddar cheese, including low-fat varieties.

Using USDA's Cheese Grades

The USDA grade shield means that the cheese has been inspected and graded by an experienced and highly trained government grader. And it means the cheese was produced in a USDA-approved plant, under sanitary conditions. It is your guarantee of consistent and dependable quality

USDA Grade AA Cheese

Cheddar cheese meeting the U.S. Grade AA is the highest quality. It meets exacting USDA standards, has a fine, highly pleasing flavor, a smooth, compact texture, uniform color, and attractive appearance.

To earn this grade, cheese must be produced with special care—in the quality of the milk, cheese-making skill, curing or ripening process, and packaging.

The AA shield is assurance of consistently fine Cheddar flavor and texture in every package.

USDA Grade A Cheese

Cheddar cheese meeting the U.S. Grade A is also of good quality, but not as high as AA. The flavor is pleasing. However, there may be more variation in flavor and texture between packages.

USDA "Quality Approved" Cheese

Cheese and cheese products not covered by a U.S. grade standard may be inspected and bear the USDA "Quality Approved" inspection shield on the label. Pasteurized process cheese, cheese food and spreads, and cottage cheese are examples of cheese products receiving USDA inspection.

To carry the "Quality Approved" shield, the product must be manufactured in a plant meeting the USDA sanitary specifications for plants and equipment.

Labels

Labels on natural cheese, pasteurized process cheese, and related products carry important descriptive information. The name of a natural cheese will appear as the variety, such as "Cheddar cheese," "Swiss cheese," or "Blue cheese."

Pasteurized process cheese labels will always include the words "pasteurized process," together with the name of the variety or varieties of cheese used—for example, "pasteurized process American cheese" or "pasteurized process Swiss and American cheese."

Cheese food also contains ingredients other than cheese and therefore is labeled as "pasteurized process cheese food." Cheese spreads have a different composition from cheese foods and are labeled as "pasteurized process cheese spread." All the ingredients used in the preparation of these products are listed on the respective labels along with the kinds or varieties of cheese used in the mixture. Also, the milkfat and moisture content may be shown.

Coldpack cheese and coldpack cheese food are labeled in the same manner as other cheese and cheese foods, except that the names "club cheese" or "comminuted cheese" may be substituted for the name "coldpack cheese."

Check the Cure

The age or degree of curing is very important label information on certain varieties of natural cheese. For example, Cheddar cheese may be labeled as "mild," "medium" or "mellow," and "aged" or "sharp." In some cases, pasteurized process cheese may be labeled to indicate a sharp flavor when a much higher proportion of sharp or aged cheese was used in its preparation.

Check the Name

Look for the name of the cheese item. Don't confuse the brand name with the name of the cheese. For some purposes, you may want natural cheese, for others, process cheese or cheese food. For still others, pasteurized process cheese spread or coldpack cheese may best serve your needs. In many cases, products may be packaged alike. but the names on the labels will be different.

Making Natural Cheese

Cheesemaking is a centuries old art. It consists of separating most of the milk solids from the milk by curdling with rennet or bacterial culture or both. The curd is then separated from the whey by heating, stirring, and pressing.

Most cheeses in this country are made from whole milk. For certain types of cheese, both milk and cream are used. For other types, skim milk, whey or mixtures of all of these are used.

456

The distinctive flavor, body and texture characteristics of the various cheeses are due to: 1) the kind of milk used; 2) the method used for curdling the milk and for cutting, cooking, and forming the curd; 3) the type of bacteria or molds used in ripening; 4) the amount of salt or other seasonings added; and 5) ripening conditions such as temperature, humidity, and length of time. Sometimes only minor differences in the procedures followed may make the difference between one variety of cheese and another.

After the cheese has been formed into its characteristic shape, it is coated with wax or other protective coating or wrapping, then cured or aged for varying lengths of time, depending upon the kind or variety of cheese being made.

When the cheese has reached its proper curing stage, it is often cut or sliced from larger blocks or wheels into smaller sizes. The refrigerated showcase in a modern food market is most enticing with its display of various shapes and sizes of cheese packages such as wedges, oblongs, segments. cubes. slices. blocks. and cut portions.

Care in the Home

All natural cheese should be refrigerated. When possible store the cheese in its original wrapper or covering. To store opened cheeses for any extended period, wrap them tightly in clinging plastic wrap to keep all air and moisture away from the surface. The following storage times are guidelines for maintaining the quality of cheese in the refrigerator after purchase:

Soft unripened cheeses: cottage—10-30 days; creamed and neufchatel—opened 2 weeks; ricotta— 5 days.

Ripened or cured cheeses: hard and wax coated Cheddar, Edam, Gouda, Swiss, brick, etc.—unopened 3-6 months, opened 3-4 weeks, sliced 2 weeks.

- Mold formed on natural, hard, block cheeses is not harmful and may be removed; just cut off at least an inch around and below the mold spot, keeping the knife out of the mold itself. The particular mold in the interior of cheeses such as Blue, Gorgonzola, Roquefort, or Stilton has been carefully developed to produce the characteristic color and distinctive flavor of those varieties and is consumed as part of the cheese.

457

- Ends or pieces of cheese that have become dried out and hard may be grated and kept refrigerated in a clean, airtight container, and used for garnishing or accenting.

- Store aromatic cheeses such as Limburger in tightly sealed containers. These cheeses are fast-curing and are best when used soon after purchase.

- Normally, frozen cheese will lose its characteristic body and texture, becoming crumbly and mealy. However, small pieces (1 pound or less, not over 1 inch thick) of certain varieties may be frozen for as long as 6 months—if they are handled and stored properly. To prevent evaporation, cut cheese should be tightly wrapped in foil or other moistureproof freezer wrapping, then frozen immediately. Freeze the product quickly, at a temperature setting of 0 °F. or lower.

- Cheese varieties that can be successfully frozen in small pieces are: Brick, Cheddar, Edam, Gouda, Muenster, Port du Salut, Swiss, Provolone, Mozzarella, and Camembert. Small cheeses, such as Camembert, can be frozen in their original packages. When removed from the freezer, cheese should be thawed in the refrigerator and used as soon as possible after thawing

- Except for soft, unripened cheeses such as cottage and cream cheese, all cheese should be served unchilled to help bring out distinctive flavor and texture characteristics. This usually requires 20 minutes to 1 hour or more at room temperature. Soft and semisoft cheeses should not be kept at room temperature longer than 2 hours.

Characteristics of Some Popular Varieties of Natural Cheeses

Kind or Name Place of Origin	Kind of Milk Used in Manufacture	Ripening or Curing Time	Flavor	Body and Texture	Color	Retail Packaging	Uses
Soft, Unripened Varieties							
Cottage, plain or creamed (Unknown)	Cow's milk skimmed; plain curd, or plain curd with cream added	Unripened	Mild, acid	Soft, curd particles of varying size	White to creamy white	Cup-shaped containers, tumblers, dishes	Salads, with fruits vegetables, sandwiches, dips, cheese cake
Cream, plain (U.S.A.)	Cream from cow's milk	Unripened	Mild, acid	Soft and Smooth	White	3- to 8-oz. packages	Salads, dips, sandwiches snacks, cheese cake, desserts
Neufchatel (Nū-shä-těl') (France)	Cow's milk	Unripened	Mild, acid	Soft, smooth similar to cream cheese but lower in milk fat	White	4- to 8-oz. packages	Salads, dips, sandwiches, snacks, cheese cake, desserts

Characteristics of Some Popular Varieties of Natural Cheeses-Continued

Kind or Name Place of Origin	Kind of Milk Used in Manufacture	Ripening or Curing Time	Flavor	Body and Texture	Color	Retail Packaging	Uses
Ricotta (Rĭ-cŏl-ta) (Italy)	Cow's milk, whole or partly skimmed, or whey from cow's milk with whole or skim milk added. In Italy, whey from sheep's milk	Unripened	Sweet, nut-like	Soft, moist or dry	White	Pint and quart paper and plastic containers, 3 lb. metal cans	Appetizers, salads, snacks, lasagne, ravioli, noodles and other cooked dishes, grating, desserts
Firm, Unripened Varieties							
Gjetost,[1] (Yĕt-ôst) (Norway)	Whey from goat's milk or a mixture of whey from goat's and cow's milk	Unripened	Sweetish, Caramel	Firm, buttery consistency	Golden brown	Cubical and rectangular	Snacks, desserts, served with dark breads, crackers, biscuits or muffins

[1]Imported only

Characteristics of Some Popular Varieties of Natural Cheeses-Continued

Kind or Name Place of Origin	Kind of Milk Used in Manufacture	Ripening or Curing Time	Flavor	Body and Texture	Color	Retail Packaging	Uses
Myost (Müs-ôst) also called Primost (Prē m-ôst) (Norway)	Whey from cow's milk	Unripened	Sweetish, caramel	Firm, buttery consistency	Light brown	Cubical, cylindrical, pie-shaped wedges	Snacks, desserts, served with dark breads
Mozzarella (Mō-tsa-rel'la) also called Scamorza (Italy)	Whole or partly Skimmed cow's milk; originally made in Italy, from buffalo's milk	Unripened	Delicate, mild	Slightly firm, plastic	Creamy white	Small round or braided form, shredded, sliced	Snacks, toasted sandwiches, cheeseburgers, cooking, as in meat loaf, or topping for lasagne, pizza, and casseroles
Soft, Ripened Varieties							
Brie (Brē) (France)	Cow's milk	4 to 8 weeks	Mild to pungent	Soft, smooth when ripened	Creamy yellow interior; edible brown and white crust	Circular, pie-shaped wedges	Appetizers, sandwiches, snacks; good with crackers and fruit, dessert

461

Characteristics of Some Popular Varieties of Natural Cheeses-Continued

Kind or Name Place of Origin	Kind of Milk Used in Manufacture	Ripening or Curing Time	Flavor	Body and Texture	Color	Retail Packaging	Uses
Camembert (Kăm´ĕm-bar) (France)	Cow's milk	4 to 8 weeks	Mild to pungent	Soft, smooth; very soft when fully ripened	Creamy yellow interior; edible thin white, or gray-white crust	Small circular cakes and pieshaped portions	Appetizers, sandwiches, snacks; good with crackers and fruit such as pears and apples, dessert
Limburger (Belgium)	Cow's milk	4 to 8 weeks	Highly pungent, very strong	Soft, smooth when ripened; usually contains small irregular openings	Creamy white interior; yellow surface	Cubical, rectangular	Appetizers, snacks, good with crackers, rye or other dark breads, dessert

Characteristics of Some Popular Varieties of Natural Cheeses-Continued

Kind or Name Place of Origin	Kind of Milk Used in Manufacture	Ripening or Curing Time	Flavor	Body and Texture	Color	Retail Packaging	Uses
Bel Paese[2] (Bel Pä´-a-zě) (Italy)	Cow's milk	6 to 8 weeks	Mild to moderately robust	Soft to medium firm, creamy	Creamy yellow interior; slightly gray or brownish surface, sometimes covered with yellow wax coating	Small Wheels, wedges, segments	Appetizers; good with crackers, snacks, sandwiches, dessert
Brick (U.S.A.)	Cow's milk	2 to 4 months	Mild to moderately sharp	Semisoft to medium firm, elastic, numerous small openings	Creamy yellow	Loaf, brick, slices, cut portions	Appetizers, sandwiches, snacks, dessert
Muenster (Mŭn´stěr) (Germany)	Cow's milk	1 to 8 weeks	Mild to mellow	Semisoft, numerous small openings. Contains more moisture than brick	Creamy White interior; yellow tan surface	Circular cake, blocks, wedges, segments, slices	Appetizers, sandwiches, snacks, dessert

[2]Italian trademark-licensed for manufacture in U.S.A.; also imported.

463

Characteristics of Some Popular Varieties of Natural Cheeses-Continued

Kind or Name Place of Origin	Kind of Milk Used in Manufacture	Ripening or Curing Time	Flavor	Body and Texture	Color	Retail Packaging	Uses
Por du Salut (Por dü Sa-lü´) (France)	Cow's milk	6 to 8 weeks, robust	Mellow to robust	Semisoft, smooth, buttery, small openings	Creamy yellow	Wheels and Wedges	Appetizers, snacks, served with raw fruit, dessert
Firm, Ripened Varieties							
Cheddar (England)	Cow's milk	1 to 12 months or more	Mild to very sharp	Firm, smooth, some openings	White to medium yellow-orange	Circular, cylindrical, loaf, pie-shaped wedges, oblongs, slices, cubes, shredded, grated	Appetizers, sandwiches, sauces, on vegetables, in hot dishes, toasted sandwiches, grating, cheeseburgers, dessert
Colby (U.S.A.)	Cow's milk	1 to 3 months	Mild to mellow	Softer and more open than Cheddar	White to medium yellow-orange	Cylindrical, pie-shaped wedges	Sandwiches, snacks, cheeseburgers

Characteristics of Some Popular Varieties of Natural Cheeses-Continued

Kind or Name Place of Origin	Kind of Milk Used in Manufacture	Ripening or Curing Time	Flavor	Body and Texture	Color	Retail Packaging	Uses
Caciocavallo (Kä´-cho-kä-val´lö) (Italy)	Cow's milk. (In Italy, cow's milk or mixtures of sheep's, goat's, and cow's milk)	3 to 12 months	Piquant, similar to Provolone but not smoked	Firm, lower in milkfat and moisture than Provolone	Light or white interior; clay or tan colored surface	Spindle or ten-pin shaped, bound with cord, cut pieces	Snacks, sandwiches, cooking, dessert; suitable for grating after prolonged curing
Edam (Ḗd-ăm) (Netherlands)	Cow's milk, partly skimmed	2 to 3 months	Mellow, nut-like	Semisoft to firm, smooth; small irregularly shaped or round holes; lower milkfat than Gouda	Creamy yellow or medium yellow-orange interior; surface coated with red wax	Cannon ball shaped loaf, cut pieces, oblong	Appetizers, snacks, salads, sandwiches, seafood sauces, dessert
Gouda (Gou´-dä) (Netherlands)	Cow's milk, whole or partly skimmed	2 to 6 months	Mellow, nut-like	Semisoft to firm, smooth; small irregularly shaped or round holes; higher milkfat than Edam	Creamy yellow or medium yellow-orange interior; may or may not have wax coating	Ball-shaped with flattened top and bottom	Appetizers, snacks, salads, sandwiches, seafood sauces, dessert

465

Characteristics of Some Popular Varieties of Natural Cheeses-Continued

Kind or Name Place of Origin	Kind of Milk Used in Manufacture	Ripening or Curing Time	Flavor	Body and Texture	Color	Retail Packaging	Uses
Provolone (Prō-vō-lō-ne´), also smaller sizes and shapes called Provolette, provolocini (Italy)	Cow's milk	2 to 12 months or more	Mellow to sharp, smoky salty	Firm, smooth	Light, creamy interior; light brown or yellow surface	Pear shaped, sausage and salami shaped, wedges, slices	Appetizers, sandwiches, snacks, souffle, macaroni and spaghetti dishes, pizza; suitable for grating when fully cured and dried
Swiss, also called Emmentaler (Switzerland)	Cow's milk	3 to 9 months	Sweet, nut-like	Firm, smooth with large round eyes	Light yellow	Segments, pieces, slices	Sandwiches, snacks, sauces, fondue, cheeseburgers
Parmesan (Pär´mē-zan), also called Reggiano (Italy)	Partly Skimmed cow's milk	14 months to 2 years	Sharp, piquant	Very hard, granular, lower moisture and milkfat than Romano	Creamy white	Cylindrical, wedges, shredded, grated	Grated for season-ing in soups, or vegetables, spaghetti, ravioli, breads, popcorn; used extensively in pizza and lasagne

Characteristics of Some Popular Varieties of Natural Cheeses-Continued

Kind or Name Place of Origin	Kind of Milk Used in Manufacture	Ripening or Curing Time	Flavor	Body and Texture	Color	Retail Packaging	Uses
Romano (Rō-mä´-nō), called Sardo Romano or Pecorino Romano (Italy)	Cow's milk. In Italy, sheep's milk (Italian law)	5 to 12 months	Sharp, piquant	Very hard, granular	Yellowish-interior, greenish-black surface	Round with flat ends, wedges, shredded, grated	Seasoning in soups, casserole dishes, ravioli, sauces, breads; suitable for grating when cured for about 1 year
Sap Sago[1] (Sáp´-sä-go) (Switzerland)	Skimmed cow's milk	5 months or more	Sharp, pungent clover-like	Very hard	Light green by addition of dried, powdered clover leaves	Conical, shakers	Grated to flavor soups, meats, macaroni, spaghetti, hot vegetables; mixed with butter makes a good spread on crackers or bread
Blue-Vein Mold Ripened Varieties							
Blue, spelled Bleu on imported cheese, (France)	Cow's milk	2 to 6 months	Tangy, peppery	Semisoft, pasty, sometimes crumbly	White interior, marbled or streaked with blue veins of mold	Cylindrical, wedges, oblongs, squares, cut portions	Appetizers, salads, dips, salad dressing, sandwich spreads; good with crackers, dessert

[1]Imported only

467

Characteristics of Some Popular Varieties of Natural Cheeses-Continued

Kind or Name Place of Origin	Kind of Milk Used in Manufacture	Ripening or Curing Time	Flavor	Body and Texture	Color	Retail Packaging	Uses
Gorgonzola (Gôr-gŏn-zō-là) (Italy)	Cow's milk. In Italy, cow's milk or goat's milk or mixtures of these	3 to 12 months	Tangy, peppery	Semisoft, pasty, sometimes crumbly, lower moisture than Blue	Creamy white interior, mottled or streaked with blue-green veins of mold. Clay-colored surface	Cylindrical, wedges, oblongs	Appetizers, snacks, salads, dips, sandwich spreads; good with crackers, dessert
Roquefort[1] (Rŏk´-fêrt) or (Rŏk-fôr´)	Sheep's milk	2 to 5 months or more	Sharp, slightly peppery	Semisoft, pasty, sometimes crumbly	White or creamy white interior, marbled or streaked with blue veins of mold	Cylindrical, wedges	Appetizers, snacks salads, dips, sandwich spreads; good with crackers, dessert
Stilton[1] (England)	Cow's milk	2 to 6 months	Piquant, milder than Gorgonzola or Roquefort	Semisoft, flaky; slightly more crumbly than blue	Creamy white interior, streaked with blue-green veins of mold	Circular, wedges, oblongs	Appetizers, snacks, salads, dessert

[1]Imported only

468

Ripening Classifications

Unripened Varieties

The soft, unripened varieties such as cottage cheese contain relatively high moisture and do not undergo any curing or ripening. They are consumed fresh—soon after manufacture. Firm, unripened cheeses such as Gjetost and Mysost also may be used soon after manufacture; but, because they contain very low moisture, they may be kept for several weeks or months.

Soft, Ripened Varieties

In the soft, ripened cheeses, curing progresses from the outside, or rind of the cheese, towards the center. Particular molds and bacterial cultures that grow on the surface of some cheeses contribute to their characteristic flavor, body, and texture. Curing continues as long as the temperature is favorable. These cheeses usually contain more moisture than semisoft, ripened varieties.

Semisoft, Ripened Varieties

These cheeses ripen from the interior as well as from the surface. The process begins soon after the cheese is formed, with the aid of a characteristic mold or bacterial culture, or both. Curing continues as long as the temperature is favorable. These cheeses contain higher moisture than the firm, ripened varieties.

Firm, Ripened Varieties

These cheeses ripen with the aid of a bacterial culture distributed throughout the entire cheese. Ripening continues as long as the temperature is favorable. The rate and degree of curing is also closely related to the moisture content. Therefore, being lower in moisture than softer varieties, they usually require a longer curing time.

Very Hard, Ripened Varieties

These cheeses also are cured with the aid of a bacterial culture and enzymes. The rate of curing, however, is much slower because of the very low moisture and higher salt content

469

Blue-Vein Mold Ripened

Curing is accomplished by the aid of bacteria, but more particularly by the use of a characteristic mold culture that grows throughout the interior of the cheese to produce the familiar appearance and characteristic flavor.

Kinds of Cheese

The charts in this pamphlet will help you in learning some of the more popular and generally available varieties of natural cheese, their general classification, principal characteristics, and some of their uses.

Pasteurized Process Cheese

Pasteurized process cheese is a blend of fresh and aged natural cheeses that have been shredded, mixed and heated (pasteurized), after which no further ripening occurs. It melts easily when reheated. The blend may consist of one or more varieties of natural cheese and may contain pimentos, fruits, vegetables, or meats. Smoked cheese or smoke flavor may also be added.

The flavor of pasteurized process cheese depends largely on the flavor of the cheese used, and may be modified by flavorings added. Pasteurized Gruyere cheese has a nutsweet flavor, somewhat similar to Swiss.

Other available varieties are pasteurized process American cheese, pasteurized process Swiss cheese, pasteurized process Swiss cheese blended with American, and pasteurized Process Brick cheese.

Process cheese is packaged in slices, 1/2-, 1-, 2-, and 5-pound loaves, and cut portions. It may be used in main dishes, for snacks and cheeseburgers, with cold cuts and salads, on grilled or toasted sandwiches, in numerous sandwich combinations, and in casseroles. All pasteurized process cheese products should be kept refrigerated after opening.

Pasteurized Process Cheese Food

Pasteurized process cheese food is prepared in much the same manner as process cheese, except that it contains less cheese, with nonfat dry milk, or whey solids and water added. This results in a lower milkfat content and more moisture than in process cheese. Pasteurized process cheese food also may contain pimentos, fruits, vegetables or meats or may have a smoked flavor.

Cheese food has milder flavor and softer texture. It spreads more easily and melts more quickly than process cheese. The most popular variety is pasteurized process American cheese food, packaged in slices, rolls, links and loaves. It may be used any place where process cheese is used, although it is not likely to add as much cheese flavor.

Pasteurized Process Cheese Spread

Pasteurized process cheese spread is made in much the same manner as pasteurized process cheese food, but generally contains higher moisture, and the milkfat content is usually lower. A stabilizer is used in this product to prevent separation of ingredients. It is normally more spreadable than cheese food. Cheese spread also may contain pimentos, fruits, vegetables or meats, or may have a smoked flavor.

The flavor of pasteurized process cheese spread depends largely on the flavor of the cheese used and may be modified by added flavorings. Some available varieties are pasteurized process American cheese spread, pasteurized process pimento cheese spread, pasteurized process pineapple cheese spread, and pasteurized process Blue cheese spread.

Spreads are packaged in jars and loaves. They are convenient for use as snacks, in stuffing celery stalks, in deviled eggs, and as an ingredient in noodle casseroles, meatballs, hot vegetables, sandwiches, sauces, and dressings.

Coldpack Cheese

Coldpack cheese, or Club cheese, is a blend of one or more varieties of fresh and aged natural cheese. Coldpack cheese is similar to process cheese, except that it is mixed into a uniform product without heating. It may have a smoked flavor.

Coldpack American cheese and Coldpack Swiss cheese are the principal varieties. Their flavor, usually aged or sharp, is the same as the natural cheese used. The body is softer than natural cheese and it spreads easily.

Coldpack cheese is packed in jars, rolls, or links. It is especially good as an appetizer, snack, or dessert. Always refrigerate coldpack cheese products after opening.

471

Coldpack Cheese Food

Coldpack cheese food is prepared in the same manner as Coldpack cheese but includes dairy ingredients used in process cheese food. In addition, sweetening agents such as sugar or corn syrup may be added.

Coldpack cheese food may contain pimentos, fruits, vegetables, or meats, or may have a smoked flavor. The flavor resembles the cheese from which it is made but is milder. It is softer than natural cheese and spreads more easily due to the added ingredients and higher moisture content. It is packaged the same way as Coldpack cheese and may be served in the same manner.

For more information about nutrition, write:

U.S. Department of Agriculture
Center for Nutrition Policy and Promotion
1120 20th Street NW, Suite 200 North
Washington, DC 20036

Section 2

How to Buy Dairy Products

The many kinds of milk and dairy products on the market today give consumers a tempting variety of delicious foods from which to choose.

Points to Consider

Wholesomeness . . . quality . . . nutritive value . . . convenience . . . and informative labeling are some of the points to consider when purchasing dairy products.

Wholesomeness

Before grading or inspection of a dairy product is provided, the processing plant must meet the U.S. Department of Agriculture's specifications for quality and sanitation. A USDA dairy inspector checks the plant, incoming raw products, and processing and packaging techniques.

Nutritive Value

Milk products provide varying amounts of protein, fat, saturated fat, cholesterol, carbohydrate, vitamins, and minerals. Of all milk products, milk, yogurt, and cheese are the best sources of calcium.

Agricultural Marketing Service Home and Garden Bulletin No. 255

Some milk products contain added sugars. Some are high in sodium or fat, especially saturated fat, while others are low. Although butter is made from cream, nutritionally it is a fat and is not in the milk group of the Food Guide Pyramid. Use the Nutrition Facts panel on each individual product label to learn about the nutrient content of that food and how it fits into an overall daily diet.

Choose a diet low in fat, saturated fat, and cholesterol to help reduce the risk of getting certain diseases and to help maintain a healthy weight. The Dietary Guidelines for Americans suggest choosing a diet containing 30 percent or less of calories from fat and less than 10 percent of calories from saturated fatty acids. Also, some health authorities suggest that dietary cholesterol be limited to an average of 300 milligrams or less per day.

The Food Guide Pyramid suggests 2 to 3 servings each day of food from the milk, yogurt, and cheese group. Count as a serving: 1 cup of milk or yogurt, 1 1/2 ounces of natural cheese, or 2 ounces of process cheese.

Tips: Skim milk and plain nonfat yogurt are lowest in fat, saturated fat, and cholesterol; contain no added sugars; and should be chosen often. "Part skim" or lowfat cheeses and lower fat milk desserts, such as lowfat ice cream or frozen yogurt, are available. When you choose a higher fat milk product, balance your fat intake by choosing other foods that are low in fat.

Marks of Quality

USDA has established U.S. grade standards to describe different grades of quality in butter; Cheddar, Colby, Monterey, and Swiss cheese; and instant nonfat dry milk. FDA has established the Grade A designation for fluid milk products, yogurt, and cottage cheese.

Manufacturers use the grade standards to identify levels of quality, to have a basis for establishing prices at wholesale, and to provide consumers with a choice of quality levels.

USDA also provides inspection and grading services which manufacturers, wholesalers, or other distributors may request. A fee is charged to cover the cost of the service. Only products that are officially graded may carry the USDA grade shield.

Fat Content of Milk Products

Selected products	Total fat (grams)	Saturated (grams)	Cholesterol fatty acids (milligrams)
1 cup milk,			
skim	trace	trace	4
1 percent	3	2	10
2 percent	5	3	18
whole	8	5	33
1 cup yogurt			
nonfat plain	trace	trace	4
lowfat plain	4	2	15
½ cup cottage cheese,			
lowfat, 1% fat	1	1	5
creamed	5	3	16
1 oz. cheese,			
mozzarella, part skim milk	5	3	15
natural Cheddar	9	6	29
½ cup vanilla frozen dessert			
lowfat ice cream	3	2	9
ice cream	7	4	27
frozen yogurt	2	1	8

How USDA's Dairy Grading Program Works

The U.S. Grade AA or Grade A shield is most commonly found on butter and sometimes on Cheddar cheese.

U.S. Extra Grade is the grade name for instant nonfat dry milk of high quality. Processors who use USDA's grading and inspection service may use the official grade name or shield on the package.

475

The "Quality Approved" shield may be used on other dairy products (for example, cottage cheese) or other cheeses for which no official U.S. grade standards exist if the products have been inspected for quality under USDA's grading and inspection program.

Dairy Facts

- Milk available in stores today is usually pasteurized and homogenized. Very little raw milk is sold today.

- In pasteurizing, milk is heated briefly to kill pathogens and harmful bacteria. Then, it is rapidly chilled.

- Homogenized milk has been processed to reduce the size of the milkfat globules so the cream does not separate and the product stays uniform throughout.

- Depending on its milkfat content, fluid milk is labeled milk, lowfat milk, or skim milk (nonfat milk). Vitamin D may be added to any of these milks, and the milk is then so labeled. If added, the vitamin D content must be increased to at least 400 International Units (I.U.) per quart.

- Lowfat and skim (nonfat) milk are fortified with vitamin A (at least 2,000 I.U. per quart), usually providing more vitamin A than whole milk. The protein and other vitamin and mineral content of milks with reduced milkfat are equivalent to that of whole milk.

- Federal, State, and local laws or regulations control the composition, processing, and handling of milk. Federal laws apply when packaged or bottled milk is shipped interstate. Raw milk is prohibited from being sold interstate.

- The Pasteurized Milk Ordinance of the Food and Drug Administration (FDA) requires that all packaged or bottled milk shipped interstate be pasteurized to protect consumers. Milk can be labeled "Grade A" if it meets FDA or State standards under the Pasteurized Milk Ordinance.

- The Grade A rating designates wholesomeness or safety rather than a level of quality. According to the standards recommended in the ordinance, Grade A pasteurized milk must come from healthy cows and be produced, pasteurized, and handled under strict sanitary controls which are enforced by State and local milk sanitation officials.

- The following storage times are guidelines for maintaining the quality of milk and cream in the refrigerator at home after purchase: Fresh milk —5 days; buttermilk—10-30 days; condensed or evaporated milk—opened 4-5 days; half and half, light cream, and heavy cream—10 days; sour cream— 2-4 weeks.

Dairy Dictionary

In the definitions that follow, the composition or milkfat content given for each product (except for butter) is required under FDA regulations. State laws or regulations may differ somewhat from FDA's. The milkfat content of butter is set by a Federal law. FDA has established a regulation that allows a product to deviate from the standard composition in order to qualify for a nutrient content claim. Products such as nonfat sour cream, light eggnog, reduced fat butter, and nonfat cottage cheese fall into this category.

Milk

n   **Whole Milk:** Whole milk is usually homogenized and fortified with vitamin D. For shipment in interstate commerce, it must contain a minimum of 3.25 percent milkfat and 8.25 percent milk solids not fat (MSNF). The milk must also meet minimum milkfat requirements set by the State or municipality where it is sold.

n   **Lowfat Milk:** Lowfat milk has between 0.5 and 2 percent milkfat, contains 8.25 percent MSNF, and is fortified with vitamin A. The addition of vitamin D is optional.

Tip on Lowfat Milk: Lowfat milk can be made at home by mixing half whole milk with half skim milk or reconstituted instant nonfat dry milk.

n   **Skim milk:** (nonfat milk) must have less than 0.5 percent milkfat, contain 8.25 percent MSNF, and must be fortified with vitamin A. The addition of vitamin D is optional.

Tip on Skim Milk: The flavor and food value of skim milk can be improved by adding a teaspoonful of instant nonfat dry milk to each glass.

n **Flavored Milks:** Flavored milks are made by adding fruit, fruit juice, or other natural or artificial food flavorings such as strawberry, chocolate syrup, or cocoa to pasteurized milk.

Tips on Chocolate-Flavored Milk: Regular, lowfat, or skim chocolate-flavored milk can be heated for quick and easy hot chocolate. Use chocolate-flavored milk in cookie or cake recipes that call for both milk and chocolate or cocoa.

n **Buttermilk:** All commercially sold buttermilk is cultured. This means that a safe lactic acid-producing bacterial culture is added to freshly pasteurized skim or lowfat milk to produce the buttermilk. It is much thicker than skim milk and is higher in sodium than other milk. Buttermilk is a good thirst quencher.

Tips on Buttermilk: Always keep cultured buttermilk chilled. If it is allowed to warm, it may separate. If it does separate, just stir it. Dried buttermilk, a byproduct of buttermaking, is used in pancake mixes and bakery products.

n **Dry Whole Milk:** Dry whole milk is pasteurized whole milk with the water removed. It has limited retail distribution—mainly for use in infant feeding and for people without access to fresh milk, such as campers. Dry whole milk is usually sold to chocolate and candy manufacturers.

Tips on Dry Whole Milk: An opened package should be tightly sealed and stored in a cool, dry place. Dry whole milk develops off-flavors if not used soon after opening.

n **Nonfat Dry Milk:** Nonfat dry milk, made by removing nearly all the fat and water from pasteurized milk, contains about half the calories of whole milk. "Instant" nonfat dry milk is made of larger particles that dissolve more easily in water. Some instant nonfat dry milk contains added vitamins A and D. To earn the "U.S. Extra Grade" shield, instant nonfat dry milk must have a sweet, pleasing flavor and a natural color. It must also dissolve immediately when mixed with water.

Tips on Nonfat Dry Milk: Nonfat dry milk needs no refrigeration and can be stored for several months in a cool, dry place. An opened package should be tightly resealed. After nonfat dry milk is reconstituted, refrigerate and handle as fresh milk.

Use nonfat dry milk both as a beverage and in cooking. When used as a beverage, reconstitute it several hours before serving to allow time to chill.

n   **Evaporated Milk:** Evaporated milk is prepared by heating homogenized whole milk under a vacuum to remove half its water, sealing it in cans, and thermally processing it. When evaporated milk is mixed with an equal amount of water, its nutritive value is about the same as whole milk. Evaporated skim milk is also available.

Tips on Evaporated Milk: Always refrigerate after opening. Used full strength, evaporated milk adds extra nutritive value to the diet. Evaporated milk, with an equal amount of water added, may replace fresh milk in recipes. It can also be used in coffee or on hot or cold cereal.

n   **Sweetened Condensed Milk:** This concentrated canned milk is prepared by removing about half the water from whole milk. Often used in candy and dessert recipes, sweetened condensed milk has at least 40 percent sugar by weight.

Cream

FDA sets standards of composition for milk and different types of cream. These standards give minimum milkfat requirements, which must be met if the product is to be shipped in interstate commerce.

n   **Light Cream:** Light cream, also called coffee cream or table cream, must have at least 18 percent milkfat, but less than 30 percent.

Tips on Light Cream: For maximum shelf life, do not return unused cream from a pitcher to its original container. Store it separately in the refrigerator. Try to pour only as much from the original container as is needed at one time.

n **Half-and-Half:** Half-and-half is made by homogenizing a mixture of milk and cream. It must contain at least 10.5 percent milkfat, but not more than 18 percent.

Tip on Half-and-Half: Half-and-half can be mixed at home using equal parts homogenized whole milk and light cream.

n **Light Whipping Cream:** Light whipping cream must have at least 30 percent milkfat, but less than 36 percent

Tip on Light Whipping Cream: To whip this kind of cream, both the bowl and cream should be well chilled.

n **Heavy Cream:** Heavy cream must have at least 36 percent milkfat.

Tips on Heavy Cream: Although heavy cream is more easily whipped than light whipping cream, it will whip still more easily if the cream and the bowl are well chilled. Don't over-whip heavy cream; it may become grainy.

n **Sour Cream:** Sour cream is made by adding a special bacterial culture to light cream. The bacteria produce lactic acid, which sours the cream. Sometimes manufacturers use food-grade acid instead of bacteria to make sour cream. The product must be labeled "acidified sour cream" if this process is used. Acidified sour cream has the same wholesomeness as sour cream; the only difference is in the manufacturing process. Both sour cream and acidified sour cream are smooth and thick, and meet the milkfat requirements for light cream.

n **Sour Half-and-Half:** A bacterial culture or a food-grade acid is used to make sour half-and-half. FDA standards of identity require the product to be labeled acidified sour half-and-half if food-grade acid is used.

Tip on Sour Half-and-Half: Use sour half-and-half instead of sour cream for less fat.

Butter

Butter is made by churning pasteurized cream. Federal law requires that it contain at least 80 percent milkfat. Salt and coloring may be added. Nutritionally, butter is a fat; one tablespoon contains 12 grams total fat, 7 grams saturated fatty acids, 31 milligrams cholesterol, and 100 calories.

Whipped butter is regular butter whipped for easier spreading. Whipping increases the amount of air in butter and increases the volume of butter per pound.

The USDA grade shield on butter packages means that butter has been tested and graded by experienced government graders. In addition to checking the quality of the butter, the graders also test its keeping ability.

n   **U.S. Grade AA Butter:** has a delicate sweet flavor, with a fine, highly pleasing aroma, is made from fresh sweet cream, and has a smooth, creamy texture with good spreadability

n   **U.S. Grade A Butter:** has a pleasing flavor, is made from fresh cream, and is fairly smooth in texture

Tip on Butter: Unsalted butter may be labeled "sweet" or "unsalted" butter. Some people prefer its flavor.

When using whipped butter in place of regular butter in recipes, use 1/3 to 1/2 more than the recipe calls for if the measurement is by volume (1 cup, 1/2 cup, etc.). If the measurement is by weight (1/4 pound, 1/2 pound, etc.), use the amount called for.

Store butter in its original wrapper or container so it won't pick up flavors from other foods.

Butter thinly spread in sandwiches adds moisture and flavor, and keeps the filling from soaking the bread.

Cheese—(see Section 1)

Yogurt

Milk is cultured with a special bacteria to make custard-like yogurt. Yogurt is usually made from homogenized, pasteurized lowfat milk, and may be enriched with nonfat dry milk solids. Because it is slightly more concentrated, it is higher in several nutrients (such as calcium) than an equal amount of milk.

Tips on Yogurt: If separation occurs, just stir the liquid back into the yogurt.

Sweetened and fruit-flavored yogurt is available in sundae-style with the fruit at the bottom, and Swiss-style with the fruit distributed throughout the yogurt.

Frozen Desserts

n   **Ice Cream:** Ice cream is made from cream, milk, sweeteners, flavorings, stabilizers, and emulsifiers. To be shipped in interstate commerce, it must contain at least 10 percent milkfat.

n   **Frozen Custard:** (French Ice Cream) Frozen custard, also called French ice cream or New York ice cream, has egg yolks added.

n   **Lowfat Ice Cream:** Lowfat ice cream, or ice milk, is made from milk, stabilizers, sweeteners, and flavorings, and contains not more than 3 grams of fat per 4-ounce serving. Ice creams advertised as "reduced fat" or "light" must have a lower fat content than "regular" ice cream, but may not meet the standard for "lowfat." Soft-serve frozen desserts are similar to lowfat ice cream, but are specially processed.

n   **Sherbet:** Sherbet, made from milk, fruit or fruit juice, stabilizers, and sweeteners, has about twice as much sweetener as ice cream. It must have 1 to 2 Percent milkfat.

n   **Frozen Yogurt:** Frozen yogurts, containing sweeteners and flavorings, are available in regular and lowfat varieties.

Tips on Frozen Dessert: Keep frozen desserts in tightly closed cartons. If you store them in the freezer of your refrigerator, try to use them within a week. Frozen desserts stored in a deep freezer at temperatures below 0 °F. will keep about a month. Hard freezing prevents formation of ice crystals.

Frozen desserts are easier to serve if placed in the refrigerator before serving—about 10 minutes for a pint and 20 minutes for a half gallon.

Milk Products and Calcium

The following milk products provide the same amount of calcium as 1 cup of skim milk, but many also contain more fat and calories:

1 cup 2% fat milk

1 cup whole milk

1 cup 2% fat chocolate milk

8 ounces plain nonfat yogurt

8 ounces plain lowfat yogurt

8 ounces lowfat vanilla yogurt

8 ounces lowfat fruited yogurt

1 1/2 ounces natural cheese

2 ounces process American cheese

Note: Cottage cheese has less calcium than most other cheeses. One cup of cottage cheese contains only as much calcium as 1/2 cup of milk.

For more information about nutrition, write:

U.S. Department of Agriculture
Center for Nutrition Policy and Promotion
1120 20th Street NW, Suite 200 North
Washington, DC 20036

Section 3

How to Buy Dry Beans, Peas and Lentils

Dry beans, peas, and lentils—delicious, nutritious, low-cost foods that can be served in so many ways. But how much do you really know about these foods? For example, what is a lentil? What is the difference between black-eye peas and black-eye beans? What quality factors should you bear in mind when buying beans, peas, and lentils? How do you store and prepare them? Which need soaking and which do not before cooking? What are the varieties of beans and peas available? These are some of the factors a smart shopper should consider when buying these products.

Dry beans, and their close cousins, dry peas and lentils, are food bargains. They are an excellent source of protein—in fact, dry beans provide more protein for your money than most other foods. And the protein derived from these foods, when combined with protein from meats and other foods of animal origin, makes an unbeatable "protein team" which the body needs to build and repair vital organs and tissues.

Dry beans, peas, and lentils provide a wealth of energy and nutrition at a cost per pound that is nominal. They contain B vitamins, such as thiamin, and riboflavin, and some are a good source of calcium. They are real nuggets of mineral value for the iron they provide. A 3/4 cup serving of dried beans or dry peas, for example, provides about a third of the iron recommended daily for an adult male.

The dry bean sometimes is considered a building food, an energy food, and to some extent a protective food. Peas and lentils also fall

Agricultural Marketing Service Home and Garden Bulletin No. 177

into these same categories, and since their fat content is low they are useful in some special diets.

Buying Tips

Although there are many varieties of dry beans, peas, and lentils available in the stores. the following buying tips apply for all of them:

Federal-State Grades—

Nearly all peas and lentils and about one-third of all beans are officially inspected before or after processing. However, retail packages of beans, peas, or lentils seldom carry the Federal or State grade.

Developed by the U.S. Department of Agriculture's Agricultural Marketing Service, Federal grades for beans, peas, and lentils are generally based on the following factors: shape, size, color, damage, and foreign material. The more uniform the color and size of the product, the higher the Federal grade will be. Beans, peas, and lentils in the lower grades usually contain more foreign matter and more kernels of uneven size and off-color. Lower qualities are not usually sold through retail stores.

The Federal grades for beans, peas, and lentils you may see on the grocery shelf are normally the highest grades. Some of these higher grades are:

U.S. No. 1—for dry whole or split peas, lentils, and black-eye peas (beans).

U.S. No. 1 Choice Hand-picked, or Hand-picked—for Great Northern, pinto, and pea beans.

U.S. Extra No. 1—for lima beans, large or small.

Instead of the Federal grade on beans, you might find a State grade which is based on quality factors similar to those for Federal grades.

Quality factors—

If you do not find packages of beans, peas, or lentils marked with Federal or State grades, you can be your own "grader" in a way by looking for the same factors a Federal grader considers.

First, try to buy your beans, peas, or lentils in cellophane bags or other "see through" types of packages, such as cardboard boxes with a cellophane "window." Then, consider these factors:

Brightness of color—Beans, peas, and lentils should have a bright uniform color. Loss of color usually indicates long storage, lack of freshness, and a product that will take longer to cook. Eating quality, however, is not affected.

Uniformity of size—Look for beans, peas, or lentils of uniform size. Mixed sizes will result in uneven cooking, since smaller beans cook faster than larger ones.

Visible defects—Cracked seed coats, foreign material, and pinholes caused by insect damage are signs of a low quality product.

Read the label—

In addition to the Federal or State grade, the package label can provide other important buying information. By law, the label must contain at least the following basic information: the name and address of the manufacturer, packer, or distributor, the common or usual name of the product (pea beans, Great Northern beans, etc.), and the weight (given in pounds and ounces).

Other information on the label might include a picture of a suggested way to serve beans, peas, or lentils, and instructions on how to prepare and serve them, including recipes.

In summary, look for beans, peas, and lentils in cellophane or other clear packages which carry a Federal or State grade. If you can't find graded packages, look for a product with a bright color, beans of uniform size, and no visible damage. Read the label carefully—it may give you important instructions for preparing the product.

STORAGE TIPS

Dry beans, peas, and lentils should be kept in tightly covered containers and stored in a dry, cool place (50 to 70 degrees Fahrenheit). Stored in this manner, they will keep their quality for several months.

After opening a package, don't mix the contents with that of other packages bought at separate times, particularly several months apart.

Mixing packages will result in uneven cooking since older beans take longer to cook than fresher ones. Keep the product in the original package until opened. Then store it in a glass or metal jar or a container with a tight-fitting lid.

Preparation Tips

- Wash beans, peas, and lentils first.

- Dry beans and whole peas should be soaked before cooking to reduce the time required for cooking. Split peas used in soup and lentils may be boiled without soaking. Split peas used for other purposes hold their shape better if soaked for a short time.

- A quick and effective way to soak beans and whole peas is to start by boiling them in water for two minutes. Remove from heat, soak one hour, and they are ready to cook. Soak split peas only 1/2 hour before cooking them.

- If beans or peas are to be soaked overnight, it is still advantageous to start with the two minute boil because this will mean fewer hard skins. If the beans or peas are to be soaked overnight in a warm room, the brief boil will keep them from souring.

- A teaspoon of salt for each cup of dry beans, peas, or lentils will suit the average taste. For special flavor, add onions, herbs, or meat. Add salt and flavoring only after soaking since salt toughens the surface of the beans and increases cooking time.

- Boil gently and stir very little in order to prevent breaking of skins.

- If preferred, some dry beans and peas—including Great Northern, kidney, large lima, black, cranberry, pea (navy), and pinto beans and whole peas—can be pressure cooked in from 3-10 minutes, depending on variety. Fill pressure cooker no more than one-third full of food and water to allow for expansion. Beans and peas which normally cook in short periods of time should not be pressure-cooked. These include black eye peas (beans), lentils, and split peas.

- Always remember to allow for expansion of beans, peas, and lentils when cooking. For example, depending on the kind, one cup of the dried beans yields 2 to 2 1/2 cups of cooked beans.

The following specific information about beans, peas, and lentils should help you decide which product to buy.

Beans

Beans are among the oldest of foods and today are considered an important staple for millions of people.

They once were considered to be worth their weight in gold—the jeweler's "carat" owes its origin to a pea-like bean on the east coast of Africa.

Beans also once figured very prominently in politics. During the age of the Romans, balloting was done with beans. White beans represented a vote of approval and the dark beans meant a negative vote. Today, beans still play an active role in politics—bean soup is a daily "must" in both the Senate and the House dining rooms in the Nation's Capitol.

Beans undergo rather extensive processing before reaching the consumer. They are delivered to huge processing plants where they are cleaned to remove pods, stems, and other debris. Special machines separate debris by weight (gravity), and then screen the beans by size. Discolored beans are removed by machines equipped with photosensitive electric eyes.

Many varieties of beans may be found on the grocery shelf. Although you will not find all of them, here are some of the more popular varieties, and their uses:

Black beans (or black turtle soup beans)— They are used in thick soups and in Oriental and Mediterranean dishes.

Black-eye peas (also called black-eye beans or "cow peas")—These beans are small, oval-shaped, and creamish white with a black spot on one side. They are used primarily as a main dish vegetable. Black-eye peas are beans. There is no difference in the product, but different names are used in some regions of the country.

Garbanzo beans—Known as "chick-peas," these beans are nut-flavored and commonly pickled in vinegar and oil for salads. They can also be used as a main dish vegetable, in the "unpickled" form. Similar beans are cranberry and yellow-eye beans.

Great Northern beans—Larger than but similar to pea beans, these beans are used in soups, salads, casserole dishes, and home baked beans.

Kidney beans—These beans are large and have a red color and kidney shape. They are popular for chili con carne and add zest to salads and many Mexican dishes.

Lima beans—Not widely known as dry beans, lima beans make an excellent main dish vegetable and can be used in casseroles. They are broad and flat. Lima beans come in different sizes, but the size does not affect the quality.

Navy beans—This is a broad term which includes Great Northern, pea, flat small white, and small white beans.

Pea beans—Small, oval, and white, pea beans are a favorite for home baked beans, soups, and casseroles. They hold their shape even when cooked tender.

Pinto beans—These beans are of the same species as the kidney and red beans. Beige-colored and speckled, they are used mainly in salads and chili.

Red and pink beans—Pink beans have a more delicate flavor than red beans. Both are used in many Mexican dishes and chili. They are related to the kidney bean.

Peas

Dry peas are an interesting and versatile food group that add variety to meals. Dry peas may be green or yellow and may be bought either split or whole.

Green dry peas—This type of dry pea has a more distinct flavor than yellow dry peas. Green dry peas enjoy their greatest popularity in the United States, England, and North European countries and are gaining in popularity in Japan.

Yellow dry peas—This type of dry pea has a less pronounced flavor than other types of peas but is in popular demand in the Southern and Eastern parts of the country. They are also preferred in Eastern Canada, the Caribbean, and South America.

Dry split peas—These peas have had their skins removed and they are mainly used for split pea soup. Dry split peas also combine well with many different foods. How do split peas get split? Specially grown whole peas are dried and their skins are removed by a special machine. A second machine then breaks the peas in half.

Dry whole peas—These peas are used in making soups, casseroles, puddings, vegetable side dishes, dips, and hors d'oeuvres.

Green and yellow whole peas and green and yellow split peas, although they vary in taste a little, are used interchangeably in many recipes and in making soups. Individual preference is the deciding factor here. Remember, though, there is a difference in soaking procedure for whole and split peas.

Dry peas are served in many ways—"just plain boiled" and served with butter, for example, they serve as a welcome dish with meats, fish, poultry, and game. They can also be served as a puree and they can be made into dips, patties, croquettes, stuffed peppers, and even soufflés.

Lentils

The lentil is an old world legume that is disc-shaped, about the size of a pea. Thousands of years old, lentils were perhaps the first of the convenience foods. With no coddling at all, they cook to puffed tenderness in a mere half hour. With such a short cooking time, the use of a pressure cooker is not advised. If the cooked lentils are to be drained, as in making salad, save the cooking liquid (which is loaded with nutrients) for a cup of luncheon soup or to use in gravies and stews.

Lentils are an excellent partner with many foods—fruits, vegetables, and meat. To cook, place 2 cups of lentils in a heavy saucepan, and add 5 cups of cold or warm water and 2 teaspoons salt. Bring to boiling point, reduce heat, cover tightly, and boil gently for 30 minutes.

Coldpack Cheese Food

Coldpack cheese food is prepared in the same manner as Coldpack cheese but includes dairy ingredients used in process cheese food. In addition, sweetening agents such as sugar or corn syrup may be added.

Coldpack cheese food may contain pimentos, fruits, vegetables, or meats, or may have a smoked flavor. The flavor resembles the cheese from which it is made but is milder. It is softer than natural cheese and spreads more easily due to the added ingredients and higher moisture content. It is packaged the same way as Coldpack cheese and may be served in the same manner.

For more information about nutrition, write:

U.S. Department of Agriculture
Center for Nutrition Policy and Promotion
1120 20th Street NW, Suite 200 North
Washington, DC 20036

Section 4

How to Buy Eggs

Eggs are easy to prepare in a variety of ways. They are key ingredients in many recipes, they go well with other foods, and they are economical.

Points to Consider

Wholesomeness . . . grade . . . size . . . nutritive value . . . cost and convenience should be considered when buying eggs.

Wholesomeness

Packers who use USDA's voluntary shell egg grading service have their facilities and procedures federally approved and monitored to ensure that they meet USDA's rigid sanitary requirements. Other packers operate according to State laws.

Nutritive Value

Eggs provide protein, vitamin A, riboflavin, and other vitamins and minerals. The yolk contains all the fat, saturated fat, and cholesterol in an egg. In 1 large egg, the yolk contains 5 grams total fat, 2 grams saturated fatty acids, 213 milligrams cholesterol, and 60 calories. The egg white contains 15 calories. Use the Nutrition Facts panel on each

Agricultural Marketing Service Home and Garden Bulletin No. 264

individual product label to learn about the nutrient content of that food and how it fits into an overall daily diet.

Choose a diet low in fat, saturated fat, and cholesterol to help reduce the risk of getting certain diseases and to help maintain a healthy weight. The Dietary Guidelines for Americans suggest choosing a diet containing 30 percent or less of calories from fat, and less than 10 percent of calories from saturated fatty acids. Also, some health authorities suggest that dietary cholesterol be limited to an average of 300 milligrams or less per day.

The Food Guide Pyramid (see Chapter 2) suggests 2 to 3 servings each day of food from the meat group, the equivalent of 5 to 7 ounces of cooked lean meat, poultry, or fish. Because egg protein is of high quality, eggs are an alternative to lean meat, poultry, and fish. Count one whole egg as 1/3 serving, and remember that egg yolks should be limited to four per week.

Tips: Substitute 2 egg whites for each whole egg in muffins, cookies, puddings, and pie fillings. Some specialty egg products are available, such as liquid whole eggs that are lower in fat and cholesterol, liquid products made without yolks, and dried whites for cake decorators. When you choose a whole egg, balance your cholesterol intake by choosing other foods that are low in cholesterol.

Quality and Weight (Size) Assurance

Most eggs are packed according to official U.S. quality grade standards and weight (size) classes. The grade and weight (size) are printed on the egg carton.

The USDA grade shield on the carton means that the eggs were graded for quality and checked for weight (size) under the supervision of a technically trained USDA grader. USDA's grading service is voluntary; egg packers who request it, pay for it. Compliance with grade, weight (size), and sanitary requirements is monitored by USDA.

Egg packers who do not use the USDA grading service will put terms such as "Grade A" on their egg cartons without the shield. Their compliance with grade, weight (size), and other requirements is monitored by State agencies.

Select by Weight (Size) (U.S. Weight Class)

Size tells you the minimum required net weight per dozen eggs. It does not refer to the dimensions of an egg or how big it looks. Eggs of any weight (size) class may differ in quality. Most published recipes are based on large-size eggs.

Size or weight class	Minimum net weight per dozen
Jumbo	30 ounces
Extra Large	27 ounces
Large	24 ounces
Medium	21 ounces
Small	18 ounces
Peewee	15 ounces

Select by U.S. Grade (Quality)

There are three consumer grades for eggs: U.S. Grade AA, A, and B. The grade is determined by the interior quality of the egg and the appearance and condition of the egg shell. Eggs of any quality grade may differ in weight (size).

U.S. Grade AA eggs have whites that are thick and firm; yolks that are high, round, and practically free from defects; and clean, unbroken shells.

U.S. Grade A eggs have whites that are reasonably firm; yolks that are high, round, and practically free from defects; and clean, unbroken shells. This is the quality most often sold in stores.

U.S. Grade B eggs have whites that may be thinner and yolks that may be wider and flatter than eggs of the higher grades; the shells must be unbroken, but may show slight stains. This quality is seldom found in retail stores.

U.S. Grade AA and A eggs are good for all purposes, but especially for poaching and frying where appearance is important. U.S. Grade B eggs, if available, are fine for general cooking and baking.

The Parts of an Egg

1—Shell

Outer covering of egg, composed mainly of calcium carbonate. May be white or brown depending on breed of chicken. Color does not affect quality, flavor, cooking characteristics, nutritional value, or shell thickness.

2—Shell Membranes

Two membranes—outer and inner—just inside the shell surrounding the albumen (white). Provide protective barrier against bacterial penetration. Air cell forms between membranes.

3—Air Cell

Pocket of air usually found at large end of the egg between shell membranes. Caused by contraction of contents while egg cools after laying. Increases in size with age.

4—Outer Thin Albumen (White)

Nearest to the shell. Spreads around thick white of high-quality egg.

5—Firm or Inner Thick Albumen (White)

Excellent source of riboflavin and protein. In high-quality eggs, stands higher and spreads less than thin white. In low-quality eggs, appears like thin white.

6—Chalazae

Twisted, cord-like strands of egg white. Anchor yolk in center of thick white. Prominent, thick chalazae indicate high quality and freshness.

7—Vitelline (Yolk) Membrane

Colorless membrane surrounding yolk.

8—*Yolk*

Yellow portion of egg. Color varies with feed of the hen; does not indicate nutritional content. Major source of vitamins, minerals almost half of the protein, and all of the fat and cholesterol. Germinal disc; slight depression barely noticeable on side of yolk.

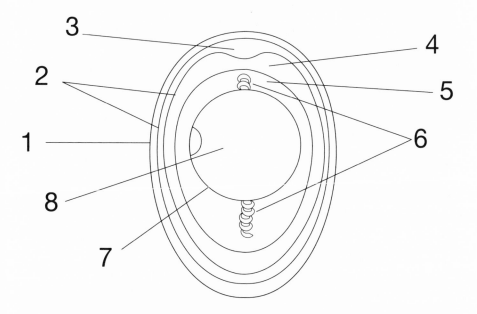

Buying and Storing Tips

Only buy refrigerated eggs with clean, unbroken shells.

It is best not to wash eggs before storing or using them. Washing is a routine part of commercial egg processing and the eggs do not need to be rewashed.

At home, keep raw eggs in their original carton on an inside shelf in the refrigerator (40 °F). For best quality, use within 5 weeks after bringing them home.

Keep hard-cooked eggs (in the shell or peeled) in the refrigerator (40 °F). Use within 1 week after cooking.

Most eggs sold today are infertile; roosters are not housed with the laying hens. Shell color depends on the breed of the hen. Yolk color depends on the feed the hen consumes. There is no nutritional difference between fertile and infertile eggs, brown- and white-shelled eggs, or pale or dark egg yolks.

Safe Handling

Wash hands, utensils, equipment, and work areas with hot, soapy water before and after they come in contact with eggs and egg-containing foods.

Remove only the number of eggs needed from the carton and return the carton to the refrigerator.

Cook eggs until the white is completely firm and the yolk begins to thicken but is not hard. Scrambled eggs should be cooked until no visible liquid remains. Fried eggs should be cooked on both sides or in a covered pan.

Take care when preparing egg-containing foods that are not cooked or are only lightly cooked before serving, such as ice cream, eggnog, mayonnaise, caesar salad, hollandaise sauce, or bearnaise sauce. Only use recipes that start with a stirred egg custard base that is first cooked to 160 °F.

If a recipe calls for adding raw eggs to a previously cooked dish, the dish must be cooked further until it reaches 160 °F.

When preparing any recipe that contains eggs, resist the temptation to taste-test the mixture during preparation. Egg-containing foods should be thoroughly cooked before eating.

When preparing and serving eggs and egg-rich foods, keep them out of the refrigerator no more than 2 hours total, not including cooking time.

If hot egg-rich foods are not going to be served immediately after cooking, put the hot foods into shallow containers and refrigerate at once so they will cool quickly.

For information about egg safety, call USDA's Meat and Poultry Hotline. The national toll-free number is 800-535-4555. In the Washington, DC, area, call (202) 720-3333.

For more information about nutrition, write:

U.S. Department of Agriculture
Center for Nutrition Policy and Promotion
1120 20th Street NW, Suite 200 North
Washington, DC 20036

Section 5

How to Buy Fresh Fruits

Walk into today's food store and you'll see fresh fruits available in fairly constant supply during the entire year. Fresh fruits add color and variety to any meal. Because of their natural sweetness, they are great for dessert and are a good lowfat snack alternative.

Points to Consider

Wholesomeness. . . quality. . . nutritive value. . . convenience. . . methods of use . . .and informative labeling are some of the points to consider when purchasing fresh fruits.

Wholesomeness

Do it yourself. There is no substitute for your own experience in choosing the right quality of fresh fruit for different uses. Tips in this section can help you achieve satisfaction and save money.

Don't buy just because of low price. It seldom pays to buy perishable fruits merely because the price is low. Unless the lower price is a result of overabundance of the fruit at the time, the so-called bargain may be undesirable.

Buy only what you need. Home refrigeration makes it possible to keep an adequate supply of most perishable fruits on hand, but never buy more than you can properly refrigerate and use without waste—even if the product is cheaper in quantity.

Agricultural Marketing Service Home and Garden Bulletin No. 260

Keep on the lookout for deterioration. Even with the most modern handling methods, product quality can decline rapidly on display. Sometimes, this off-quality fruit can be bought for less money, but the waste in preparation may offset the price reduction.

Appearance and quality are closely associated in many respects, but fine appearance does not always denote fine quality. Often a very attractive fruit may not taste good because of a varietal characteristic, or because of some internal condition such as over maturity. On the other hand, a fruit with poor appearance due to poor color or superficial blemishes may be delicious

Buy in season. Quality is usually higher and prices are more reasonable when fruit is in season. Out-of-season produce is generally more expensive.

When you must handle a fruit to judge its quality, use thoughtful care to prevent injury. Rough handling causes spoilage and waste. The consumer pays for carelessness in the long run.

Nutritive Value

Fresh fruits and fruit juices contain many vitamins and minerals, they are low in fat (except avocados) and sodium, and they provide dietary fiber. USDA nutritionists recommend 2 to 4 servings from the fruit group each day. Count as a serving an individual unit (one medium apple, pear, banana, orange), a fraction of a unit (grapefruit half, melon wedge), ½ cup berries, ½ cup chopped or cooked fruit, or ¾ cup fruit juice. Whole, unpeeled fruit is higher in fiber than peeled fruit or fruit juice.

Labeling

Under federal guidelines, a substantial number of retailers must provide nutrition information for the 20 most frequently eaten raw fruits. These fruits are: bananas, apples, watermelons, oranges, cantaloupes, grapes, grapefruit, strawberries, peaches, pears, nectarines, honeydew melons, plums, avocados, lemons, pineapples, tangerines, sweet cherries, kiwifruit, and limes. Information about other fruits may also be provided. The nutritional information may appear on posters, brochures, leaflets, or stickers near the fruit display. It may include serving size; calories per serving; amount of protein, total carbohydrates, total fat, and sodium per serving; and percent of the U.S. Recommended Daily Allowances for iron, calcium, and vitamins A and C per serving.

Quality

Some fruits are labeled with a USDA quality grade. The quality of most fresh fruits can be judged reasonably well by their external appearance. Therefore, by following the guide provided here, consumers usually can make a good selection of fresh fruits from retail display counters even without the help of a grade mark or other identification of quality.

Quality Grades For Fresh Fruit

The U.S. Department of Agriculture has established grade standards for most fresh fruits. The grades are used extensively as a basis for trading among growers, shippers, wholesalers, and retailers. Grade standards are used to a limited extent in sales from retailers to consumers.

Use of U.S. grade standards is voluntary. In most cases, however, some State laws and Federal marketing programs require grading and grade labeling of certain fruits.

Most packers grade their fruits, and some mark consumer packages with the grade. If a package carries a grade, the packer is legally obligated to make the contents measure up to official grade requirements. Some shippers, wholesalers, and distributors use USDA or State grading services.

Grade designations are most often seen on packages of pears and apples. Other fruits occasionally carry the grade designations.

U.S. Fancy Fancy means premium quality. Only a small percentage of fruits are packed in this grade.

U.S. No. 1 U.S. No. 1 means good quality and is the most commonly used grade for most fruits.

U.S. No. 2 and U.S. No. 3 U.S. No. 2 is noticeably superior to U.S. No. 3 which is the lowest grade practical to pack under normal commercial conditions.

A Consumer's Guide to Buying Fruit

The following alphabetical list of fruits is designed as a reference to help you shop more intelligently. Some of the terms used (such as "mature" and "ripe") have special meanings in the produce field. A brief glossary in the back of this section will help you understand these terms.

Apples

The many varieties of apples differ widely in appearance, flesh characteristics, seasonal availability, and suitability for different uses.

For good eating as fresh fruit, the commonly available varieties are: Red Delicious, McIntosh, Granny Smith, Empire, and Golden Delicious. For making pies and applesauce, use tart or slightly acid varieties such as Gravenstein, Grimes Golden, Jonathan, and Newtown.

For baking, the firmer fleshed varieties—Rome Beauty, Northern Spy, Rhode Island Greening, Winesap, and York Imperial—are widely used.

Look for: Firm, crisp, well-colored apples. Flavor varies in apples, and depends on the stage of maturity at the time that the fruit is picked. Apples must be mature when picked to have a good flavor, texture, and storing ability. Immature apples lack color and are usually poor in flavor. They may have a shriveled appearance after being held in storage.

Most apples are marketed by grade, and consumer packages show the variety, the grade, and the size. U.S. grades for apples are: U.S. Extra Fancy, U.S. Fancy, U.S. No. 1, and combinations of these grades. U.S. Utility is a less desirable grade. Apples from the far Western States are usually marketed under State grades which are similar to the U.S. grades.

Avoid: Overripe apples (indicated by a yielding to slight pressure on the skin, and soft, mealy flesh) and apples affected by freeze (indicated by internal breakdown and bruised areas). Scald on apples (irregularly shaped tan or brown areas) may not seriously affect the taste.

Apricots

Most fresh apricots are marketed in June and July, but a limited supply of imported apricots is available in large cities during December and January. Domestic apricots are grown principally in California, Washington, and Utah.

Apricots develop their flavor and sweetness on the tree, and should be mature but firm at the time that they are picked.

Look for: Apricots that are plump and juicy looking, with a uniform, golden-orange color. Ripe apricots will yield to gentle pressure on the skin.

Avoid: Dull-looking, soft, or mushy fruit, and very firm, pale yellow, or greenish-yellow fruit. These indicate overmaturity or immaturity, respectively.

Avocados

Avocados, grown in California and Florida, are available all year. Two general types, and a number of varieties of each, are grown. Depending upon type and variety, avocados vary greatly in shape, size, and color. Most tend to be pear-shaped, but some are almost spherical. Fruits weighing under ½ pound are most commonly available. Some have rough or leathery textured skin, while others have smooth skin. The skin color of most varieties is some shade of green, but certain varieties turn maroon, brown, or purplish-black as they ripen

Despite this variation in appearance, avocados are of good eating quality when they are properly ripened, becoming slightly soft. This ripening process normally takes from 3 to 5 days at room temperature for the quite firm avocados usually found in food stores. Ripening can be slowed by refrigeration.

Look for: For immediate use, select slightly soft avocados which yield to gentle pressure on the skin. For use in a few days, buy firm fruits that do not yield to the squeeze test. Leave them at room temperature to ripen.

Irregular light-brown markings are sometimes found on the outside skin. These markings generally have no effect on the flesh of the avocado.

Avoid: Avocados with dark sunken spots in irregular patches or cracked or broken surfaces. These are signs of decay.

An extra tip: When preparing avocados, to avoid the browning of avocado flesh when exposed to air, immediately place the peeled fruit in lemon juice until ready for use.

Bananas

Unlike most other fruits, bananas develop their best eating quality after they are harvested. This allows bananas to be shipped great distances. Almost our entire supply of bananas, available year-round, is imported from Central and South America. Bananas are sensitive to cool temperatures and will be injured in temperatures below 55 °F. For this reason, they should never be kept in the refrigerator. The ideal temperature for ripening bananas is between 60 and 70 °F. Higher temperatures cause them to ripen too rapidly.

Look for: Bananas which are firm, bright in appearance, and free from bruises or other injury. The state of ripeness is indicated by skin color. Best eating quality has been reached when the solid yellow color is specked with brown. At this stage, the flesh is mellow and the flavor is fully developed. Bananas with green tips or with practically no yellow color have not developed their full flavor potential.

Avoid: Bruised fruit (indicating rapid deterioration and waste); discolored skins (a sign of decay); a dull, grayish, aged appearance (showing that the bananas have been exposed to cold and will not ripen properly).

Occasionally, the skin may be entirely brown and yet the flesh will still be in prime condition.

Blueberries

Fresh blueberries are on the market from May through September. Generally, the large berries are cultivated varieties and the smaller berries are wild varieties.

Look for: A dark blue color with a silvery bloom is the best indication of quality. This silvery bloom is a natural, protective, waxy coating. Buy blueberries that are plump, firm, uniform in size, dry, and free from stems or leaves

Avoid: Soft, mushy, or leaking berries.

Cherries

Excellent as dessert fruit, most sweet cherries found in the food store are produced in the Western States and are available from May through August. Red tart cherries, also called sour or pie cherries and used mainly in cooked desserts, have a softer flesh, lighter red color, and a tart flavor. They generally are shipped to processing plants and are sold frozen or canned.

Look for: A very dark color is your most important indication of good flavor and maturity in sweet cherries. Bing, Black Tartarian, Schmidt, Chapman, and Republican varieties should range from deep maroon or mahogany red to black for richest flavor. Lambert cherries should be dark red. Rainier cherries should be straw-colored. Good cherries have bright, glossy, plump-looking surfaces and fresh-looking stems.

Avoid: Overmature cherries lacking in flavor, indicated by shriveling, dried stems, and a generally dull appearance. Decay is fairly common at times on sweet cherries, but because of the normal dark color, decayed areas are often inconspicuous. Soft, leaking flesh, brown discoloration, and mold growth are indications of decay.

Cranberries

A number of varieties of fresh cranberries are marketed in large volume from September through January. They differ considerably in size and color, but are not identified by variety names in your food store.

Look for: Plump, firm berries with a lustrous color provide the best quality. Duller varieties should at least have some red color.

Avoid: Brown or dark, discolored berries and soft, spongy, or leaky berries should be sorted out before cooking, because they may produce an off-flavor.

Grapefruit

Grapefruit is available all year, with most abundant supplies from January through May. While Florida is the major source of fresh grapefruit, there also is substantial production in Texas, California, and Arizona. Several varieties are marketed, but the principal distinction at retail is between those which are "seedless" (having few or no seeds) and the "seeded" type. Another distinction is color of flesh. Pink- or red-fleshed fruit is most common, but white-fleshed varieties are also available.

Grapefruit is picked "tree ripe" and is ready to eat when you buy it in the store.

Look for: Firm fruits, heavy for their size, are usually the best eating. Thin-skinned fruits have more juice than coarse-skinned ones. If a grapefruit is pointed at the stem end, it is likely to be thick-skinned. Rough, ridged, or wrinkled skin can also be an indication of thick skin, pulpiness and lack of juice.

Grapefruit often have skin defects such as scale, scars, thorn scratches, or discoloration. This usually does not affect how the fruit tastes.

Avoid: Soft, water-soaked areas, lack of bright color, and soft, tender peel that breaks easily with finger pressure are symptoms of decay.

Grapes

Most table grapes available in food stores are of the European type, grown principally in California and Arizona. Only small quantities of Eastern-grown American-type grapes are sold for table use.

European types are firm-fleshed and generally have high sugar content. Common varieties are Thompson seedless (an early, green grape), Red seedless (an early, red grape), Tokay and Cardinal (early, bright-red, seeded grapes), and Emperor (late, deep-red, seeded grapes). These all have excellent flavor when well-matured.

American-type grapes have softer flesh and are juicier than European types. The outstanding variety for flavor is the Concord, which is blue-black when fully matured. Delaware and Catawba are also popular.

Look for: Well-colored, plump grapes that are firmly attached to the stem. White or green grapes are sweetest when the color has a yellowish cast or straw color, with a tinge of amber. Red varieties are better when good red predominates on all or most of the berries. Bunches are more likely to hold together if the stems are predominantly green and pliable.

Avoid: Soft or wrinkled grapes, or bunches of grapes with stems that are brown and brittle; these are the effects of freezing or drying. Also avoid grapes with bleached areas around the stem ends (indicating injury and poor quality), and leaking berries (a sign of decay).

Kiwifruit

The kiwifruit is a relatively small, ellipsoid-shaped fruit with a bright green, slightly acid-tasting pulp surrounding many small, black, edible seeds, which in turn surround a pale heart. The exterior of the kiwifruit is unappealing to some, being somewhat "furry" and light to medium brown in color. (While the furry skin is edible, some prefer to peel the fruit before eating.) Domestic kiwifruit is produced primarily in California, but imported kiwifruit is also commonly marketed.

Look for: Plump, unwrinkled fruit, either firm or slightly yielding. Kiwifruit is fully ripe when it is yielding to the touch but not soft. Firm kiwifruit can be ripened at home in a few days by leaving it at room temperature. Use of a ripening bag or bowl will speed the process.

Avoid: Fruit that shows signs of shriveling, mold, or excessive softening, all of which indicate spoilage. Some kiwifruit may appear to have a "water-stained" exterior. This is perfectly normal for the fruit and does not affect interior quality in any way.

Note: Kiwifruit contains an enzyme, actinidin, similar to papain in papayas, that reacts chemically to break down proteins. (It has been used as a "secret ingredient" to tenderize meat.) Actinidin prevents gelatin from setting, so if you are going to serve kiwifruit in a gelatin dish, cook the fruit for a few minutes before adding it to the gelatin.

Lemons

Most of the Nation's commercial lemon supply comes from California and Arizona, and is available year round.

Look for: Lemons with a rich yellow color, reasonably smooth-textured skin with a slight gloss, and those which are firm and heavy. A pale or greenish yellow color means very fresh fruit with slightly higher acidity. Coarse or rough skin texture is a sign of thick skin and not much flesh.

Avoid: Lemons with a darker yellow or dull color, or with hardened or shriveled skin (signs of age), and those with soft spots, mold on the surface, and punctures of the skin (signs of decay).

Limes

Most limes sold at retail are produced in Florida or imported from Mexico, and are marketed when mature. Imported limes are mostly the smaller "seeded" lime.

Look for: Limes with glossy skin and heavy weight for the size.

Avoid: Limes with dull, dry skin (a sign of aging and loss of acid flavor), and those showing evidence of decay (soft spots, mold, and skin punctures.)

Melons

Selection of melons for quality and flavor is difficult, challenging the skill of even the most experienced buyer. Although no absolute formula exists, considering several factors when judging a melon will increase the likelihood of success.

Cantaloupe (Muskmelons)

Cantaloupe, generally available from May through September, are produced principally in California, Arizona, and Texas. Some are also imported early in the season.

Look for: There are three major signs of full maturity. First, the stem should be gone, leaving a smooth symmetrical, shallow base called a "full slip." If all or part of the stem base remains, or if the stem scar is jagged or torn, the melon is probably not fully matured. Second, the netting, or veining, should be thick, coarse, and corky, and should stand out in bold relief over some part of the surface. Third, the skin color (ground color) between the netting should have changed from green to yellowish-buff, yellowish-gray, or pale yellow.

Signs of ripeness: A cantaloupe might be mature, but not ripe. A ripe cantaloupe will have a yellowish cast to the rind, have a pleasant cantaloupe aroma, and yield slightly to light thumb pressure on the blossom end of the melon.

Most cantaloupe are quite firm when freshly displayed in retail stores. While some may be ripe, most have not yet reached their best eating stage. Hold them for 2 to 4 days at room temperature to allow completion of ripening. After conditioning the melons, some people like to place them in the refrigerator for a few hours before serving.

Avoid: Overripeness is indicated by a pronounced yellow rind color, a softening over the entire rind, and soft, watery, and insipid flesh. Small bruises normally will not hurt the fruit, but large bruised areas should be avoided, since they generally cause soft, water-soaked areas underneath the rind. Mold growth on the cantaloupe (particularly in the stem scar, or if the tissue under the mold is soft and wet) is a sign of decay.

Casaba

This sweet, juicy melon is normally pumpkin-shaped with a very slight tendency to be pointed at the stem end. It is not netted, but has shallow, irregular furrows running from the stem end toward the blossom end. The rind is hard with light green or yellow color. The stem does not separate from the melon, and must be cut in harvesting. The casaba melon season is from July to November. Casabas are produced in California and Arizona.

Look for: Ripe melons with a gold-yellow rind color and a slight softening at the blossom end. Casabas have no aroma.

Avoid: Dark, sunken water-soaked spots which indicate decay.

Crenshaw

Its large size and distinctive shape make this melon easy to identify. It is rounded at the blossom end and tends to be pointed at the stem end. The rind is relatively smooth with only very shallow lengthwise furrowing. The flesh is pale orange, juicy, and delicious; and generally considered outstanding in the melon family. Crenshaws are grown in California from July through October, with peak shipments in August and September.

Look for: There are three signs of ripeness. First, the rind should be generally a deep golden yellow, sometimes with small areas having a lighter shade of yellow. Second, the surface should yield slightly to moderate pressure, particularly at the blossom end. Third, the melon should have a pleasant aroma.

Avoid: Slightly sunken, water-soaked areas on the rind are signs of decay.

Honey Ball

The honey ball melon is very similar to the honey dew melon, except that it is much smaller, very round, and slightly and irregularly netted over the surface. Use the same buying tips for this melon as for the honey dew melon.

Honey Dew

The outstanding flavor characteristics of honey dews make them highly prized as a dessert fruit. The melon is large (4 to 8 lb.), bluntly oval in shape, and generally very smooth with only occasional traces of surface netting. The rind is firm and ranges from creamy white to creamy yellow, depending on the stage of ripeness. The stem does not separate from the fruit, and must be cut for harvesting.

Honey dews are available to some extent almost all year round, due in part to imports during the winter and spring. Chief sources, however, are California, Arizona, and Texas. The most abundant supplies are available from July through October.

Look for: A soft, velvety texture indicates maturity. Slight softening at the blossom end, a faint pleasant fruit aroma, and yellowish-white to creamy rind color indicate ripeness.

Avoid: Dead-white or greenish-white color and a hard, smooth feel are signs of immaturity. Large, water-soaked, bruised areas are signs of injury; and cuts or punctures through the rind usually lead to decay. Small, superficial, sunken spots do not damage the melon for immediate use, but large decayed spots will.

Persian

Persian melons resemble cantaloupe, but are more nearly round, have finer netting, and are about the same size as honey dews. The flesh is thick, fine-textured, and orange-colored. Grown primarily in California, they are available in fair supply in August and September.

Look for: The same quality and ripeness factors listed for cantaloupe apply to Persian melons.

Watermelons

Although watermelons are available to some degree from early May through September, peak supplies come in June, July, and August. Judging the quality of a watermelon is very difficult unless it is cut in half or quartered.

Look for: Firm, juicy flesh with good red color that is free from white streaks; and seeds which are dark brown or black. Seedless watermelons often contain small white, immature seeds, which are normal for this type.

Avoid: Melons with pale-colored flesh, white streaks (or "white heart"), and whitish seeds (indicating immaturity). Dry, mealy flesh, or watery stringy flesh are signs of overmaturity or aging after harvest.

If you want to buy an uncut watermelon, here are a few appearance factors which may be helpful (though not totally reliable) in guiding you to a satisfactory selection. The watermelon surface should be relatively smooth; the rind should have a slight dullness (neither shiny nor dull); the ends of the melon should be filled out and rounded; and the underside, or "belly" of the melon should have a creamy color.

Nectarines

This fruit, available from June through September from California, combines characteristics of both the peach and the plum.

Look for: Rich color and plumpness, and a slight softening along the "seam" of the nectarine. Most varieties have an orange-yellow background color between the red areas, but some varieties have a greenish background color. Bright-looking fruits which are firm to moderately hard will probably ripen normally within 2 or 3 days at room temperature.

Avoid: Hard, dull fruits or slightly shriveled fruits (which may be immature—picked too soon—and of poor eating quality) and soft or overripe fruits or those with cracked or punctured skin or other signs of decay.

Russeting or staining of the skin may affect the appearance but not detract from the internal quality of the nectarine.

Oranges

California, Florida, Texas, and Arizona produce our year-round supply of oranges.

Leading varieties from California and Arizona are the Washington Navel and the Valencia, both characterized by a rich orange skin color. The Navel orange, available from November until early May, has a thicker, somewhat more pebbled skin than the Valencia; the skin is more easily removed by hand, and the segments separate more readily. It is ideally suited for eating as a whole fruit or in segments in salads. The western Valencia orange, available from late April through October, is excellent either for juicing or for slicing in salads.

Florida and Texas orange crops are marketed from early October until late June. Parson Brown and Hamlin are early varieties, while the Pineapple orange—an important, high-quality orange for eating— is available from late November through March. Florida and Texas Valencias are marketed from late March through June. The Florida Temple orange is available from early December until early March. Somewhat like the California Navel, it peels easily, separates into segments readily, and has excellent flavor.

Oranges are required by strict State regulations to be mature before being harvested and shipped out of the producing State. Thus, skin color is not a reliable index of quality, and a greenish cast or green spots do not mean that the orange is immature. Often fully matured oranges will turn greenish (called "regreening") late in the marketing season. Some oranges are artificially colored to improve their appearance. This practice has no effect on eating quality, but artificially colored fruits must be labeled "color added."

"Discoloration" is often found on Florida and Texas oranges, but not on California oranges. This is a tan, brown, or blackish mottling or specking over the skin. It has no effect on eating quality, and in fact often occurs on oranges with thin skin and superior eating quality.

Look for: Firm and heavy oranges with fresh, bright-looking skin which is reasonably smooth for the variety.

Avoid: Light-weight oranges, which are likely to lack flesh content and juice. Very rough skin texture indicates abnormally thick skin and less flesh. Dull, dry skin and spongy texture indicate aging and deteriorated eating quality. Also avoid decay— shown by cuts or skin punctures, soft spots on the surface, and discolored, weakened areas of skin around the stem end or button.

Peaches

A great many varieties of peaches are grown, but only an expert can distinguish one from another. These varieties, available May to November, fall into two general types: freestone (flesh readily separates from the pit) and clingstone (flesh clings tightly to the pit). Freestones are usually preferred for eating fresh or for freezing, while clingstones are used primarily for canning, although they are sometimes sold fresh.

Look for: Peaches which are fairly firm or becoming a trifle soft. The skin color between the red areas (ground color) should be yellow or at least creamy.

Avoid: Very firm or hard peaches with a distinctly green ground color, which are probably immature and won't ripen properly. Also avoid very soft fruits which are overripe. Don't buy peaches with large flattened bruises (they'll have large areas of discolored flesh underneath) or peaches with any sign of decay. Decay starts as a pale tan spot which expands in a circle and gradually turns darker in color.

Pears

The most popular variety of pear is the Bartlett, which is produced in great quantities (in California, Washington, and Oregon) both for canning and for sale as a fresh fruit. With the aid of cold storage, Bartlett pears are available from early August through November.

Several fall and winter varieties of pears are grown in Washington, Oregon, and California, and shipped to fresh fruit markets. These varieties—Anjou, Bosc, Winter Nellis, and Comice—keep well in cold storage and are available over a long period, from November until May.

Look for: Firm pears of all varieties. The color depends on variety. For Bartletts, look for a pale yellow to rich yellow color; Anjou or Comice—light green to yellowish-green; Bosc—greenish-yellow to brownish-yellow (the brown cast is caused by skin russeting, a characteristic of the Bosc pear); Winter Nellis—medium to light green.

Pears which are hard when you find them in the food store will probably ripen if kept at room temperature, but it is wise to select pears that have already begun to soften—to be reasonably sure that they will ripen satisfactorily.

Avoid: Wilted or shriveled pears with dull-appearing skin and slight weakening of the flesh near the stem, which indicates immaturity. These pears will not ripen. Also avoid spots on the sides or blossom ends of the pear, which means that corky tissue may be underneath.

Pineapples

Pineapples are available all year, but are most abundant from March through June. Hawaii, Puerto Rico, and Mexico are principal suppliers. Present marketing practices, including air shipments, allow pineapples to be harvested as nearly ripe as possible. They are delivered to market near the peak of sweetness, with color ranging from green to orange and yellow. A mature green pineapple will normally turn yellow to orange within a few days at room temperature, but many are already fully colored when you find them in the food store.

Look for: Bright color, fragrant pineapple aroma, and a very slight separation of the eyes or pips—the berry-like fruitlets patterned in a spiral on the fruit core. At their mature stage, pineapples are usually dark green, firm, plump, and heavy for their size. The larger the fruit, the greater the proportion of edible flesh.

As the popular varieties ripen, the green color turns to orange and yellow. When fully colored, pineapples are golden yellow, orange-yellow, or reddish brown, depending on the variety.

Avoid: Pineapples with sunken or slightly pointed pips, dull yellowish-green color, and dried appearance—all signs of immaturity. Also avoid bruised fruit, shown by discolored or soft spots, which are susceptible to decay. Other signs of decay are traces of mold, unpleasant odor, and eyes which are dark and watery.

Plums and Prunes

Quality characteristics for both are very similar, and the same buying tips apply to both.

Plums—A number of varieties of plums are produced in California and are available from June to September. Varieties differ slightly in appearance and flavor, so you should buy and taste one to see if that variety appeals to you.

Prunes—Only a few varieties of prunes are commonly marketed, and they are all very similar. Prunes are purplish-black or bluish-black, with a moderately firm flesh which separates freely from the pit. Most commercial production is in the Northwestern States. Fresh prunes are available in food stores from August through October.

Look for: Plums and prunes with a good color for the variety, in a fairly firm to slightly soft stage of ripeness.

Avoid: Fruits with skin breaks, punctures, or brownish discoloration. Also avoid immature fruits (relatively hard, poorly colored, very tart, sometimes shriveled) and overmature fruits (excessively soft, possibly leaking or decaying)

Raspberries, Boysenberries, etc.

Blackberries, raspberries, dewberries, loganberries, and youngberries are similar in general structure. They differ from one another in shape or color, but quality factors are about the same for all.

Look for: A bright, clean appearance and a uniform good color for the species. The individual small cells making up the berry should be plump and tender but not mushy. Look for berries that are fully ripened, with no attached stem caps.

Avoid: Leaky and moldy berries. You can usually spot them through the openings in the ventilated plastic containers. Also look for wet or stained spots on wood or fiber containers, as possible signs of poor quality or spoiled berries.

Strawberries

First shipments of strawberries come from southern Florida in January, and then production increases, gradually spreading north and west into many parts of the country before tapering off in the fall. Strawberries are in best supply in May and June.

Look for: Berries with a full red color and a bright luster, firm flesh, and the cap stem still attached. The berries should be dry and clean, and usually medium to small strawberries have better eating quality than large ones.

Avoid: Berries with large uncolored areas or with large seedy areas (poor in flavor and texture), a full shrunken appearance or softness (signs of overripeness or decay), or those with mold, which can spread rapidly from one berry to another.

Note: In most containers of strawberries you will likely find a few that are less desirable than others. Try to look at some berries lower in the container to be sure that they are reasonably free from defects or decay.

Tangerines

Florida is the chief source of tangerines. Considerable quantities of tangerines and similar types of oranges are produced in California and Arizona, some in Texas, and few are imported. Tangerines are available from late November until early March, with peak supplies in December and January. The Murcott, a large, excellent variety of orange resembling the tangerine, is available from late February through April.

Look for: Deep yellow or orange color and a bright luster is your best sign of fresh, mature, good-flavored tangerines. Because of the typically loose nature of tangerine skins, they will frequently not feel firm to the touch

Avoid: Very pale yellow or greenish fruits, which are likely to be lacking in flavor (although small green areas on otherwise high-colored fruit are not bad), and tangerines with cut or punctured skins or very soft spots (all signs of decay, which spreads rapidly).

A Consumer's Glossary of Fruit Terms

Blossom end—The opposite end from the stem end. The stem end will have a scar or remains of the stem. The blossom end is often more rounded.

Breakdown of tissue—Decomposition or breaking down of cells due to pressure (bruise) or age (internal breakdown).

Decay—Decomposition of the fruit due to bacteria or fungus infection.

Ground Color—The basic or background color of a fruit before the sun's rays cause the skin to redden. The ground color may be seen beneath and between the red blush of the fruit.

Degree of Ripeness—The terms "hard," "firm," and "soft" are subjective terms used to describe the degrees of maturity or ripeness of a fruit. A "hard" texture will not give when pressed. A "firm" texture will give slightly to pressure. A "soft" texture will be soft to the touch.

Mature—Describes a fruit that is ready to be picked, whether or not it is ripe at this time. If a fruit is picked when mature, it can ripen properly, but if picked when immature, it cannot ripen properly.

Netting—The vein-like network of lines running randomly across the rinds of some melons.

Ripe—Describes a fruit that is ready to be eaten.

Russeting—A lacy, brownish, blemish-type coating on top of the skin.

For information about nutrition, write:

U.S. Department of Agriculture,
Human Nutrition Information Service,
6505 Belcrest Road,
Hyattsville, MD 20782.

517

Section 6

How to Buy Canned And Frozen Fruits

Canned and frozen fruits, preserved at the peak of goodness, are ready to serve straight from the container and are delicious ingredients in salads, sauces, desserts, and other dishes. They are convenient to use and are always available.

Points to Consider

Nutritive value . . . wholesomeness . . . quality . . . convenience . . . methods of use . . . and informative labeling are some of the points to consider when purchasing canned and frozen fruits.

Nutritive Value

Canned and frozen fruits and fruit juices contain many vitamins and minerals, they are low in fat and sodium. Fruits provide dietary fiber. USDA nutritionists recommend 2 to 4 servings from the fruit group each day. Count as a serving ½ cup canned or frozen fruit or ¾ cup fruit juice. Canned and frozen fruits processed in juice have fewer calories than products in heavy syrups or with added sweeteners. Count only 100 percent fruit juice as fruit.

Agricultural Marketing Service Home and Garden Bulletin No. 261

Wholesomeness

When buying canned fruit, avoid cans that show signs of bulging or swelling at the ends, or of leakage. Small dents in a can usually will not harm the contents unless the dents have pierced the metal or loosened the can seam. Badly dented cans, however, should always be avoided.

Fruits sold in glass jars with twist-off lids are tightly sealed to preserve the contents. If you find any indication that the lid has been tampered with, return the jar to the store and report it to the store manager.

Frozen fruits should be frozen solid. If fruits in a package are not firm, they may have lost quality. Avoid buying frozen fruit with stains on the package since this may indicate that the fruit was defrosted at some time during marketing. To ensure the quality of frozen fruits, pick them up as the last item while shopping, take them home in an insulated bag and store in a freezing compartment immediately.

Grades for Canned and Frozen Fruits

Processed fruits vary in quality based on taste, texture, appearance, and how they are prepared. They are usually priced according to their quality. Because different qualities of fruits are suited to different uses, you can make better buys by choosing processed fruits of the quality that fits your needs.

The U.S. Department of Agriculture's Agricultural Marketing Service has established U.S. grade standards as measures of quality for many canned and frozen fruits. USDA provides an inspection service which certifies the quality of processed fruits on the basis of these U.S. grade standards. The inspection service is voluntary and paid for by the user. Under the program, processed fruits are inspected by highly trained specialists during all phases of preparation, processing, and packaging.

Many processors, wholesalers, buyers for food retailers, and others use the USDA grade standards to establish the value of a product described by the grades. If you've been selecting canned or frozen fruits by habit, or can't tell which can or package would be best for the use you have in mind, here's some information that can help you make a wise choice.

U.S. Grade A Grade A fruits are the very best, with an excellent color and uniform size, weight, and shape. Having the proper ripeness and few or no blemishes, fruits of this grade are excellent to use for special purposes where appearance and flavor are important.

This highest grade of fruits is the most flavorful and attractive, and therefore, usually the most expensive. They are excellent to use for special luncheons or dinners, served as dessert, used in fruit plates, or broiled or baked to serve with meat entrees.

U.S. Grade B Grade B fruits make up much of the fruits that are processed and are of very good quality. Only slightly less perfect than Grade A in color, uniformity, and texture, Grade B fruits have good flavor and are suitable for most uses.

Grade B fruits, which are not quite as attractive or tasty as Grade A, are of good quality. They have many uses: as breakfast fruits, in gelatin molds, fruit cups or compotes, topping for ice cream, or as side dishes.

U.S. Grade C Grade C fruits may contain some broken and uneven pieces. While flavor may not be as sweet as in higher qualities, these fruits are still good and wholesome. They are useful where color and texture are not of great importance, such as in puddings, jams. and frozen desserts.

Grade C fruits vary more in taste and appearance than the higher grades and they cost less. They are useful in many dishes, especially where appearance is not important; for example, in sauces for meats, in cobblers, tarts, upside-down cakes, frozen desserts, jams, or puddings.

Other names are often used to describe the quality grades of canned and frozen fruits—Grade A as "Fancy," Grade B as "Choice," and Grade C as "Standard."

The brand name of a frozen or canned fruit may also be an indication of quality. Producers of nationally advertised brand name products spend considerable effort to maintain the same quality for a particular brand, year after year. Unadvertised brands may offer an assurance of a specific quality level, often at a slightly lower price. Many stores, particularly chain stores, carry two or more qualities under their own name labels (private labels).

Labels

When a product has been officially graded under continuous inspection, labels may carry the official grade name and the statement "Packed under continuous inspection of the U.S. Department of Agriculture." The grade name and the statement may also appear within shields or without shields.

You may find the USDA grade shield on cans or packages of fruits that have been packed under continuous USDA inspection.

The grade name, such as "Fancy" or "Grade A," is sometimes shown on the label without "U.S." in front of it. If the grade name alone appears on a container, the contents should meet the quality for the grade shown, even though the product may not have been officially inspected for grade.

Federal regulations require that the following information be included on the front panel of the label of a can or package:

- The common or usual name of the fruit.

- The form (or style) of fruit, such as whole, slices, or halves. If the form is visible through the package, it need not be stated.

- For some fruits, the variety or color.

- Liquid in which a fruit is packaged must be listed near the name of the product.

- The total contents (net weight) must be stated in ounces for containers holding 1 pound or less. Weight must be given both in total ounces and in pounds and ounces (or pounds and fractions of a pound) for products containing a net weight of 1 to 4 pounds.

The net weight shown on a label includes both fruit and liquid. For the best buy, figure out the cost per ounce. Large containers often cost less per ounce, but not always.

Other information required on the label, although not on the front panel, is:

- Ingredients, such as spices, flavoring, coloring.

- Special sweetener, if used.

- Any special type of treatment.

- The packer's or distributor's name and place of business.

- Nutritional information.

- Labels may also give the quality or grade, count, size, and maturity of the fruit, cooking directions and recipes or serving ideas.

For information about nutrition, write:

U.S. Department of Agriculture,
Human Nutrition Information Service,
6505 Belcrest Road,
Hyattsville, MD 20782.

Section 7

How to Buy Meat

Consumers buy meat because they like its taste and flexibility for being prepared in a variety of ways for just about any occasion.

Points to Consider

Wholesomeness . . . quality . . . nutritive value . . . cost . . . convenience . . . and informative labeling are some of the points to consider when making meat purchase decisions.

Also consider the amount of meat that can be stored in the freezer, the amount of raw meat that can be used within a few days of purchase, and the kinds of cuts and quality preferred.

Wholesomeness

All meat processed in plants which sell their products across State lines must, under Federal law, be inspected for wholesomeness by USDA's Food Safety and Inspection Service. This mandatory inspection program is paid for by tax dollars. Many States operate their own inspection program for plants that produce meat for sale within State lines. These programs must be certified by USDA as equal to the Federal program. Federal and State inspectors supervise the cleanliness and operating procedures of meat packing and processing plants to make sure meat is not contaminated or adulterated

Agricultural Marketing Service Home and Garden Bulletin No. 265

Meat that has passed Federal inspection for wholesomeness is stamped with a round purple mark, "U.S. INSP'D & P'S'D." The mark is put on carcasses and major cuts, so it might not appear on such cuts as roasts and steaks. However, meat that is packaged in an inspected facility will have an inspection legend which identifies the plant on the label.

Labeling for Safety

Meat inspection procedures are designed to minimize the likelihood of harmful bacteria being present in meat products. However, some bacteria could be present and could become a problem if the meat is not handled properly. That's why it's important to handle meat properly during storage and preparation. USDA requires that safe handling and cooking instructions be put on all packages of raw meat. This includes any meat product not considered "ready to eat."

Safe Handling Instructions

This product was inspected for your safety. Some animal products may contain bacteria that could cause illness if the product is mishandled or cooked improperly. For your protection, follow these safe handling instructions.

Keep refrigerated or frozen. Thaw in refrigerator or microwave.

Keep raw (meats or poultry) separate from other foods. Wash working surfaces (including cutting boards), untensils, and hands after touching raw (meat or poultry).

Cook thoroughly.

Refrigerate leftovers within 2 hours.

Processed meat products that are considered "ready-to-eat"—such as hot dogs, luncheon meats, or canned ham—are also perishable. They should be refrigerated and handled with care to prevent spoilage.

Information about meat inspection and safety should be directed to USDA's Meat and Poultry Hotline. The national toll free number is 800-535-4555. In the Washington, DC, area, call (202) 720-3333.

Nutritive Value

Meat is a source of protein, niacin, vitamins B_6 and B_{12}, iron, phosphorus, and zinc. Fat, saturated fat, and cholesterol are also present in all meat; the amount varies depending on the species, the cut of meat, and the amount of marbling (fat) that is distributed within the lean. Use the Nutrition Facts panel on each individual product label to learn about the nutrient content of that food and how it fits into an overall daily diet. The nutrition Facts panel must appear on all processed meat products, while its use is voluntary on single-ingredient raw meat.

Choose a diet low in fat, saturated fat, and cholesterol to help reduce the risk of getting certain diseases and to help maintain a healthy weight. The Dietary Guidelines for Americans suggests choosing a diet containing 30 percent or less of calories from fat, and less than 10 percent of calories from saturated fatty acids. Also, some health authorities suggest that dietary cholesterol be limited to an average of 300 milligrams or less per day.

The Food Guide Pyramid (see Chapter 2) suggests 2 to 3 servings each day of food from the meat group, the equivalent of 5 to 7 ounces of cooked lean meat, poultry, or fish. Count as a serving 2 to 3 ounces of cooked lean meat, about the size of an average hamburger or a deck of playing cards.

Tips: Buy lean cuts of meat, those with less marbling (fat) distributed within the lean. Most of the visible fat is trimmed before meat is sold to consumers, and any remaining visible fat can be trimmed off. Ground beef can contain variable amounts of fat. To reduce fat in cooked meats, broil, roast, bake, simmer, or microwave meat rather than fry. Drain and discard any fat that accumulates during cooking. Organ meats are high in cholesterol and should only be eaten occasionally. When you select cuts of meat with a higher fat content, balance your fat intake by choosing other foods that are low in fat.

Fat Content of Typical Retail Meat Products

Selected meat products, 3 ounces	Total fat (grams)	Saturated fatty acids (grams)	Cholesterol (milligrams)	Calories (Kcal)
Beef eye or round, roasted, 1/4" trim				
lean only				
USDA Select	3	1	59	136
USDA Choice	5	2	59	149
lean and fat				
USDA Select	10	4	61	184
USDA Choice	12	5	62	205
Beef ribeye steak, broiled 0" trim				
lean only				
USDA Select	7	3	68	168
USDA Choice	10	4	68	191
lean and fat				
USDA Select	17	7	70	242
USDA Choice	19	8	70	265
Ground beef patty, cooked				
extra lean	14	5	71	215
regular	17	7	76	245
Pork center loin, roasted				
lean only	8	3	67	150
lean and fat	11	4	68	180
Beef liver, braised	4	2	331	135

Quality

Quite apart from the wholesomeness of meat is its quality—its tenderness, juiciness, and flavor. Consumers can be assured of always getting the quality of meat they expect by looking for the USDA grade shield on raw meat packages. The shield-shaped USDA grade mark is a guide to the quality of meat. It's also your assurance that the meat is wholesome because only meat that has first passed inspection for wholesomeness may be graded. USDA's quality grading program is voluntary and paid for by user fees.

USDA's Meat Grading Program

USDA has quality grades for beef, veal, lamb, yearling mutton, and mutton. It also has yield grades for beef, pork, and lamb. Although there are USDA quality grades for pork, these do not carry through to the retail level as do the grades for other kinds of meat.

USDA meat grades are based on nationally uniform Federal standards of quality. They are applied by experienced USDA graders, who are routinely checked by supervisors who travel throughout the country to make sure that all graders are interpreting and applying the standards in a uniform manner. A USDA Choice rib roast, for example, must have met the same grade criteria no matter where or when you buy it.

When meat is graded, a shield-shaped purple mark is stamped on the carcass. With today's close trimming at the retail level, however, you may not see the USDA grade shield on meat cuts at the store. Instead, retailers put stickers with the USDA grade shield on individual packages of meat. In addition, grade shields and inspection legends may appear on bags containing larger wholesale cuts.

Using USDA Meat Grades

Since many cuts of meat—such as steaks, chops, and roasts - are labeled with a USDA grade, you don't have to be a meat expert to identify the quality you want.

Just look in the meat counter or case until you find the cut you want. Then, look for the USDA quality shield on the package to make sure you're getting the quality you want.

Some meat counters may contain meat that isn't USDA graded. Instead, it may be labeled with a company's private quality label or sold without a grade. Where this occurs, you will need to become familiar with the purchase specifications of each company to be sure of the quality you are buying.

Sometimes a store will advertise that it sells USDA-graded meat, but the individual packages don't bear a USDA grade shield. When this happens, you can ask to see some of the boxes of untrimmed wholesale cuts to determine if the meat has actually been graded by USDA and what the quality is.

Buying Beef

Regardless of their quality grade, some cuts of meat are naturally more tender than others. Cuts from the less-used muscles along the back of the animal—the rib and loin sections - will always be more tender than those from the more active muscles such as the shoulder, flank, and leg.

Since the most tender cuts make up only a small proportion of a beef or lamb carcass, they are in greatest demand and usually command a higher price than other cuts.

Each USDA beef quality grade is a measure of a distinct level of quality - and it takes eight grades to span the range. They are USDA Prime, Choice, Select, Standard, Commercial, Utility, Cutter, and Canner.

USDA Prime, Choice, Select, and Standard grades come from younger beef. The highest grade, USDA Prime, is used mostly by hotels and restaurants, but a small amount is sold at retail markets. The grade most widely sold at retail is USDA Choice. However, consumer preference for leaner beef has increased the popularity of the Select grade of beef. Select grade can now be found at most meat counters.

Standard and Commercial grade beef frequently is sold as ungraded or as "brand name" meat.

The three lower grades - USDA Utility, Cutter, and Canner - are seldom, if ever, sold at retail but are used instead to make ground beef and manufactured meat items such as frankfurters.

Following are photographs of rib steaks in the top three beef grades, together with a description of the level of quality that can be expected in each of these grades.

USDA Prime:

Prime grade beef is the ultimate in tenderness, juiciness, and flavor. It has abundant marbling—flecks of fat within the lean—which enhances both flavor and juiciness. Prime roasts and steaks are unexcelled for dry-heat cooking (roasting and broiling).

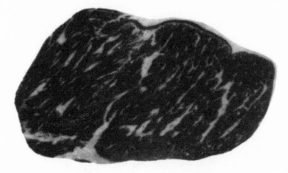

USDA Choice:

Choice grade beef has less marbling than Prime, but is of very high quality. Choice roasts and steaks from the loin and rib will be very tender, juicy, and flavorful and are, like Prime, suited to dry-heat cooking. Many of the less tender cuts, such as those from the rump, round, and blade chuck, can also be cooked with dry heat.

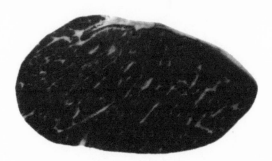

531

USDA Select:

Select grade beef is very uniform in quality and somewhat leaner than the higher grades. It is fairly tender, but, because it has less marbling, it may lack some of the juiciness and flavor of the higher grades. Only the tender cuts should be cooked with dry heat. Other cuts should be marinated before cooking or cooked with moisture to obtain maximum tenderness and flavor.

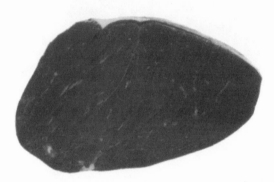

Buying Lamb

Lamb is produced from animals less than a year old. Since the quality of lamb varies according to the age of the animal, it is advisable to buy lamb that has been USDA-graded.

USDA Prime:

Prime grade lamb is very high in tenderness, juiciness, and flavor. It has moderate marbling, which enhances both flavor and juiciness. Prime chops and roasts are excellent for dry-heat cooking (broiling and roasting).

USDA Choice:

Choice grade lamb has slightly less marbling than Prime, but still is of very high quality. Choice chops and roasts also are very tender, juicy, and flavorful and suited to dry-heat cooking. Lower grades of lamb and mutton (USDA Good, Utility, and Cull) are seldom marked with the grade if sold at retail.

Most cuts of USDA Prime and Choice lamb—including shoulder cuts—are tender and can be oven roasted, broiled, or pan broiled. A leg of lamb graded Choice or Prime, for example, is delectable when oven roasted.

The less tender cuts - the breast, riblets, neck, and shank - can be braised slowly to make excellent (and tender) lamb dishes.

Meat from older sheep is called yearling mutton or mutton and, if it is graded, these words will be stamped on the meat along with the shield-shaped grade mark. Grades for yearling mutton and mutton are the same as for lamb, except that mutton does not qualify for the Prime grade and the Cull grade applies only to mutton.

The best way to identify lamb cuts is with the lamb carcass chart shown on the following pages. These terms are generally recognized throughout the meat industry.

Buying Pork

Like lamb, pork is generally produced from young animals and is, therefore, less variable in tenderness than beef. However, there is another reason why pork is less variable. Producers have responded to consumer demand by actually changing their feeding and management programs. They've even changed the genetic makeup of their breeding stock to consistently produce leaner carcasses. Also, most visible fat is trimmed off at the processing plant. Because of these changes, today's fresh pork products have considerably less fat than they did just a decade ago.

Because of this consistency, USDA grades for pork reflect only two levels of quality—Acceptable and Unacceptable. Acceptable quality pork is also graded for yield, i.e., the yield ratio of lean to waste. Unacceptable quality pork—which includes meat that is soft and watery—is graded U.S. Utility.

In buying pork, look for cuts with a relatively small amount of fat over the outside and with meat that is firm and grayish pink color. For best flavor and tenderness, meat should have a small amount of marbling.

The Versatility of Pork

Pork's consistency makes it suitable for a variety of cooking styles. However, like beef and lamb, the cut affects the cooking method.

Following are some of the more popular pork cuts and suggested methods of cooking:

Pork chops come in a variety of cuts - center loin, rib chops, sirloin chops, boneless or bone-in. They can be prepared by pan broiling, grilling, baking, braising, or sauteing. Thin chops (1/4 - 3/8 inch) are best sauteed. Boneless chops cook more quickly than bone-in chops

Ribs are available as spareribs, back ribs, and country-style ribs. Spareribs come from the belly portion, while back ribs and country-style ribs come from the loin. All three styles can be braised or roasted in the oven or on the barbecue grill. Slow cooking yields the most tender and flavorful results.

Tenderloins are considered to be the most tender and tasty cut of pork. Extremely lean, tenderloins can be roasted whole, cut into cubes for kabobs or into strips for stir-fry, and sliced for scaloppini or medallions.

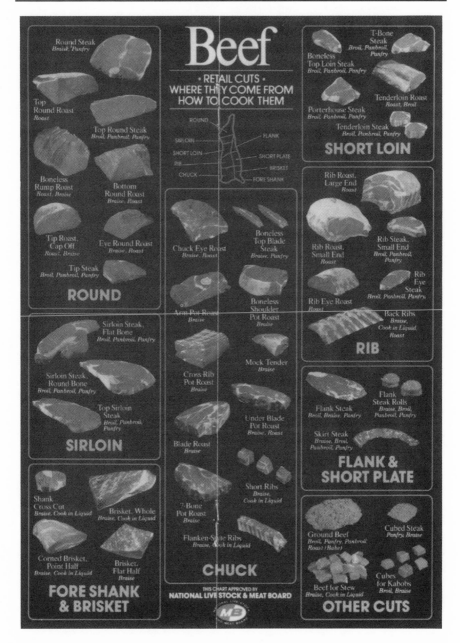

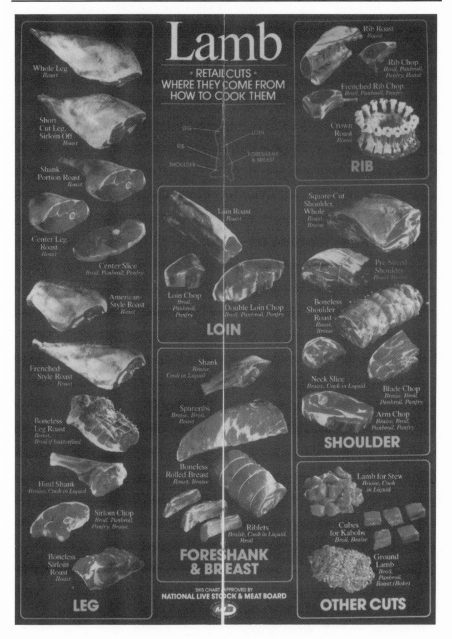

536

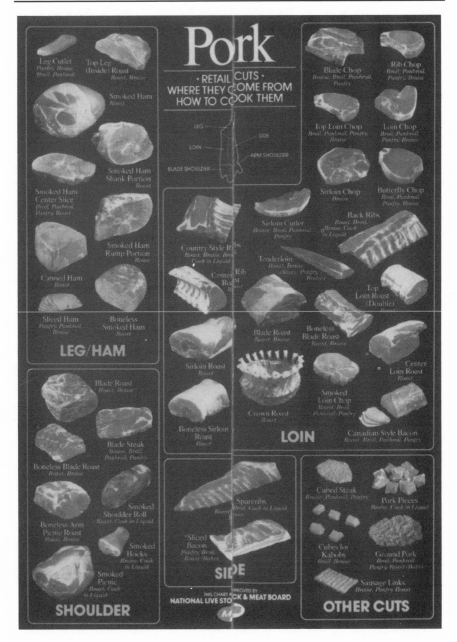

Storing Meat

Properly wrapped meat cuts, frozen at 0 °F, or lower, will maintain their quality for several months. This varies, however, with the kind of meat. The following table shows a range within which you can store meat with reasonable expectation that it will maintain its quality. Meats can be kept safely frozen for longer periods than indicated, but they are apt to lose quality.

Suggested Storage Times for Raw Meat

Product	Freezer (0 °F)	Refrigerator (40 °F)
Beef, roasts and steaks	6-12 months	3-5 days
Lamb, roasts and chops	6-9 months	3-5 days
Pork, roasts and chops	4-6 months	3-5 days
Beef and lamb, ground	3-4 months	1-2 days
Pork, sausage	1-2 months	1-2 days

On the average, 1 cubic foot of freezer space will accommodate 35 to 40 pounds of cut and wrapped meat, slightly less if the meat is packaged in odd shapes.

Meat should be initially frozen at -10 °F, or lower, and as quickly as possible. If you are freezing it yourself, allow some space for air to circulate between the packages.

Buying Meat in Quantity

How much meat you should buy at any one time depends, of course, on your food budget, the amount of storage space in your refrigerator or freezer, and how much your household will consume.

There are two ways to buy meat in quantity. You can purchase multiple retail packages of meats, or you can purchase carcasses, sides, or wholesale cuts of meat.

In determining whether or not you can save money by buying carcasses or wholesale cuts of meat over what it would cost to buy retail cuts, you will have to take into account several factors: the yield of meat you will get from the carcass or wholesale cut; the quality of the meat; and the costs of cutting, wrapping, and quick-freezing. When buying bulk meat, you should find out whether these costs are included in the price per pound, or if you'll have to pay additional for these services.

If you're thinking of buying a pork carcass or side, you'll want to get it from an establishment that is equipped to cure the bacon, hams, and other cuts that you may not want to use fresh. If you cannot obtain this service, you would probably find it better to buy retail cuts or the wholesale cuts such as shoulders, loins, and hams.

Using USDA Yield Grades: The yield of usable meat from a carcass or wholesale cut can vary greatly regardless of the grade. This variation is caused, primarily, by differences in the amount of fat on the outside of the carcass. USDA has grades to measure this yield. Yield Grade 1 denotes the highest ratio of lean to fat, and Yield Grade 5 the lowest yield ratio.

Cutting, Wrapping, and Freezing: For large meat purchases, it is usually best to get the freezing done by an establishment properly equipped to do the job. Quick freezing causes less damage to the meat fibers. Slower freezing causes more of the cells to rupture, due to formation of large ice crystals, so that more meat juices are lost when the meat is thawed.

Proper wrapping of meat for the freezer is as important as proper storage. Use a moisture-vapor-proof wrap such as heavy aluminum foil, heavily waxed freezer paper, etc. Wrap the meat closely, eliminating all air if possible. Double thicknesses of waxed paper should be placed between chops and steaks to prevent their sticking together. Seal the packages well and mark them with the date. The rule in using frozen meat should be "first in, first out."

Improperly wrapped packages will allow air to enter and draw moisture from the meat, resulting in "freezer burn" or meat which is dry and less flavorful.

Know Your Dealer

When buying meat in quantity, know your dealer. Although most businesses are honest, some will take advantage of the uninformed.

There are a few practices that you should be particularly on guard against:

Bait & Switch: Meat will be offered at a very low price, sometimes advertised as USDA-graded. When the customer arrives at the establishment, the dealer will show the "advertised" carcass, which will be over-fat and wasteful. Then, the customer is shown another carcass—one which is leaner, more appealing, and offered at a much higher price. The customer might also be assured that, although there is no USDA grade mark on the carcass, it qualifies for some likely sounding "USDA grade" name. Remember, the only official USDA grades for meat are those listed in this pamphlet. And, if the meat has been graded, the grade mark will be on the carcass.

Substituting Cuts: Wholesale cuts will be advertised at a "real deal." The customer will buy a more expensive wholesale cut, say a hindquarter or loin, but end up with cuts from the forequarter or shoulder. Consult the carcass charts in this pamphlet to know which cuts come from which part of the carcass.

In general, beware of ads that are too good to be true. They usually are. **If you encounter such practices, call USDA's Grain Inspection, Packers and Stockyards Administration at (202) 720-7363 to report the incidence.**

For more information about nutrition, write:

U.S. Department of Agriculture
Center for Nutrition Policy and Promotion
1120 20th Street NW, Suite 200 North
Washington, DC 20036

Section 8

How to Buy Poultry

Poultry's popularity is growing as consumers seek foods that are versatile, quick-to-fix, economical, and nutritious.

Points to Consider

Wholesomeness . . . quality . . . class . . . nutritive value . . . cost . . . convenience. . . and informative labeling are some of the points to consider when purchasing poultry.

Wholesomeness

All poultry must be officially inspected to ensure that it is wholesome, properly labeled, and not adulterated. The processing plant's premises, facilities, equipment, and procedures must be inspected. And, the inspection stamp must appear on the label. This mandatory inspection is done by USDA's Food Safety and Inspection Service. It must be done before poultry can be rated for quality.

Labeling for Safety

Poultry inspection procedures are designed to minimize the likelihood of harmful bacteria being present in poultry products. However, some bacteria could be present and could become a problem if the poultry is not handled properly during preparation. USDA requires

Agricultural Marketing Service Home and Garden Bulletin No. 263

541

that safe handling and cooking instructions be put on all packages of raw poultry; this includes any poultry product not considered "ready to eat."

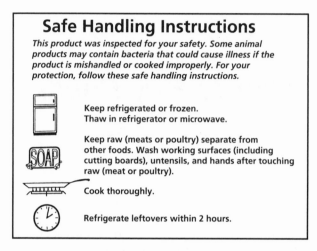

Processed poultry products considered "ready to eat"—such as poultry hotdogs, luncheon meats, and turkey ham—are also perishable. They, too, should be kept refrigerated and handled with care to prevent spoilage.

For information about poultry inspection and safety, call USDA's Meat and Poultry Hotline. The national toll-free number is 800-535-4555. In the Washington, DC, area, call (202)720-3333.

Quality Assurance

Grading involves evaluating poultry in terms of quality standards. Quality standards reflect factors that affect the inherent properties of poultry, factors that determine its relative degree of excellence or value. The highest quality is U.S. Grade A, the only grade you are likely to see in the store. U.S. Grades B and C may be sold at retail, but are usually used in further-processed products where the poultry meat is cut up, chopped, or ground.

The official grade shield certifies that the poultry has been graded for quality by a technically trained government grader. USDA's Agricultural Marketing Service provides the grading service, on a voluntary basis, to poultry processors and others who request it and pay a fee for it.

Poultry That is Graded

U.S. grades apply to six kinds of poultry: chicken, turkey, duck, goose, guinea, and pigeon.

The USDA grade shield may be found on the following ready-to-cook poultry products, whether chilled or frozen:

- whole poultry carcasses,

- poultry parts—with or without the skin, bone-in or boneless,

- poultry roasts, and poultry tenderloins.

- There are no grade standards for poultry necks, wing tips, tails, giblets, or poultry meat that is diced, shredded, or ground.

U.S. Grade A Poultry

Grade A poultry whole carcasses and bone-in parts

- are fully fleshed and meaty; have a good conformation, a normal shape; are free of disjointed or broken bones;

- have a well-developed and well-distributed layer of fat in the skin;

- are free of pinfeathers, exposed flesh, and discolorations; and,

- in the case of whole carcasses, have no missing parts.

Grade A boneless poultry products are free of bone, cartilage, tendons, bruises, and blood clots.

Grade A poultry products that are frozen must be free of freezing defects such as dehydration or excess moisture.

Select by Class

The class of poultry indicates the age of the bird. Age affects the tenderness of poultry meat and dictates the cooking method to use for maximum flavor and tenderness. Poultry meat from young birds is more tender than poultry meat from older birds.

543

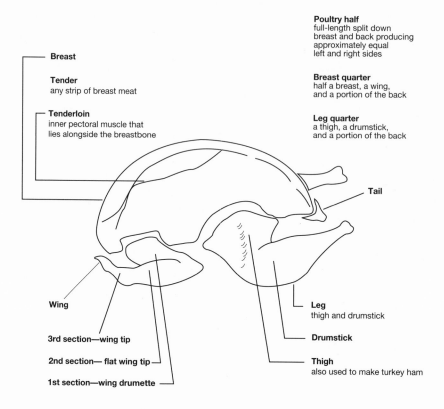

Poultry half
full-length split down
breast and back producing
approximately equal
left and right sides

Breast

Tender
any strip of breast meat

Breast quarter
half a breast, a wing,
and a portion of the back

Tenderloin
inner pectoral muscle that
lies alongside the breastbone

Leg quarter
a thigh, a drumstick,
and a portion of the back

Tail

Wing

3rd section—wing tip

2nd section— flat wing tip

1st section—wing drumette

Leg
thigh and drumstick

Drumstick

Thigh
also used to make turkey ham

Young birds provide tender-meated poultry that is suitable for all cooking methods, especially broiling, barbecuing, roasting, or frying. They may be labeled as:

Chicken: young chicken, Rock Cornish game hen, broiler, fryer, roaster, or capon.

Turkey: young turkey, fryer-roaster, young hen, or young tom

Duck: duckling, young duckling, broiler duckling, fryer duckling, or roaster duckling.

Goose and guinea: young goose or guinea.

Pigeon: squab.

Mature birds provide less tender-meated poultry that is suitable for moist-heat cooking such as stewing or baking, and may be preferred for use in soups, casseroles, salads, or sandwiches. They may be labeled as:

Chicken: mature chicken, hen, fowl, baking chicken, or stewing chicken.

Turkey: mature turkey, yearling turkey, or old turkey.

Duck, goose, and guinea: mature or old duck, goose, or guinea.

Pigeon: pigeon.

Safe Handling

Wash hands, cutting board, utensils, and work surface with hot, soapy water before and after handling raw and cooked poultry.

Keep raw poultry in the refrigerator (40 °F). Cook within 1 to 2 days, or freeze it.

Keep frozen poultry in the freezer (O °F). Cook promptly after thawing. Thaw in the refrigerator; in cold water, changing the water every 30 minutes; or in a microwave oven.

Keep cooked poultry in the refrigerator. Use within 4 days, or freeze it.

Completely cook poultry at one time. Never partially cook, then store and finish cooking later.

Whole birds should be stuffed just before cooking. Mix dry ingredients with other ingredients (for example, margarine, onion, and broth) just before stuffing the bird. Remove stuffing from the bird immediately after cooking. Store stuffing separately in the refrigerator.

When serving poultry, never leave it out of the refrigerator more than 2 hours.

Put cooked poultry on a clean plate, never on a plate that held raw poultry and had not yet been thoroughly washed.

Nutritive Value

Poultry provides protein, niacin, vitamins B6 and B12, iron, zinc, and phosphorus. Fat, saturated fat, and cholesterol are also present in all poultry, with most of the fat being in the skin. Use the Nutrition Facts panel on each individual product label to learn about the nutrient content of that food and how it fits into an overall daily diet. The Nutrition Facts panel must appear on all processed poultry products, while its use is voluntary on single-ingredient raw poultry.

Choose a diet low in fat, saturated fat, and cholesterol to help reduce the risk of getting certain diseases and to help maintain a healthy weight. The Dietary Guidelines for Americans suggest choosing a diet containing 30 percent or less of calories from fat and less than 10 percent of calories from saturated fatty acids. Also, some health authorities suggest that dietary cholesterol be limited to an average of 300 milligrams or less per day.

The Food Guide Pyramid (see Chapter 2) suggests 2 to 3 servings each day of food from the meat group, the equivalent of 5 to 7 ounces of cooked lean meat, poultry, or fish. Count as a serving 2 to 3 ounces of cooked poultry, about the amount of poultry meat on a medium chicken breast half.

Tips: To reduce fat in cooked poultry, broil, roast, bake, simmer, or microwave poultry rather than fry. Cook whole birds on a rack. Drain and discard any fat that accumulates during cooking. Remove the skin before eating. When you choose poultry dishes that are higher in fat, balance your fat intake by choosing other foods that are low in fat.

Fat Content of Chicken

Chicken, light and dark meat, roasted, 3 oz.	Without skin	With skin
Fat total (grams)	6	12
Saturated fatty acids (grams)	2	3
Cholesterol (milligrams)	75	74
Calories	160	200

For more information about nutrition write:

U.S. Department of Agriculture
Center for Nutrition Policy and Promotion
1120 20th Street NW, Suite 200 North
Washington, DC 20036

Section 9

How To Buy Fresh Vegetables

In nearly every U.S. supermarket, today's consumer can find an abundant supply of fresh vegetables year-round. Fresh vegetables add color and variety to any meal.

Points to Consider

Wholesomeness . . . quality . . . nutritive value . . . convenience . . . methods of use . . . and informative labeling are some of the points to consider when purchasing fresh vegetables.

Wholesomeness

Demand freshness! Check the characteristic signs of freshness such as bright, lively color and crispness. Vegetables are usually at their best quality and price at the peak of their season

Use thoughtful care to prevent injury to vegetables. Some vegetables are more hardy than others, but bruising and damage can be prevented by just being careful. The consumer pays for carelessness in the long run.

Don't buy because of low price alone. It doesn't pay to buy more vegetables than you can properly store in your refrigerator or use without waste. Most fresh vegetables can be stored for 2 to 5 days, except for root vegetables, which can be stored from 1 to several weeks.

Agricultural Marketing Service Home and Garden Bulletin No. 258

547

Avoid decay. It's a waste of money to buy fresh vegetables affected by decay. Even if you do trim off the decayed area, rapid deterioration is likely to spread to the salvaged area. Paying a few cents extra for vegetables in good condition is a good investment.

Nutritive Value

Fresh vegetables provide a variety of vitamins and minerals, they are low in fat, and they provide fiber. USDA nutritionists recommend 3 to 5 servings from the vegetable group each day. Count as a serving 1 cup raw leafy vegetables, 1/2 cup of other vegetables that are cooked or chopped raw, or 3/4 cup of vegetable juice. Go easy on the fat and salt added during cooking or at the table in the form of spreads, sauces, dressings, toppings, and seasonings.

Quality

Differences in quality mean differences in appearance, amount of waste (from decay or defects), and price. This section can help you choose vegetables of good quality.

Some vegetables are labeled with a USDA quality grade. The quality of most fresh vegetables can be judged reasonably well by their external appearance. Therefore, consumers can usually make a good selection of vegetables from retail display counters even without the help of a grade mark or other identification of quality. Vegetables are available year-round from both domestic production and imports from other countries

Quality Grades For Fresh Vegetables

USDA has established grade standards for most fresh vegetables. The standards are used extensively as a basis for trading between growers, shippers, wholesalers, and retailers. They are used to a limited extent in sales from retailers to consumers.

Use of U.S. grade standards is voluntary in most cases. However, some State laws and Federal marketing programs require official grading and grade labeling of certain vegetables.

Most packers grade their vegetables and some mark the consumer packages with the grade. If a package carries a grade, the packer is legally obligated to make the contents measure up to the official grade.

Some packers, wholesalers, and distributors use official USDA or Federal-State grading services.

Grade designations are most often seen on packages of potatoes and onions. Other vegetables occasionally carry the grade name.

U.S. No. 1 No. 1 is the grade that you will most often see. Vegetables of this grade should be tender and fresh-appearing, have good color, and be relatively free from bruises and decay.

U.S. Fancy U. S. Fancy vegetables are of more uniform shape and have fewer defects than U.S. No. 1.

U.S. No. 2 and No. 3 While U.S. No. 2 and No. 3 have lower quality requirements than Fancy or No. 1, all grades are nutritious. The differences are mainly in appearance, waste, and preference.

Labeling

Under federal guidelines, a substantial number of retailers must provide nutrition information for the 20 most frequently eaten raw vegetables. These vegetables are: potatoes, iceberg lettuce, tomatoes, onions, carrots, celery, sweet corn, broccoli, green cabbage, cucumbers, bell peppers, cauliflower, leaf lettuce, sweet potatoes, mushrooms, green onions, green (snap) beans, radishes, summer squash, and asparagus. Information about other vegetables may also be provided. The nutritional information may appear on posters, brochures, leaflets, or stickers near the vegetable display. It may include serving size; calories per serving; amount of protein, total carbohydrates, total fat, and sodium per serving; and percent of the U.S. Recommended Daily Allowances for iron, calcium, and vitamins A and C per serving.

A Consumer's Guide To Fresh Vegetables

There are no set rules for buying vegetables because they all have individual characteristics and values. Experience in personal selection is the best teacher. The following alphabetical list is designed as a handy reference to help you make your selections.

Artichokes

The globe artichoke is the large, unopened flower bud of a plant belonging to the thistle family. The many leaf-like parts making up the bud are called "scales." Produced domestically only in California, the peak of the crop comes in April and May.

Look for: Plump, globular artichokes that are heavy in relation to size, and compact with thick, green, fresh-looking scales. Size is not important with respect to quality.

Avoid: Artichokes with large areas of brown on the scales and with spreading scales (a sign of age, indicating drying and toughening of the edible portions), grayish-black discoloration (caused by bruises), mold growth on the scales, and worm injury.

Asparagus

California, New Jersey, Washington, and Michigan are the chief sources of domestically grown asparagus.

Look for: Closed, compact tips; smooth, round spears; and a fresh appearance. A rich green color should cover most of the spear. Stalks should be almost as far down as the green extends.

Avoid: Tips that are open and spread out, moldy or decayed tips, or ribbed spears (spears with up-and-down ridges or that are not approximately round). Those are all signs of aging, and indicate tough asparagus and poor flavor. Also avoid excessively sandy asparagus, because sand grains can lodge beneath the scales or in the tips of the spears and are difficult to remove in washing.

Beans (Snap)

Snap beans, produced commercially in many States, are available throughout the year. Most beans found in the food store will be the common green podded varieties, but large green pole beans and yellow wax beans are occasionally available.

Look for: A fresh, bright appearance with good color for the variety. Get young, tender beans with pods in a firm, crisp condition.

Avoid: Wilted or flabby bean pods, serious blemishes, and decay. Thick, tough, fibrous pods indicate overmaturity.

Beets

Beets, available year-round, are grown in most parts of the Nation. Many beets are sold in bunches with the tops still attached, while others are sold with the tops removed.

Look for: Beets that are firm, round, with a slender tap root (the large main root), a rich, deep red color, and smooth over most of the surface. If beets are bunched, you can judge their freshness fairly accurately by the condition of the tops. Badly wilted or decayed tops indicate a lack of freshness, but the roots may be satisfactory if they are firm.

Avoid: Elongated beets with round, scaly areas around the top surface—these will be tough, fibrous, and strong-flavored. Also avoid wilted, flabby beets—they have been exposed to the air too long.

Broccoli

A member of the cabbage family, and a close relative of cauliflower, broccoli is available throughout the year.

California is the heaviest producer, although other States also produce large amounts of broccoli.

Look for: A firm, compact cluster of small flower buds, with none opened enough to show the bright-yellow flower. Bud clusters should be dark green or sage green—or even green with a decidedly purplish cast. Stems should not be too thick or too tough.

Avoid: Broccoli with spread bud clusters, enlarged or open buds, yellowish-green color, or wilted condition, which are all signs of overmaturity. Also avoid broccoli with soft, slippery, water-soaked spots on the bud cluster. These are signs of decay.

Brussels Sprouts

Another close relative of the cabbage, Brussels sprouts develop as enlarged buds on a tall stem, one sprout appearing where each main leaf is attached. The "sprouts" are cut off and, in most cases, are packed in small consumer containers, although some are packed loose, in bulk. Although they are often available about 10 months of the year, peak supplies appear from October through December.

Look for: A fresh, bright-green color, tight fitting outer leaves, firm body, and freedom from blemishes.

Avoid: Elongated beets with round, scaly areas around the top surface—these will be tough, fibrous, and strong-flavored. Also avoid wilted, flabby beets —they have been exposed to the air too long.

Cabbage

Three major groups of cabbage varieties are available: smooth-leaved green cabbage; crinkly-leaved green Savoy cabbage; and red cabbage. All types are suitable for any use, although the Savoy and red varieties are more in demand for use in slaw and salads.

Cabbage may be sold fresh (called "new" cabbage) or from storage. Cabbage is available throughout the year, since it is grown in many States. California, Florida, and Texas market most new cabbage. Many Northern States grow cabbage for late summer and fall shipment or to be held in storage for winter sale.

Look for: Firm or hard heads of cabbage that are heavy for their size. Outer leaves should be a good green or red color (depending on type), reasonably fresh, and free from serious blemishes. The outer leaves (called "wrapper" leaves) fit loosely on the head and are usually discarded, but too many loose wrapper leaves on a head cause extra waste.

Some early-crop cabbage may be soft or only fairly firm, but is suitable for immediate use if the leaves are fresh and crisp. Cabbage out of storage is usually trimmed of all outer leaves and lacks green color, but is satisfactory if not wilted or discolored.

Avoid: New cabbage with wilted or decayed outer leaves or with leaves turned decidedly yellow. Worm-eaten outer leaves often indicate that the worm injury penetrates into the head.

Storage cabbage with badly discolored, dried, or decayed outer leaves probably is over-aged. Separation of the stems of leaves from the central stem at the base of the head also indicates over-age.

Carrots

Freshly harvested carrots are available year round. Most are marketed when relatively young, tender, well-colored, and mild-flavored—an ideal stage for use as raw carrot sticks. Larger carrots are packed separately and used primarily for cooking or shredding. California and Texas market most domestic carrots, but many other States produce large quantities.

Look for: Carrots which are well formed, smooth, well colored, and firm. If tops are attached, they should be fresh and of a good green color.

Avoid: Roots with large green "sunburned" areas at the top (which must be trimmed) and roots which are flabby from wilting or show spots of soft rot.

Cauliflower

Although most abundant from September through January, cauliflower is available during every month of the year. California, New York, and Florida are major sources. The white edible portion is called "the curd" and the heavy outer leaf covering is called "the jacket leaves." Cauliflower is generally sold with most of the jacket leaves removed, and is wrapped in plastic film.

Look for: White to creamy-white, compact, solid, and clean curds. A slightly granular or "ricey" texture of the curd will not hurt the eating quality if the surface is compact. Ignore small green leaflets extending through the curd. If jacket leaves are attached, a good green color is a sign of freshness.

Avoid: A spreading of the curd—a sign of aging or overmaturity. Also avoid severe wilting or discolored spots on the curd. A smudgy or speckled appearance of the curd is a sign of insect injury, mold growth, or decay, and should be avoided.

Celery

Celery, a popular vegetable for a variety of uses, is available throughout the year. Production is concentrated in California, Florida,

Michigan and New York. Most celery is of the so-called "Pascal" type, which includes thick-branched, green varieties.

Look for: Freshness and crispness in celery. The stalk should have a solid, rigid feel and leaflets should be fresh or only slightly wilted. Also look for a glossy surface, stalks of light green or medium green, and mostly green leaflets.

Avoid: Wilted celery and celery with flabby upper branches or leaf stems. You can freshen celery somewhat by placing the butt end in water, but badly wilted celery will never become really fresh again.

Celery with pithy, hollow, or discolored centers in the branches also should be avoided. Celery with internal discoloration will show some gray or brown on the inside surface of the larger branches near where they are attached to the base of the stalk.

Also avoid celery with blackheart, a brown or black discoloration of the small center branches; insect injury in the center branches or the insides of outer branches; and long, thick seed stems in place of the usually small, tender heart branches.

Chard (See Greens)

Chinese Cabbage

Primarily a salad vegetable, Chinese cabbage plants are elongated, with some varieties developing a firm head and others an open, leafy form.

Look for: Fresh, crisp, green plants that are free from blemishes or decay.

Avoid: Wilted or yellowed plants.

Chicory, Endives, Escarole

These vegetables, used mainly in salads, are available practically all year-round, but primarily in the winter and spring. Chicory or endive has narrow, notched edges, and crinkly leaves resembling the dandelion leaf. Chicory plants often have "blanched" yellowish leaves in the center which are preferred by many people. Escarole leaves are much broader and less crinkly than those of chicory.

Look for: Freshness, crispness, tenderness, and a good green color of the outer leaves.

Avoid: Plants with leaves which have brownish or yellowish discoloration or which have insect injury.

Note: Witloof or Belgian endive is a compact, cigar-shaped plant which is creamy white from blanching. The small shoots are kept from becoming green by being grown in complete darkness.

Collards (See Greens)

Corn

Sweet corn is available practically every month of the year, but is most plentiful from early May until mid-September. Yellow-kernel corn is the most popular, but some white-kernel and mixed-color corn is sold. Sweet corn is produced in a large number of States during the spring and summer, but most mid-winter supplies come from south Florida.

For best quality, corn should be refrigerated immediately after being picked. Corn will retain fairly good quality for a number of days, if it has been kept cold and moist since harvesting. Therefore, it should be refrigerated as soon as possible and kept moist until used.

Look for: Fresh, succulent husks with good green color, silk-ends that are free from decay or worm injury, and stem ends (opposite from the silk) that are not too discolored or dried.

Select ears that are well-covered with plump, not-too-mature kernels. Sweet corn is sometimes sold husked in overwrapped film trays.

Avoid: Ears with under-developed kernels which lack yellow color (in yellow corn), old ears with very large kernels, and ears with dark yellow or dried kernels with depressed areas on the outer surface. Also avoid ears of corn with yellowed, wilted, or dried husks, or discolored and dried-out stem ends.

Cucumbers

Although cucumbers are produced at various times of the year in many States, and imported during the colder months, the supply is most plentiful in the summer months.

Look for: Cucumbers with good green color that are firm over their entire length. They should be well developed, but not too large in diameter.

Avoid: Overgrown cucumbers that are large in diameter and have a dull color, turning yellowish. Also avoid cucumbers with withered or shriveled ends —signs of toughness and bitter flavor.

Eggplants

Eggplant is most plentiful during late summer, but is available all year. Although the purple eggplant is more common, white eggplant is occasionally seen in the marketplace.

Look for: Firm, heavy, smooth, and uniformly dark purple eggplants.

Avoid: Those which are poorly colored, soft, shriveled, cut, or which show decay in the form of irregular dark-brown spots.

Endive, Escarole (See Chicory)

Greens

A large number of widely differing species of plants are grown for use as "greens." The better known kinds are spinach, kale, collard, turnip, beet, chard, mustard, broccoli leaves, chicory, endive, escarole, dandelion, cress, and sorrel. Many others, some of them wild, are also used to a limited extent as greens.

Look for: Leaves that are fresh, young, tender, free from defects, and that have a good, healthy, green color. Beet tops and red chard show reddish color.

Avoid: Leaves with coarse, fibrous stems, yellowish-green color, softness (a sign of decay), or a wilted condition. Also avoid greens with evidence of insects—especially aphids—which are sometimes hard to see and equally hard to wash away.

Kale (See Greens)

Lettuce

Among the leading U.S. vegetables, lettuce owes its prominence to the growing popularity of salads in our diets. It's available throughout the year in various seasons from California, Arizona, Florida, New York, New Jersey, and other States. Four types of lettuce are generally sold: iceberg, butter-head, Romaine, and leaf.

Iceberg lettuce is the major type. Heads are large, round, and solid, with medium-green outer leaves and lighter green or pale-green inner leaves.

Butter-head lettuce, including the Big Boston and Bibb varieties, has a smaller head than iceberg. This type will have soft, succulent light-green leaves in a rosette pattern in the center.

Romaine lettuce plants are tall and cylindrical with crisp, dark-green leaves in a loosely folded head.

Leaf lettuce includes many varieties—none with a compact head. Leaves are broad, tender, succulent, and fairly smooth, and they vary in color according to variety.

Look for: Signs of freshness in lettuce. For iceberg lettuce and Romaine, the leaves should be crisp. Other lettuce types will have a softer texture, but leaves should not be wilted. Look for a good, bright color— in most varieties, medium to light green. Some varieties have red leaves.

Avoid: Heads of iceberg type which are very hard and which lack green color (signs of overmaturity). Such heads sometimes develop discoloration of the inner leaves and midribs, and may have a less desirable flavor. Also avoid heads with irregular shapes and hard bumps on top, which indicate the presence of overgrown central stems.

Check the lettuce for tip burn, a tan or brown area around the margins of the leaves. Look for tip burn of the edges of the head leaves. Slight discoloration of the outer or wrapper leaves will usually not hurt the quality of the lettuce, but serious discoloration or decay definitely should be avoided.

Mushrooms

Grown in houses, cellars, or caves, mushrooms are available year-round in varying amounts. Most come from Pennsylvania, but many are produced in California, New York, Ohio, and other States.

We usually describe mushrooms as having a cap (the wide portion on top), gills (the numerous rows of paper-thin tissue seen underneath the cap when it opens), and a stem.

Look for: Young mushrooms that are small to medium in size. Caps should be either closed around the stem or moderately open with pink or light-tan gills. The surface of the cap should be white or creamy, or uniform light brown if of a brown type.

Avoid: Overripe mushrooms (shown by wide-open caps and dark, discolored gills underneath) and those with pitted or seriously discolored caps.

Okra

Okra is the immature seed pod of the okra plant, generally grown in Southern States.

Look for: Tender pods (the tips will bend with very slight pressure) under 4-1/2 inches long. They should be bright green color and free from blemishes.

Avoid: Tough, fibrous pods, indicated by tips which are stiff and resist bending, or by a very hard body of the pod, or by pale, faded green color.

Onions

The many varieties of onions grown commercially fall into three general classes, distinguished by color: yellow, white, and red.

Onions are available year-round, either fresh or from storage.

Major onion-growing States are California, New York, Texas, Michigan, Colorado, Oregon, and Idaho.

Look for: Hard or firm onions which are dry and have small necks. They should be reasonably free from green sunburn spots or other blemishes.

Avoid: Onions with wet or very soft necks, which usually are immature or affected by decay. Also avoid onions with thick, hollow, woody centers in the neck or with fresh sprouts.

Onions (Green), Leeks

Onions and leeks (sometimes called scallions) are similar in appearance, but are somewhat different in nature.

Green onions are ordinary onions harvested very young. They have very little or no bulb formation, and their tops are tubular.

Leeks have slight bulb formation and broad, flat, dark-green tops.

Sold in small, tied bunches, they are all available to some extent throughout the entire year, but are most plentiful in spring and summer.

Look for: Bunches with fresh, crisp, green tops. They should have portions extending two or three inches up from the root end.

Avoid: Yellowing, wilted, discolored, or decayed tops (indicating flabby, tough, or fibrous condition of the edible portions). Bruised tops will not affect the eating quality of the bulbs, if the tops are removed.

Parsley

Parsley is generally available the year-round. It is used both as a decorative garnish and to add its own unique flavor.

Look for: Fresh, crisp, bright-green leaves, for both the curled-leaf and the flat-leaf types of parsley. Slightly wilted leaves can be freshened by trimming off the ends of the stems and placing them in cold water

Avoid: Yellowing, discolored, or decayed leaves.

Parsnips

Although available to some extent throughout the year, parsnips are primarily late-winter vegetables because the flavor becomes sweeter and more desirable after long exposure to cold temperatures, below 40 °F.

Look for: Parsnips of small or medium width that are well formed, smooth, firm, and free from serious blemishes or decay.

Avoid: Large, coarse roots (which probably have woody, fibrous, or pithy centers) and badly wilted and flabby roots (which will be tough when cooked).

Peppers

Most of the peppers that you'll find are the sweet green peppers, available in varying amounts throughout the year, but most plentiful during late summer. (Fully matured peppers of the same type have a bright red color.) A variety of colored peppers are also available, including white, yellow, orange, red, and purple.

Look for: Peppers with deep, characteristic color, glossy sheen, relatively heavy weight, and firm walls or sides.

Avoid: Peppers with very thin walls (indicated by lightweight and flimsy sides), peppers that are wilted or flabby with cuts or punctures through the walls, and pepper with soft watery spots on the sides (evidence of decay).

Potatoes

For practical purposes, potatoes can be put into three groups, although the distinctions between them are not clear-cut, and there is much overlapping.

"New potatoes" is a term most frequently used to describe those potatoes freshly harvested and marketed during the late winter or early spring. The name is also widely used in later crop producing areas to designate freshly dug potatoes which are not fully matured. The best uses for new potatoes are boiling or creaming. They vary widely in size and shape, depending upon variety, but are likely to be affected by "skinning" or "feathering" of the outer layer of skin. Skinning usually affects only their appearance.

"General purpose potatoes" include the great majority of supplies, both round and long types, offered for sale in markets. With the aid of air-cooled storage, they are amply available throughout the year. As the term implies, they are used for boiling, frying, and baking, although many of the common varieties are not considered to be best for baking.

Potatoes grown specifically for their baking quality also are available. Both variety and area where grown are important factors affecting baking quality. A long variety with fine, scaly netting on the skin, such as the Russet Burbank, is commonly used for baking.

Look for: With new potatoes, look for firm potatoes that are free from blemishes and sunburn (a green discoloration under the skin). Some amount of skinned surface is normal, but potatoes with large skinned and discolored areas are undesirable. For general-purpose and baking potatoes, look for reasonably smooth, firm potatoes free from blemishes, sunburn, and decay.

Avoid: Potatoes with large cuts, bruises, or decay (they'll cause waste in peeling) and sprouted or shriveled potatoes.

Also avoid green potatoes. The green portions, which contain the alkaloid solanin, may penetrate the flesh and cause bitter flavor.

Radishes

Radishes, available the year-round, are most plentiful from May through July. California and Florida produce most of our winter and spring supplies, while several Northern States provide radishes the rest of the year.

Look for: Medium-size radishes—3/4 to 1 inch in diameter—that are plump, round, firm, and of a good, red color.

Avoid: Very large or flabby radishes (likely to have pithy centers). Also avoid radishes with yellow or decayed tops (sign of over-age)

Rhubarb

This highly specialized vegetable is used like a fruit in sweetened sauces and pies. Very limited supplies are available during most of the year, with best supplies available from January to June.

Look for: Fresh, firm rhubarb stems with a bright, glossy appearance. Stems should have a large amount of pink or red color, although many good-quality stems will be predominantly light green. Be sure that the stem is tender and not fibrous.

561

Avoid: Either very slender or extremely thick stems, which are likely to be tough and stringy. Also avoid rhubarb that is wilted and flabby.

Rutabagas (See Turnips)

Spinach (See Greens)

Squash (Summer)

Summer squash includes those varieties which are harvested while still immature and when the entire squash is tender and edible. They include the yellow Crookneck, the large Straightneck, the greenish-white Patty Pan, and the slender green Zucchini. Some of these squash are available at all times of the year.

Look for: Squash that are tender and well developed, firm, and fresh-appearing. You can identify a tender squash, because the skin is glossy instead of dull, and it is neither hard nor tough.

Avoid: Stale or overmature squash, which will have a dull appearance and a hard, tough surface. Such squash usually have enlarged seeds and dry, stringy flesh. Also avoid squash with discolored or pitted areas.

Squash (Fall and Winter)

Winter squash are those varieties which are marketed only when fully mature. Some of the most important varieties are the small corrugated Acorn (available all year-round), Butternut, Buttercup, green and blue Hubbard, green and gold Delicious, and Banana. Winter squash is most plentiful from early fall until late winter

Look for: Full maturity, indicated by a hard, tough rind. Also look for squash that is heavy for its size (meaning a thick wall and more edible flesh). Slight variations in skin color do not affect flavor.

Avoid: Squash with cuts, punctures, sunken spots, or moldy spots on the rind. These are indications of decay. A tender rind indicates immaturity, which is a sign of poor eating quality in winter squash varieties.

Sweet Potatoes

Two types of sweet potatoes are available in varying amounts the year-round. Moist sweet potatoes, sometimes called yams, are the most common type. They have orange-colored flesh and are very sweet. (The true yam is the root of a tropical vine which is not grown commercially in the United States.)

Dry sweet potatoes have pale-colored flesh and are low in moisture.

Most sweet potatoes are grown in the Southern tier and some Eastern States, in an area from Texas to New Jersey. California also is a major producer.

Look for: Firm sweet potatoes with smooth, bright, uniformly colored skins, free from signs of decay. Because they are more perishable than white potatoes, extra care should be used in selecting sweet potatoes.

Avoid: Sweet potatoes with worm holes, cuts, grub injury, or any other defects which penetrate the skin; this causes waste and can readily lead to decay. Even if you cut away the decayed portion, the remainder of the potato flesh may have a bad taste.

Decay is the worst problem with sweet potatoes and is of three types: wet, soft decay; dry, firm decay which begins at the end of the potato, making it discolored and shriveled; and dry rot in the form of sunken, discolored areas on the sides of the potato.

Sweet potatoes should not be stored in the refrigerator.

Tomatoes

Extremely popular and nutritious, tomatoes are in moderate to liberal supply throughout the year. Florida, California, and a number of other States are major producers, but imports supplement domestic supplies.

The best flavor usually comes from locally grown tomatoes produced on nearby farms. This type of tomato is allowed to ripen completely before being picked. Many areas, however, now ship tomatoes which are picked right after the color has begun to change from green to pink.

If your tomatoes need further ripening, keep them in a warm place but not in direct sunlight. Unless they are fully ripened, do not store tomatoes in a refrigerator—the cold temperatures might keep them from ripening later on and ruin the flavor.

Look for: Tomatoes which are smooth, well ripened, and reasonably free from blemishes.

For fully ripe fruit, look for an overall rich, red color and a slight softness. Softness is easily detected by gentle handling.

For tomatoes slightly less than fully ripe, look for firm texture and color ranging from pink to light red.

Avoid: Soft, overripe, or bruised tomatoes, and tomatoes with sunburn (green or yellow areas near the stem scar), and growth cracks (deep brown cracks around the stem scar). Also avoid decayed tomatoes which will have soft, water-soaked spots, depressed areas, or surface mold.

Turnips

The most popular turnip has white flesh and a purple top (reddish-purple tinting of upper surface). It may be sold "topped" (with leaves removed) or in bunches with tops still on, and is available in some food stores most of the year.

Look for: Small or medium-size, smooth, fairly round, and firm vegetables. If sold in bunches, the tops should be fresh and should have a good green color.

Avoid: Large turnips with too many leaf scars around the top and with obvious fibrous roots.

Rutabagas are distinctly yellow-fleshed, large-sized relatives of turnips. They are available generally in the fall and winter, but cold-storage rutabagas are often available in the spring. Late winter storage rutabagas are sometimes coated with a thin layer of paraffin to prevent loss of moisture and shriveling. The paraffin is readily removed with the peeling before cooking.

Look for: Heavy weight for their size, generally smooth, round or moderately elongated shape, and firmness.

Avoid: Rutabagas with skin punctures, deep cuts, or decay.

Watercress

Watercress is a small, round-leaved plant that grows naturally (or it may be cultivated) along the banks of freshwater streams and ponds. It is prized as an ingredient of mixed green salads and as a garnish, because of its spicy flavor. Watercress is available in limited supply through most of the year.

Look for: Watercress that is fresh, crisp, and has a rich green color.

Avoid: Bunches with yellow, wilted, or decayed leaves.

For information about nutrition, write:

U.S. Department of Agriculture,
Human Nutrition Information Service,
6505 Belcrest Road,
Hyattsville, MD 20782.

Section 10

How to Buy Canned And Frozen Vegetables

Canned and frozen vegetables, preserved at the peak of goodness, can be used as an entree . . . as a side dish in a main meal . . . or included in salads, soufflés, and other tasty dishes. They are convenient to use and are always available.

Points to Consider

Nutritive value. . . wholesomeness. . . quality. . . convenience. . . informative labeling. . . and methods of use are some of the points to consider when purchasing canned and frozen vegetables.

Nutritive Value

Canned and frozen vegetables provide a variety of vitamins and minerals, they are low in fat, and they provide fiber. USDA nutritionists recommend 3 to 5 servings from the vegetable group each day. Count as a serving ½ cup cooked vegetable or ¾ cup vegetable juice. Salt is usually added when vegetables are canned, but some salt-free products are available. Both canned and frozen vegetables are available in butter or cream sauces, which may be high in fat or salt. Go easy on the fat and salt added during cooking or at the table in the form of spreads. sauces, dressings, seasonings, and toppings.

Agricultural Marketing Service Home and Garden Bulletin No. 259

Wholesomeness

When you buy canned vegetables, be sure the cans are not leaking, or bulged at either end. Bulging or swelling cans indicate spoilage. Do not taste the contents. Badly dented cans should always be avoided. Small dents in cans, however, usually do not harm the contents.

Packages of frozen vegetables should be firm. Vegetables should be used immediately after defrosting to avoid loss of quality. Purchases of packages that are limp, wet, or sweating should be avoided. These are signs that the vegetables have defrosted or are in the process of defrosting. Packages stained by the contents or with ice on the outside may have been defrosted and refrozen at some stage in the marketing process. The contents may be safe to eat, but refrozen vegetables will normally not taste as good as freshly frozen vegetables.

Grades for Canned and Frozen Vegetables

All canned and frozen vegetables are wholesome and nutritious, but they can differ in quality. The difference in quality may mean a difference in taste, texture and appearance of the vegetable, and its price. Because different qualities of vegetables are suited to different uses, you can make better buys by choosing processed vegetables of the quality that fits your needs.

The U.S. Department of Agriculture's Agricultural Marketing Service has established U.S. grade standards as measures of quality for many canned and frozen vegetables. USDA also provides an inspection service which certifies the quality of processed vegetables based on these U.S. grade standards. The inspection service is voluntary and paid for by the user. Under the program, processed vegetables are inspected by highly trained specialists during all phases of preparation, processing, and packaging.

The grade standards are used extensively by processors, buyers, and others in wholesale trading to establish the value of a product described by the grades. If you've been selecting canned or frozen vegetables by habit, or can't tell which can or package would be best for the use you have in mind, here's some information that can help you make a wise choice.

U.S. Grade A Grade A vegetables are carefully selected for color, tenderness, and freedom from blemishes. They are the most tender, succulent, and flavorful vegetables produced. The term "fancy" may appear on the label to reflect the Grade A product.

U.S. Grade B Grade B vegetables are of excellent quality but not quite as well selected for color and tenderness as Grade A. They are usually slightly more mature and therefore have a slightly different taste than the more succulent vegetables in Grade A.

U.S. Grade C Grade C vegetables are not so uniform in color and flavor as vegetables in the higher grades, and they are usually more mature. They are a thrifty buy when appearance is not too important, for instance, if you are using the vegetable as an ingredient in a soup, stew, or casserole.

Other names may be used to describe the quality grades of canned or frozen vegetables—Grade A as "Fancy," Grade B as "Extra Standard," and Grade C as "Standard."

The brand name of a frozen or canned vegetable may also be an indication of quality. Producers of nationally advertised products spend considerable money and effort to maintain the same quality for their brand labels year after year. Unadvertised brands may also offer an assurance of quality, often at a slightly lower price. Many stores, particularly chain stores, carry two or more qualities under their own name labels (private labels).

Labels

When a product has been officially graded under continuous inspection, labels may carry the official grade name and the statement "Packed under continuous inspection of the U.S. Department of Agriculture." The grade name and the statement may also appear with shields or without shields.

You may find USDA grade shields on cans or packages of vegetables that have been packed under continuous USDA inspection.

Sometimes the grade name, such as "Grade A," is indicated on the label without the "U.S." in front of it. A canned or frozen vegetable with this designation must measure up to the quality stated, even if it has not been officially inspected for grade.

Federal regulations require that the following information be included on the label of a can or package:

- The common or usual name of the vegetable.

- The form (or style) of vegetable, such as whole, slices, or halves. If the form is visible through the package, it need not be stated.

- For some vegetables, the variety or color.

- Liquid in which a vegetable is packaged must be listed near the name of the product.

- The total contents (net weight) must be stated in ounces for containers holding 1 pound or less. Weight must be given in both total ounces and in pounds and ounces (or pounds and fractions of a pound) for products containing a net weight of 1 to 4 pounds

The net weight shown on a label includes both vegetables and liquid. For the best buy, figure out the cost per ounce. Large containers often cost less per ounce, but not always. Other information required on the label, although not on the front Panel, is:

- Ingredients, such as spices, flavoring, coloring, or special sweetener, if used.

- Any special type of treatment.

- The packer's or distributor's name and place of business.

- Nutritional information.

- Labels may also give the quality or grade, count, size, and maturity of the vegetables, cooking directions, and recipes or serving ideas. If the label lists the number of servings per container, the law requires that the size of the serving be given in common measures, such as ounces or cups.

For information about nutrition, write:

U.S. Department of Agriculture,
Human Nutrition Information Service,
6505 Belcrest Road
Hyattsville, MD 20782.

Section 11

For Oyster And Clam Lovers, The Water Must Be Clean

Oysters Rockefeller, clams casino, moules (mussels) marinieres. These are mollusks with all the trimmings: laid on a bed of spinach, topped with bread crumbs and bacon, or mixed with white wine and parsley.

Most molluscan shellfish commonly eaten in the United States are bivalves—that is, they have two valves, or shells, hinged together. Single-shelled mollusks, or univalves, such as snails and whelks, are found more often on European menus. Bivalve mollusks include oysters, clams, mussels, scallops and cockles.

Although some clams live in fresh water and some deep in the ocean, most mussels, clams and oysters thrive in estuaries that contain mixtures of seawater and fresh water from rivers. These mollusks get food and oxygen from their surroundings by pumping large quantities of water across their complex gill systems (see diagram). Oysters can process about four quarts an hour, clams about three quarts.

They also take in whatever bacteria, viruses, chemical contaminants and other impurities are in the water. Perhaps it is a peculiar form of revenge on their human predators, but mollusks are quite happy and healthy with a gutful of organisms that are toxic, and sometimes deadly, to Homo sapiens. The bacteria that cause cholera and gastroenteritis, the virus that causes hepatitis A, the toxin responsible for paralytic shellfish poisoning—these are all baneful to humans but don't even give a mollusk heartburn.

HHS publication No. (FDA) 85-2200

What's worse for humans, mollusks have an extremely efficient method of filtration and will concentrate microorganisms at much higher levels in their guts than are found in their habitat. The level of harmful bacteria in a mollusk can be from three to twenty times that found in the water from which it was taken.

The job of ensuring that shellfish are harvested from clean waters falls to the states. Under the terms of the National Shellfish Sanitation Program (an organization comprising the Food and Drug Administration, state regulatory agencies, and the shellfish industry) state agencies prohibit shellfish harvesting in areas that are contaminated by sewage or industrial wastes or that have a high level of the organisms that cause paralytic shellfish poisoning. These areas are patrolled by state officials.

Monitoring these growing areas has been effective. Typhoid fever, once the disease most commonly caused by mollusk consumption, is rarely transmitted by shellfish today. Similarly, few cases of cholera are transmitted by mollusks because only shellfish harvested from sewage-contaminated beds become carriers.

However, once mollusks enter commerce, the consumer can take some protective measures. To guard against eating mollusks that contain harmful organisms, consumers can take these precautions:

Obtain shellfish only from approved sources. Shellfish shippers that meet federal standards are certified by state shellfish control authorities, and a list of such shippers is published each month by FDA. One way to help ensure that shellfish come from a certified shipper is to buy them from a name grocery store. Roadside hucksters with "bargain" prices are chancey.

Shellfish that have been illegally harvested from polluted waters are the most frequent cause of shellfish-related illness; outbreaks of hepatitis A caused by shellfish consumption, in particular, almost always are traced to illegally harvested products. The mollusks become carriers of this virus when their beds are contaminated by untreated sewage containing the virus, which is quite likely to cause illness since it is not always killed by cooking and never by freezing.

Obey posted warnings when harvesting shellfish. This is particularly important when the warnings are about paralytic shellfish poisoning (PSP), frequently referred to as a "Red Tide." The neurotoxin that causes PSP blocks nerve impulses, causing paralysis of the respiratory muscles and extremities. It is so poisonous that consumption of even one contaminated mussel could be fatal.

Cleaning will not neutralize PSP toxin, nor will cooking or freezing. The best thing to do with mollusks that have been exposed to this toxin is to throw them away. There is no antidote for the toxin, and a person believed to have consumed toxic shellfish should go immediately to the hospital.

The toxin that causes PSP is produced by microscopic organisms called dinoflagellates, sometimes called plankton (see below), that belong to the species Gonyaulax. The West Coast and New England states facing on the Atlantic Ocean monitor shellfish for these toxic dinoflagellates and post warnings when concentrations in the shellfish make them dangerous to eat.

Another neurotoxin that can cause mollusks to be an unhealthy dish is that produced by a species of dinoflagellate called Ptychodiscus brevis, which inhabits the Gulf of Mexico. Perennially affected areas off Florida are monitored by that state's Department of Natural Resources; consumers who want to go oystering on their own should contact this department and ask about safe shellfish harvesting areas.

Even people who don't eat shellfish, however, can get an unhealthy dose of this toxin from activities in or near the water. In rough surf the toxin is airborne in spray; when inhaled, it can cause irritation of the upper respiratory tract.

Keep all seafood chilled—between 32 and 40 degrees Fahrenheit (0 to 5 degrees Celsius). All raw seafood contains some bacteria, which can proliferate rapidly at temperatures above 40 F. Salmonella bacteria, which can get into mollusk beds from sewage, are not killed by cold temperatures, but the cold will prevent the bacteria from proliferating.

Do not store seafood for prolonged periods. Even under ideal storage conditions, fish and shellfish will deteriorate, permitting harmful bacteria to multiply.

Observe proper sanitation when preparing seafood. Human skin is covered with bacteria, such as Staphylococcus, that can contaminate many foods, including mollusks. It is especially important to wash the hands before preparing seafoods meant to be eaten raw.

Cook shellfish thoroughly if it comes from a questionable source. Most illness associated with shellfish is caused by eating the food raw. A typical example is the illness caused by Vibrio parahaemolyticus, a bacterium that occurs widely in the marine environment, including water and sediment and in both finfish and shellfish. Outbreaks of illness caused by this species occur rarely in the United States; in Japan, however, it is the most common cause of summertime food illness because in that country it is customary to eat fish products raw.

Worm-borne infections that result from mollusk consumption are found primarily in the Pacific and Far West, where fish are commonly eaten raw. Cooking kills these parasites. Transmission of parasitic diseases by shellfish is not a problem in North America or Europe.

Cooking will kill bacteria, such as Salmonella and members of the Vibrio species. However, as noted, only very high heat will destroy hepatitis A virus, and no amount of cooking will completely deactivate the toxins that cause paralytic shellfish poisoning.

Do not eat raw seafood if you have liver disease. A person whose liver is weakened by disease is particularly susceptible to a newly identified species of bacteria, Vibrio vulnificus, described as the Vibrio species most likely to kill. The bacteria can enter the body through an open wound (such as a cut from a mollusk shell) or by ingestion and usually causes mild infection; however, the infection can lead to septicemia (fever, chills and prostration) in people with liver disease. Illness caused by V. vulnificus is associated with a 40 percent mortality rate, according to an article in the Journal of the American Medical Association (January 1984). Infections tend to occur in men over 40, particularly shellfish shuckers; wounds are the usual source of transmission, but consumption of raw oysters has been linked to the infection.

Another recently identified species of bacteria particularly hazardous to those with liver disease is Vibrio cholerae non-O1. This is a relative of the bacterium that causes the disease cholera (called Vibrio cholerae-01). The non-O1 form, unlike its classic relative, is a normal part of marine flora and is widely distributed in brackish surface waters, particularly during the summer months. It can cause a variety of gastrointestinal diseases similar to cholera, but milder, in anyone exposed to it. It can also cause septicemia in those with liver disease.

Eat mollusks when the weather is cold. There may have been some wisdom in the old saying about eating clams and oysters in months with an "R" in them, which means the chillier months. Levels of bacteria and the dinoflagellates that cause PSP tend to decrease when the water gets colder. Cold water also puts a damper on the appetites of many mollusks, and thus they do not accumulate harmful organisms.

Dino Flagellates Who?

Dinoflagellates are organisms that "bloom" to create "Red Tides." They are some of the tinier denizens of the deep. If the creatures could read scientific journals, they would have a massive identity crisis because zoologists claim them as animals and botanists call them plants. They are frequently identified as a type of plankton. The confusion arises because the microscopic dinoflagellates propel themselves through the water with two whiplike appendages (flagella) and ingest solid food (animal attributes), but they're also capable of photosynthesis, using light to manufacture food (a property of plants).

Dinoflagellates are so tiny they cannot be seen unless they "bloom" in such large numbers they color the water. Much of the phosphorescence of the sea results from coloration by these plant-animals, which can be green, yellow, brown or red. The bloom ensues from a combination of factors, including a rise in water temperature, increased freshwater runoff, upwelling of nutrients, and heavy rainfall along coastal regions.

The species of dinoflagellate called Gonyaulax is responsible for most paralytic shellfish poisoning incidents in the United States.

Legend is that in the days before the arrival of Europeans in the Americas, the Mendocino Indians of California set one of their number to watch the color of the ocean, knowing that when it turned red the clams and mussels were not safe to eat. This may have been the best technique at the time, but it is not considered so good today.

For one thing, not all Red Tides are produced by toxic dinoflagellates. And when the Red Tide is produced by the dangerous Gonyaulax species, the shellfish can be toxic for several days before the color is visible. This is especially true of mussels, which seem to be the most efficient at storing the toxin and are the most common cause of paralytic shellfish poisoning. Luckily, scientific equipment now can detect low levels of these microscopic toxin-producers, so regulatory agencies monitoring chronically affected areas can determine when shellfish are toxic without depending on the visual evidence of a Red Tide.

575

Major Disease-Causing Organisms Transmitted By Shellfish

Disease-causing Agent: *Vibrio cholerae*-01 bacteria

Disease in Humans: Cholera—ranges from subclinical (a mild uncomplicated bout with diarrhea) to fatal (intense diarrhea with dehydration). Severe cases require hospitalization.

Mode of Contamination: Bacteria are found in mollusks harvested from waters contaminated with human sewage. During cholera epidemics, the bacteria may be widely distributed.

Disease-causing Agent: *Vibrio cholerae* non-01 bacteria

Disease in Humans: Gastroenteritis—diarrhea (mild to severe), vomiting, fever, abdominal cramps. Lasts 1-2 days. The bacteria can cause septicemia (chills, fever, prostration) in people with liver disease.

Mode of Contamination: The bacteria occur naturally and are widely distributed inthe environment. They are more numerous in the summer months.

Disease-causing Agent: *Vibrio parahaemolyticus* bacteria:

Disease in Humans: Parahaemolyticus gastroenteritis—lasts 24-48 hours with abdominal pain, diarrhea, nausea, headache and fever.

Mode of Contamination: Bacteria are widespread in all parts of the marine environment, in both polluted and unpolluted waters. Bacteria multiply rapidly in warm temperatures (above 37 degrees C). Large numbers of the bacteria must be present before poisoning occurs. Illness usually results from eating raw shellfish.

Disease-causing Agent: *Vibrio vulnificus* bacteria

Disease in Humans: Septicemia—abrupt onset of chills, fever and/or prostration. Usually only people with liver disease are at risk.

Mode of Contamination: The bacteria live in coastal waters and can infect humans either through open wounds or via the gastrointestinal tract (through consumption of contaminated seafood). The bacteria are more numerous in warm weather.

Disease-causing Agent: *Salmonella* bacteria (more than 1,700 kinds)

Disease in Humans: Salmonellosis—nausea, fever, headache, abdominal cramps, diarrhea and sometimes vomiting. Can be fatal in infants, the elderly, and the infirm.

Mode of Contamination: Mollusks usually acquire only small numbers of Salmonella bacteria in the water. Unsanitary handling can allow the bacteria to multiply to the point that food poisoning occurs.

Disease-causing Agent: Hepatitis A virus

Disease in Humans: Hepatitis—begins with malaise, appetite loss, nausea, vomiting and fever. After 3 to 10 days the patient develops jaundice with darkened urine. Mild cases often are mistaken for flu; severe cases can cause liver damage and death.

Mode of Contamination: Mollusks become carriers when their beds are polluted by untreated sewage. Raw shellfish are especially potent carriers, although cooking does not always kill the virus.

Disease-causing Agent: Norwalk virus

Disease in Humans: Gastroenteritis—causes transient flu-like symptoms, including nausea, vomiting, diarrhea and abdominal pain.

Mode of Contamination: The virus enters the mollusks' environment in untreated sewage. Raw shellfish are especially potent carriers.

Disease-causing Agent: *Gonyaulax,* a genus of dinoflagellate ("plankton"). Major species causing PSP in the U.S. are: *G. tamarensis* (East Coast) *G. catenella* (West Coast)

Disease in Humans: Paralytic shellfish poisoning—Symptoms occur within 30 minutes of ingestion and include tingling, numbness or burning sensation in the lips, gums, tongue and face. This progresses to muscular weakness, respiratory paralysis, and gradual paralysis of the extremities. PSP CAN BE FATAL. Medical help should be obtained immediately.

Mode of Contamination: Mollusks become poisonous after eating one of several species of dinoflagellates. The dinoflagellates produce neurotoxins that may not affect the mollusks but are deadly to humans. The organisms are especially prolific during warm weather. In great numbers they can cause the ocean to turn color in the phenomenon known as "Red Tide."

Disease-causing Agent: *Ptychodiscus brevis* (formerly (*Gymnodinium breve*), a dinoflagellate found in the Gulf of Mexico that causes Florida's Red Tides.

Disease in Humans: Neurotoxic shellfish poisoning—similar to but milder than PSP. Symptoms include tingling of the extremities, reversal of hot and cold sensation, vomiting and diarrhea.

Mode of Contamination: Contamination occurs as with paralytic shellfish poisoning. In addition, the toxins produced by the dinoflagellates can be airborne in rough surf, and when inhaled can cause respiratory irritation, including runny nose and nonproductive cough.

by Carol Ballentine

Carol Ballentine is a member of FDA's publications staff.

Section 12

Is Something Fishy Going On?

Fresh fish for dinner tonight. Twelve dollars a pound is a bit pricy to experiment with a new recipe, but on ice in the market, the fish labeled "red snapper" looks fresh and inviting. So you buy it.

But how do you know the fish really is red snapper and not rock-fish, its look-alike that generally sells for about $2 a pound? Such species substitution—selling a cheaper fish as though it were a more expensive one—is one of several kinds of economic fraud involving seafood sales that troubles consumers, reputable dealers, and the Food and Drug Administration.

Because seafood is such a high-value product, it is a particularly attractive target for fraud. Overbreading, another form of economic fraud, has consumers paying shrimp prices for bread crumbs, and overglazing charges lobster tail prices for ice. Abuses such as these hit consumers squarely in the wallet. FDA has recently begun focusing more intensely on its mandate to reduce economic fraud in the seafood industry. In 1991, the agency established the Office of Seafood, with a 60 percent increase in funding for seafood inspection, including an increase in resources for field offices.

The seafood industry doesn't like economic fraud either. A 1985 National Fisheries Institute survey report said, "There was general agreement among the industries [processing, distributing and importing firms] as well as retailers and restaurateurs that there is widespread abuse of overglazing and overbreading of fishery products, inaccurate net weights, and species substitution." In a presentation at the Atlantic Fisheries Technology Conference in 1990, the National

Publication No. (FDA) 94-2274

Marine Fisheries Service said, "No matter what the reason, industry' s desire for a level playing field to combat fraud is strong, and consumers want full value."

Though there are reported incidents, the extent of seafood fraud is not well documented. Few databases are designed specifically to track economic fraud. The ones that do usually include data from the National Marine Fisheries Service seafood inspection laboratory (which analyzes samples upon request), state-directed surveys, and weights and measure programs, such as that of the U.S. Department of Commerce.

Fraud is not always intentional. It can occur because of misunderstanding or lack of information, or it can be an honest mistake by a grocery store if the store bought a misrepresented product. Ignorance of the mislabeling does not excuse the violation, however, and FDA holds the seller responsible.

Mary Snyder, chief of the policy guidance branch of FDA' s Office of Seafood, says the agency is doing what it can to educate retailers so they can guard against fraud. FDA advises retailers to be specific when ordering seafood and encourages them to take the initiative to learn about the products. In addition, FDA has put retailers on notice about the agency's emphasis on enforcement through letters warning about economic fraud. As a result, some supermarkets advised their seafood buyers that they would report abuses to FDA.

What Species Is It?

This question doesn't have to come up if a product is properly labeled. But it does, because species substitution is likely the most widespread abuse. Speaking to the National Fisheries Institute in April 1991, FDA Commissioner David A. Kessler, M.D., said: "There is no place in the seafood industry for those who substitute a less expensive or less desirable species of fish for one that consumers value more. We will seek out those who perpetrate fraud—and we will bring them to justice."

FDA is reeling in abusers making big profits. For example, in May 1992, FDA detained 1,200 pounds of fresh rockfish from Canada, invoiced at $1.50 per pound. According to FDA's Seattle district, it was labeled red snapper, the federally recognized name for a species that comes from the southern Atlantic and the Gulf of Mexico. FDA estimates the firm could have realized an excess profit of about $12,600 on that shipment alone over what it would have received if the fish had been properly labeled. In another case in 1989, FDA' s Chicago district seized a 45,000 pound lot of oreo dory (average price $2 per pound), imported from New Zealand, bound for Ohio markets labeled as orange roughy, which also comes from New Zealand but generally sells for $6 per pound. FDA estimates the firm could have realized an unfair profit of about $150,000.

"It's not always possible to 'see' that a lesser product has been substituted for another," says Snyder, who is also FDA's species identification expert. Sometimes, FDA regulators must use laboratory verification such as identifying the fish scale and patterns, or isoelectric focusing, a technique that identifies a species by analyzing the pattern of proteins in the flesh. When charged with an electric current, the proteins form a unique pattern for each species. The pattern from the species in question is then compared with the known pattern for that species, very much like comparing fingerprints.

Many species have distinguishing marks or specific origins, and an informed consumer can watch for the marks or ask the fish market manager where the fish comes from. (See below.) Consumers can also check one of many well illustrated seafood cookbooks. These have information on what species look like, and how to tell the difference between substitutes and the real thing. Usually there's also information about the texture and taste of a species. If a product isn't as expected after it's cooked, FDA advises consumers to discuss the problem with the fish market manager where the product was purchased.

To guide species identification, FDA maintains a seafood names list, which includes shellfish. The list is used mostly by industry so it can uniformly label its products using FDA acceptable market names. Developed in cooperation with the National Marine Fisheries Service, the list includes over 1,000 species currently sold in the United States or that have a strong potential for sale here. It does not list endangered species nor those prohibited for sale. For example, escolar, a fish commonly known as "castor oil fish," was deleted from the new edition after it was reported to cause diarrhea in many consumers.

The seafood list shows the acceptable market name, the scientific name, and any regional names. Regional names can cause confusion, sometimes deliberately, other times inadvertently. For example, rockfish is called "Pacific red snapper" in California. People in California know what to expect when they see "Pacific red snapper" but in other parts of the United States, consumers only know red snapper as a highly valued fish from the Gulf of Mexico. FDA does not allow rockfish sold across state lines out of California to be called anything other than "rockfish."

Sometimes regional names for fish are "made up" to make the fish sound better or of higher value, Snyder says. She gives the example of tilapia, a common imported fish that is also bred in the United States and other countries through aquaculture (on fish farms). Because it is also found in the Sea of Galilee in Israel, it traditionally has been called "St. Peter's fish," for the biblical fisherman of the New Testament. Importers have tried bringing it into this country labeled "St. Peter's fish," but FDA has informed them that it must be labeled tilapia.

Colors Added to Fish Feed

Some aquaculturalists have begun using the color additives canthaxanthin and astaxanthin, both derived from beta carotene, a vitamin A component that imparts an orange color. Canthaxanthin is approved for use in chicken feed—the color gives chicken flesh the yellow cast that some people find desirable. Astaxanthin has not yet been approved for any food or feed use.

When used in feed for rainbow trout, these color additives turn trout flesh the color of salmon, a much higher valued species. In addition, some aquaculturalists grow the fish to larger than trout size, and then market it as "salmon trout." There is no such species and this is not an acceptable market name, Snyder says.

Color additive experts in FDA's Center for Food Safety and Applied Nutrition are aware that the regulation listing canthaxanthin to color food may lead some to think that it may be used in fish and fish feed. FDA did not intend to list this color additive for these uses. The agency is currently working on a regulation that would make it clear that the use of regulated colors in animal feed with the intention of coloring the animal flesh must have a specific listing for such use.

Water Added

Sodium tripolyphosphate (STP) is one of a family of phosphates the seafood industry may use as humectants, substances that maintain moisture in products. STP is used to process scallops, shrimp and lobster tails.

The phosphates are currently listed by FDA as "generally recognized as safe," a classification that means a food additive may be used for certain purposes. However, FDA is concerned that the seafood industry is using STP in ways that constitute economic abuse, especially in scallops. Atlantic sea scallops, for example, usually consist of 75 to 79 percent water. They can lose a considerable amount of their moisture after the shellfish are harvested and the meat is removed from the shell.

Soaking in an STP-water solution keeps scallops from losing their natural water. Prolonged soaking, however, can result in Atlantic sea scallops with excessive water, adding to the product's total weight. Inspections of processing plants by FDA's Boston and Baltimore districts showed that some scallop processors were soaking the shellfish for up to 36 hours, resulting in a 4 to 5 percent weight gain.

Consumers could be defrauded into buying water-augmented scallops at the same price per pound as scallops that are naturally larger. FDA met with industry representatives to discuss the use of STP. The industry agreed to determine the effects of various treatment times and STP concentrations on scallops, and to determine whether STP soaking provides benefits beyond restoring water loss, such as improving the texture of the scallops.

Excessive water has also been found in shelled oyster containers. FDA is concerned that this practice adulterates the product because the water is absorbed by the oysters, increasing their apparent weight. The agency is currently revising the regulation that defines the number of oysters and amount of liquid.

FDA does not object to the industry practice of using a frozen glaze of water to protect products such as frozen shrimp and lobster tails from freezer burn. Such glaze, however, cannot be part of the net weight. FDA has sent warning letters to processors and trade associations saying that the agency will take regulatory action where evidence of this practice is found.

Overbreading and Fresh Thawed

It's disappointing to open a frozen seafood package and find more breading than fish. In 1991, the Connecticut state government surveyed breaded frozen shrimp products and found an average of 33.5 percent shrimp—the rest was bread crumbs. The FDA standard for breaded shrimp requires that the product contain at least 50 percent shrimp. The method for breading is included in the standard.

FDA is taking enforcement action against processors who overbread. For example, in March 1991 in Mississippi, FDA seized

1,788 pounds of frozen breaded shrimp, valued at $5,000 ($2.80 per pound), which contained only 41.4 percent shrimp. With an 8.2 percent shortage of shrimp, FDA estimated the firm could have realized a profit excess of $300 at the consumers' expense.

Sometimes, fish in the market is labeled "previously frozen." FDA allows the sale of thawed fish that has previously been frozen, but it must be labeled as such and cannot be labeled fresh. Fish spoils more easily than most flesh foods, and even in ideal storage conditions, it has a very short shelf life in its fresh condition. Therefore, to protect the product, many processors freeze fish as soon as possible, often at sea. This can be an excellent product. However, if a fish has previously been frozen and is then thawed for sale, the label must state that the product was previously frozen.

Is It Really Caviar?

Unless it's roe (fish eggs) from the sturgeon species, it's not caviar, FDA says affairs staff in a policy established many years ago. Sturgeon roe sells for about $35 an ounce; roe from other species such as salmon or lumpfish sells for $1 an ounce. Two years ago, FDA issued a warning letter to a firm that had labeled whitefish roe as "American Golden Caviar."

FDA is working to protect consumers from fraudulent practices in the seafood industry. The agency gives talks to industry groups, displays at trade shows, and has open exchanges with state regulatory agencies, as well as increased training for its own field investigators. And a hot line is available to answer consumer questions. But FDA emphasizes that the best defense against fraud is the educated consumer.

How to Avoid Seafood Economic Fraud

To get the best value for your money when buying seafood, it's important to know what you're buying. Be wary of unusual bargains—some seafood is seasonal. If there is a considerable difference between the price of a fresh product and what you are accustomed to paying, it could be that it is from the last season's frozen inventory. Buy from a reputable dealer. And if the fish you choose looks or smells different from what you expect, discuss it with the fish market manager.

Look for firm, shiny flesh that bounces back when touched. If the head is on, the eyes should be clear and bulge, and the gills should be bright red. The fish should not smell "fishy"—it should smell like a fresh ocean breeze.

It's easy to miss the telltale signs of species substitution. Sometimes, taste or consistency is the only way to detect it. If you feel you have purchased something different from what was represented, tell your fish market manager.

Here's how to distinguish some common species:

• Haddock has a dark lateral line along the skin surface.

• Skinless cod fillets have a distinctive white papery membrane along the belly and a white line of fat along the lateral line of the fillet.

• Shark and swordfish look alike, but shark has a dark streak of flesh in the center and rough skin along the edge.

• Red snapper comes only from the southern Atlantic Ocean and the Gulf of Mexico (ask your retailer where the snapper originated).

• Orange roughy comes only from Australia or New Zealand and always arrives frozen. It may be sold thawed, but it must be labeled as previously frozen.

• Scrod is not a type of fish. The term originated in the Boston area to describe the catch of the day. It is a fish under two and a half pounds that is either cod, haddock or pollock. Such fish should be labeled in the market or listed in a restaurant as "scrod cod," "scrod haddock," or "scrod pollock."

The FDA Seafood Hotline can be reached at (1-800) FDA-4010 or (202) 205-4314 (in the Washington, D.C., area). The automated hot line and Flash Fax service is available 24 hours a day. Public affairs specialists can be reached from noon until 4 p.m. Eastern time Monday through Friday.

by Judith E. Foulke

Judith E. Foulke is a staff writer for *FDA Consumer*. Mary Alice Sudduth contributed to this article while on FDA's public affairs staff.

Appendix B

Advice on Safe Food Handling and Preparation

Section 1

Handling Eggs Safely at Home

Eggs are a perishable food and must be properly stored and cooked. raw eggs that were contaminated with Salmonella enteritidis bacteria have caused some outbreaks of foodborne illness. Most outbreaks appear to be related to pooling (commingling) of eggs, time/temperature abuse, and incomplete cooking.

Most eggs do not contain Salmonella enteritidis and the risk of contracting salmonellosis from raw or undercooked eggs is extremely small. Scientists have concluded that Salmonella enteritidis can get inside the egg shell. Just how or when this contamination occurs is still unclear, but scientists are working to better understand the problem and find solutions.

Proper refrigeration at 40°F or below limits the growth of Salmonella enteritidis and proper cooking at 140°F or above destroys the organism. Therefore, consumers must follow safe food-handling practices when preparing eggs.

Special precautions are needed when eggs are served to people who are particularly vulnerable to Salmonella enteritidis infections. High-risk groups are the very young, the elderly, pregnant women (because of risk to the fetus), and people already weakened by serious illness or whose immune systems are weakened.

United States Department of Agriculture; Food and Drug Administration; Revised January 1992, AMS-602

Consumer Guidelines

Consumers should take the following precautions when handling both raw eggs and foods in which eggs are an ingredient, such as quiche or baked custard.

1. Avoid eating raw eggs and foods containing raw eggs: homemade Caesar salad, homemade hollandaise sauce, and homemade mayonnaise, for example. Likewise, homemade ice cream and homemade eggnog should be avoided unless made with a cooked, custard-type base. Commercial forms of these products are safe to serve since they are made with pasteurized liquid eggs. Commercial pasteurization destroys Salmonella bacteria.

2. Cook eggs thoroughly until both the yolk and the white are firm. This is especially important for people most at risk for foodborne illness. Those electing not to consume hard-cooked eggs can minimize their risk by cooking the egg until the white is completely firm and the yolk begins to thicken but is not hard. Fried eggs should be cooked on both sides or in a covered pan. Scrambled eggs should be cooked until firm throughout.

3. Realize that eating lightly cooked foods containing eggs, such as meringues, and French toast, may be risky for people in high-risk groups.

Consumers should also follow the usual safe food-handling practices for eggs:

1. Buy refrigerated grade AA or A eggs with clean. uncracked shells.

2. At home, keep eggs in their original carton and refrigerate as soon as possible at a temperature no higher than 40 F. Do not wash eggs before storing or using them. Washing is a routine part of commercial egg processing and rewashing is unnecessary.

3. Use raw shell eggs within 5 weeks after bringing them home. Use hard-cooked eggs (in the shell or peeled) within 1 week after cooking. Use leftover yolks and whites within 4 days after removing them from the shell.

4. Avoid keeping raw or cooked eggs and egg-containing foods out of the refrigerator for more than 2 hours, including time for preparing and serving (but not cooking). If you hide hard-cooked eggs for an egg hunt, either follow the 2-hour rule or do not eat the eggs.

5. Wash hands, utensils, equipment, and work areas with hot, soapy water before and after they come in contact with eggs and egg-containing foods.

6. Review traditional recipes that, when served, contain raw or under-cooked eggs. Replace with recipes that, when served, contain thoroughly cooked eggs.

7. Serve cooked eggs and egg-containing foods hot, immediately after cooking; or hold for buffet-style serving at 1 40°F or higher; or refrigerate at 40°F or below for serving later. Use within 3-4 days.

8. When refrigerating a large amount of a hot egg-containing food or leftover, divide it into several shallow containers so it will cool quickly.

For more information on handling eggs safely, Call USDA's meat and poultry hotline, 1-800-535-4555; In the Washington, D.C. area call (202) 720-3333 Hours are from 10 a.m. to 4 p.m. Eastern time

Section 2

A Consumer Guide to Safe Handling and Preparation of Ground Meat and Poultry

COOL IT!

Ground meat and ground poultry are more perishable than most foods. In the danger zone between 40° and 140° F, bacteria can multiply rapidly. Since you can't see, smell or taste bacteria, keep the products cold to keep them safe.

Safe Handling

- Choose ground meat packages that are cold and tightly wrapped. The meat surface exposed to air will be red; interior of fresh meat will be dark.

- Put refrigerated and frozen foods in your grocery cart last and make the grocery store your last stop before home.

- Pack perishables in an ice chest if it will take you more than an hour to get home.

- Place ground meat and ground poultry in the refrigerator or freezer immediately.

- Defrost frozen ground meats in the refrigerator —never at room temperature. If microwave defrosting, cook immediately.

Safe Storage

- Set your refrigerator at 40° F or colder and your freezer at 0°F or colder.

- Keep uncooked ground meat and ground poultry in the refrigerator; cook or freeze within 1 to 2 days.

- Use or freeze cooked meat and poultry stored in the refrigerator within 3 to 4 days.

- For best quality, store frozen raw ground meats no longer than 3 to 4 months; cooked meats, 2 to 3 months.

CLEAN IT!

Keep EVERYTHING clean—hands, utensils, counters, cutting boards and sinks. That way, your food will stay as safe as possible.

- Always wash hands thoroughly in hot soapy water before preparing foods and after handling raw meat.

- Don't let raw meat or poultry juices touch ready-to-eat foods either in the refrigerator or during preparation.

- Don't put cooked foods on the same plate that held raw meat or poultry.

- Wash utensils that have touched raw meat with hot, soapy water before using them for cooked meats.

- Wash counters, cutting boards and other surfaces raw meats have touched. And don't forget to keep the inside of your refrigerator clean.

COOK IT!

Cooking kills harmful bacteria. Be sure ground meat and ground poultry are cooked thoroughly.

Cook it safely

- The center of patties and meat loaf should not be pink and the juices should run clear.

- Crumbled ground meats should be cooked until no pink color remains.

- Ground meat patties and loaves are safe when they reach 160°F in the center; ground poultry patties and loaves, 165°F.

Cook it evenly

- During broiling, grilling, or cooking on the stove, turn meats over at least once.

- When baking, set oven no lower than 325°F.

- If microwaving, cover meats. Midway through cooking, turn patties over and rotate the dish; rotate a meat loaf; and stir ground meats once or twice. Let microwaved meats stand to complete cooking process.

After cooking, refrigerate leftovers immediately. Separate into small portions for fast cooling.

To reheat all leftovers, cover and heat to 165° or until hot and steaming throughout.

Consumer Guidelines

Cold Storage Times: Ground Meat And Ground Poultry

Refrigerator (40°F or below)

Product	Days
Uncooked ground meat and ground poultry (bulk or patties)	1 to 2
Cooked ground meat and ground poultry (hamburgers, meat loaf and dishes containing ground meats)	3 to 4

Freezer (0° F or below)

Product	Months
Uncooked ground meat and ground poultry (bulk or patties)	3 to 4
Cooked ground meat and ground poultry (hamburgers, meat loaf and dishes containing ground meats)	2 to 3

Internal Temperatures For Safe Cooking

Product	Temperature
Uncooked ground meat	160°F
Uncooked ground poultry	165°F
All cooked leftovers, reheated	165°F

Developed by Food Marketing Institute, 800 Connecticut Avenue, Washington, DC 20006 and American Meat Institute, N.W. Post Office Box 3556, Washington, DC 20007 in cooperation with National Live Stock & Meat Board, 444 N. Michigan Avenue, Chicago, IL 60611; U.S. Department of Agriculture Food Safety and Inspection Service Extension Service 14th Street & Independence Avenue, S.W. Washington, DC 20250; U.S. Department of Health and Human Services, Food and Drug Administration, 5600 Fishers Lane Rockville, MD 20857.

For information about the safe handling and preparation of ground meat and ground poultry, call USDA's Meat and Poultry Hotline toll-free at: 1-800-53 5-4555 10 00 a.m. to 4 00 p.m. Eastern time, Monday through Friday or contact your local Cooperative Extension Service Office

Section 3

Food Irradiation Toxic to Bacteria, Safe for Humans

A measure FDA announced in the Federal Register this year may go unused because of consumer apprehension. On May 2, 1990, FDA issued a rule defining the use of irradiation as a safe and effective means to control a major source of food-borne illness—Salmonella and other food-borne bacteria in raw chicken, turkey, and other poultry. However, FDA has received written objections that it must evaluate before the rule can go into effect.

Experts believe that up to 60 percent of poultry sold in the United States is contaminated with Salmonella, according to Joseph Madden, Ph.D., acting director of FDA's division of microbiology. Madden adds that studies suggest that all chicken may be contaminated with the Campylobacter organism.

People often become ill after eating contaminated poultry. Symptoms may range from a simple stomachache to incapacitating stomach and intestinal disorders, occasionally resulting in death.

As equipment used to irradiate food is regulated as a food additive, the FDA rule is the first step in permitting irradiation of poultry. However, although the U.S. Department of Agriculture will soon propose a companion rule finalizing guidelines for commercial irradiation of poultry, industry groups cite consumer apprehension as a drawback to implementing the procedure. And reaction to FDA's new rule has elicited more questions than answers.

DHHS Publication No. (FDA) 91-2241 (November, 1991)

A Scary Word

Irradiating food to prevent illness from food-borne bacteria is not a new concept. Research on the technology began in earnest shortly after World War II, when the U.S. Army began a series of experiments irradiating fresh foods for troops in the field. Since 1963, FDA has passed rules permitting irradiation to curb insects in foods and microorganisms in spices, control parasite contamination in pork, and retard spoilage in fruits and vegetables.

But, to many people, the word irradiation means danger. It is associated with atomic bomb explosions and nuclear reactor accidents such as those at Chernobyl and Three Mile Island. The idea of irradiating food signals a kind of "gamma alarm," according to one British broadcaster. (Gamma rays are forms of energy emitted from some radioactive materials.)

But when it comes to food irradiation, the only danger is to the bacteria that contaminate the food. The process damages their genetic material, so the organisms can no longer survive or multiply.

Irradiation does not make food radioactive and, therefore, does not increase human exposure to radiation. The specified exposure times and energy levels of radiation sources approved for foods are inadequate to induce radioactivity in the products, according to FDA's Laura Tarantino, Ph.D., an expert on food irradiation. The process involves exposing food to a source of radiation, such as to the gamma rays from radioactive cobalt or cesium or to x-rays. However, no radioactive material is ever added to the product. Manufacturers use the same technique to sterilize many disposable medical devices.

Tarantino notes that in testing the safety of the process, scientists used much higher levels of radiation than those approved for use in poultry. But even at these elevated levels, researchers found no toxic or cancer-causing effects in animals consuming irradiated poultry.

Beyond the Gamma Alarm

Market tests show that once consumers learn about irradiation, they will buy irradiated food. For example, Christine Bruhn, Ph.D., of the University of California's Center for Consumer Research in Davis, Calif., reports that irradiated papayas outsold the nonirradiated product by more than 10 to 1 when in-store information was available. And, Danny Terry, Ph.D., a consumer researcher at Central Missouri State University in Warrensburg, Mo., says that a recent market test he conducted with irradiated strawberries showed that consumers who received written information about irradiation along with the fruit were slightly more interested in buying irradiated products in the future.

Nevertheless, concern about the process remains strong. Since 1989, three states (Maine, New York, and New Jersey) have either banned or issued a moratorium on the sale of irradiated foods. According to a U.S. General Accounting Office report prepared in May 1990 at the request of Rep. Douglas Bosco (D-Calif.), "officials of these states told us that their states took the actions in response to public concern by citizen groups rather than as a result of scientific evidence questioning the safety of food irradiation."

"Something quite aside from food safety appears to lie at the root of the entire controversy, which may explain why it continues to flourish in the face of all safety assurances," says Carolyn Lochhead in the August 1989 issue of *Food Technology* magazine. "Many opponents charge that the Food and Drug Administration, the World Health Organization, and the nuclear power industry are conspiring to promote the technique as a way to dispose of nuclear waste."

Lochhead discusses concerns that one source of radioactive material for food irradiation, cesium 137, is recovered from spent fuel rods in nuclear power plants. The conspiracy charge promotes unwarranted fear among consumers, says Lochhead.

"For economic, as well as other, reasons," says Department of Energy official Barbara Thomas, "the U.S. commercial nuclear power industry does not attempt to recover material, such as cesium 137, from spent fuel."

According to DOE, commercial irradiators in the United States choose their irradiation source (whether the gamma-emitting radioactive materials cesium 137 or cobalt 60, or accelerators that can produce electrons, x-rays or both) based on practical requirements, such as cost. The product to be irradiated also influences the choice. Many foods require low energy levels to kill harmful organisms, while medical supplies may need higher doses for sterilization.

However, the fallout from a falsely characterized cesium recovery plan has charged the legislative atmosphere. George Giddings, Ph.D., a consultant food scientist and expert in food irradiation matters, sees it as the "single most inciting issue in the food irradiation area." Giddings suggests that legislators are wary of supporting food irradiation measures some critics say are linked to increased nuclear activity, including the production of nuclear weapons.

601

A 1982 congressional amendment bars using spent commercial fuel for military purposes. The Department of Energy has no interest in changing this law.

Michael Colby, director of Food and Water, Inc., one of the more vocal groups lobbying against food irradiation, says the new poultry regulation will lead to nuclear hazards, including "the continued generation of radioactive wastes for which a secure isolation technology has yet to be developed." Colby submitted the comment during a 30-day objection period following publication of the final rule. In the case of food additives, FDA evaluates objections in order to determine whether any changes in the final rule are appropriate. Based on FDA's findings, those raising the objection may be entitled to a hearing before the commissioner.

FDA inspections of all irradiation plants conducted from 1986 to 1989 showed no violations of the food irradiation regulations.

Giddings contends that groups such as Food and Water play on the public's fear of nuclear energy and misrepresent the safety questions surrounding food irradiation. They frame it as a "populist" issue to legislators and pressure them to introduce legislation banning food irradiation.

Consumer Uncertainty

Other consumer groups have taken more moderate positions. The Center for Science in the Public Interest, for instance, says that "at a minimum, irradiated foods should be labeled" so that consumers know what they're buying.

Since 1966, FDA has required that irradiated foods be labeled as such. In 1986, a mandatory logo was added to this labeling requirement. The international logo, first used in the Netherlands, consists of a solid circle, representing an energy source, above two petals, which represent the food. Five breaks in the outer circle depict rays from the energy source.

Consumer surveys show mixed reactions. According to an article in the October 1989 issue of *Food Technology* magazine, which reviewed surveys conducted by various academic and consumer research groups, consumers are more concerned about chemical sprays and pesticide residues, preservatives, and food-borne illnesses than about food irradiation. A Louis Harris poll, conducted from 1984 through 1986, however, found that 76 percent of Americans consider irradiated food a hazard.

"Consumer acceptance of irradiation as a treatment for foods is showing only minimal positive change, at best," said Fred Shank, Ph.D., director of FDA's Center for Food Safety and Applied Nutrition, in a symposium on food irradiation at the 1990 annual meeting of the Institute of Food Technology. Shank said that the greatest concern about the process is its perceived association with radioactivity and nuclear power.

Another concern, raised often in comments to FDA when it proposed the use of radiation to kill microorganisms in spices and insects in fresh foods, is that irradiation may produce substances not known to be present in nonirradiated foods.

These substances, described by scientists as "radiolytic products" sound more threatening than they actually are, says George Pauli, Ph.D., an FDA food irradiation expert and policy maker. For instance, Pauli says, when we heat food it often creates new substances that produce new tastes and smells. These substances could be called thermolytic products—an intimidating word for a harmless change.

In 1979, FDA established the Bureau of Foods Irradiated Food Committee (BFIFC) to review safety assessments of irradiated food. Experiments have shown that very few of these radiolytic products are unique to irradiated foods. In fact, the BFIFC estimated that approximately 90 percent of the substances identified as radiolytic products are found in foods that have not been irradiated—including raw, heated and stored foods. Moreover, many of these substances are not well known because the foods usually have not been studied at the minute (parts per million) levels scrutinized by chemists who analyzed the irradiated foods.

Measuring Irradiation

Absorbed radiation is measured in units called "Grays." The amount of Grays refers to the level of energy absorbed by a food from ionizing radiation that passes through the food in processing.

1,000 Grays = 1 kiloGray (1 kGy)

In the past, the term "rad" was commonly used. It stands for" radiation absorbed dose."

100 rad = 1 Gy

U.S. Food Irradiation Rules

Product	Purpose of Irradiation	Dose Permitted (kGy)	Date of Rule
Wheat and wheat powder	Disinfest insects	0.2-0.5	8/21/63
White potatoes	Extend shelf life	0.05-0.15	11/1/65
Spices and dry vegetable seasoning (38 commodities)	Decontamination/ disinfest insects	30(max.)	7/5/83
Dry or dehydrated enzyme preparations	Control insects and microorganisms	10(max.)	6/10/85
Pork carcasses or fresh, non-cut processed cuts	Control *Trichinella spiralis*	0.3(min.)- 1.0(max.)	7/22/85
Fresh fruits	Delay maturation	1	4/18/86
Dry or dehydrated enzyme preparations	Decontamination	10	4/18/86
Dry or dehydrated aromatic vegetable substances	Decontamination	30	4/18/86
Poultry	Control illness-causing microorganisms	3	5/2/90

Poultry Producers Respond

With one hand, poultry producers are giving a thumbs up sign to FDA's rule permitting irradiation of poultry. With the other, they are putting its use on hold.

Stuart Proctor, executive vice president of the National Turkey Federation—which represents 95 percent of turkey growers and producers—says "we are encouraged by FDA's decision. The industry should be allowed to use any science available that makes food safe from food-borne illness and also is safe." He continues, "as soon as consumers are ready to accept the product, we'll use it."

As George Watts, president of the National Broiler Council, says, "the U.S. poultry industry has always been a consumer-driven business, demonstrated by the variety of new products developed over the years to meet the American public's demand." He says that should consumers desire irradiated food products, "the industry will respond."

Perdue Farms, Inc., a large, East Coast chicken producer, says it has no plans to use the irradiation process. Steve McCauley, a company spokesman, said that the firm sees no need for decontaminating its poultry with irradiation because Perdue tests its products stringently. He claims this keeps them safe from contamination.

The need is for consumer education. Although poultry groups say they do not have the resources for the costly campaign needed, they believe that once consumers understand more about food irradiation, they will demand it.

Proctor compares reaction to food irradiation to earlier apprehension about microwave ovens. Once consumers recognized microwave cooking as safe, desire for fast and convenient food led to a microwave revolution. He said he could foresee the same demand for irradiated food, prompted by a desire to cut down on food-borne illness, once consumers are no longer afraid of the process.

by Dale Blumenthal

Section 4

Food Safety And The Microwave

The Supermarket, Microwave, and You—a Terrific Trio!

Almost everyone uses a microwave oven these days. Its speed fits today's lifestyle. And your supermarket has kept pace with the times by providing a limitless variety of foods you can microwave.

From fresh produce and meats to microwaveable frozen convenience foods and in-store deli items, foods become meals in minutes in your microwave.

But slow down. Even though the foods in your supermarket are safe when you buy them, it's up to you to handle them properly and microwave them correctly to avoid food poisoning.

Safe Food Begins with Proper Handling

Your supermarket and food producers maintain rigid quality assurance and sanitation standards to ensure that you always receive fresh, wholesome products. Always refer to the "Sell-by" date and "Use-by" information when printed on a product.

Once you purchase food, take it home immediately and store it correctly. This is especially important for perishable foods such as meat, poultry, seafood, eggs and dairy products. Mishandled foods can lead to food poisoning.

Observe safe storage times for refrigerated foods. Keep raw fish, poultry and ground meats no longer than two days before cooking or freezing them. Larger cuts of meat can hold for four days, about the same length of time as for cooked foods.

Raw eggs can be refrigerated in their shells three to five weeks. After hard cooking, refrigerate no longer than a week.

Do not leave raw or cooked foods out of the refrigerator for more than two hours, except during cooking.

Remember, the microwave, range or other cooking appliance cannot make food safe if it is improperly handled.

Get to Know Your Microwave

It's important to become thoroughly acquainted with your microwave. It doesn't cook like your other appliances. While microwaves can get food hot enough to kill bacteria that may be present, the microwave doesn't always cook evenly. Therefore, it's up to the cook to arrange, cover, rotate, stir and turn foods so they reach a safe temperature throughout.

Read all the manufacturer's instructions before operating the appliance. Don't use it for jobs it was not designed to handle. If you have a question about information supplied with the microwave or need guidance on other items, contact the microwave oven's manufacturer.

How Foods Cook in a Microwave

Foods cook differently by microwaves than by conventional heat. In a regular oven, hot air makes both the food and its container hot, while in the microwave, the air is cool. Cooking occurs when microwaves cause food molecules to vibrate; the resulting friction creates heat.

Since microwaves go little more than one inch deep into most foods, the center cooks when heat from the outer areas travels inward.

Food continues to cook after the microwave turns off, whether the food is still in the oven or someplace else. Be patient and allow the food to stand for an additional one third of the original cooking time, or as the recipe directs.

This carry-over heat can raise the internal temperatures by several degrees and helps equalize the temperature throughout the food. Both are important to food safety because in order to be safe, food must reach a temperature hot enough and for enough time to kill bacteria.

Defrosting Foods in a Microwave

Never defrost foods on the counter at room temperature. For gradual defrosting at a safe temperature, transfer frozen foods to the refrigerator for a day or two.

If you're short of time, microwaving is a safe way to defrost foods quickly.

First, remove food from store wrap and place it in a microwave-safe dish. Consult your oven manual for recommended defrosting times and power levels.

Several times during micro-defrosting, turn and rearrange food, and rotate the dish. Separate food items when possible and remove items as they defrost.

Since areas of food can become warm as they defrost in the microwave, cook the food immediately. Food is in a danger zone at temperatures between 40°F and 140°F.

Microwave Cooking Techniques

When preparing foods to microwave, keep your hands, utensils and work areas clean. Handle food carefully to minimize the spread of foodborne bacteria. Discard any food that looks or smells spoiled.

Choose only microwave-safe cooking utensils. Never use packaging cartons for cooking unless the package directs you to do so. Many plastic containers in which foods are sold are designed for cold storage and are not suitable for cooking or reheating. Chemicals from them can be absorbed into foods at high temperatures.

Cut food into uniform sizes so it will cook evenly. If foods are different sizes, arrange them in microwaveable dishes so thick parts are toward the outside. Outer areas receive more microwaves than the center.

For optimal safety, cover the dish with its lid or heavy-duty plastic wrap turned back at one corner. Plastic wrap shouldn't touch the food. Trapped steam will help even the temperature throughout the food, promoting safe cooking.

Rotate the dish midway through cooking. If the dish is on a rotating turntable, it's still a good idea to reposition the dish on it. Stir the food and rearrange it; turn large food items over. These practices help the food cook more evenly and safely.

Consult microwave cookbooks for estimated cooking times and power levels. Use reduced power levels for longer time when microwaving large cuts of meat and whole poultry to help even the temperatures throughout.

Microwave foods for the shortest time indicated and add more time as needed. As with any cooking device, food severely overcooked can cause a fire.

Testing for Doneness

Do not test for doneness when the microwave signals the end of cooking time. Since food continues to cook after the oven turns off, wait until after the food has had standing time. Adding extra cooking time prematurely can result in overcooked foods.

After the standing time, look for visual signs of doneness and check the temperatures:

- Juices from meat and poultry should not be pink. Poultry thigh joints must move easily. Fish should look opaque and flake easily with a fork. Runny eggs require additional cooking.

- Use the oven's temperature probe or a meat thermometer to test for doneness in several places. For meat, fish and eggs, the temperature should measure 160°F. For poultry, higher temperatures are recommended: 170°F for white meat and 180°F for dark meat.

These temperatures should kill bacteria and other harmful organisms that may be present.

People with weakened or underdeveloped immune systems should never eat raw or undercooked meat, poultry, eggs, fish or seafood. These high-risk individuals include expectant mothers, children under one year old, people age sixty and older, and individuals with chronic illness.

What to Do With Leftovers

Proper storage of leftovers and other previously-cooked foods is imperative for food safety. This category includes foods from a supermarket deli or restaurant, convenience foods or a planned extra batch of a recipe. Refrigerate (40°F or lower) or freeze (0°F) leftover foods within two hours after cooking.

Divide leftovers into several shallow dishes so they will cool to a safe temperature quickly. It's permissible to put hot food directly into the refrigerator or freezer. Foods left out more than two hours should be discarded.

Use refrigerated leftovers within three to four days. Freeze quantities that can't be used by then. Since bacteria can't grow at freezer temperatures, generally food is safe indefinitely while frozen. However, use frozen foods in a reasonable length of time for best quality.

Reheating Foods Safely

There's no doubt about it: the microwave is America's favorite reheater. But careless reheating can contribute to foodborne illness.

First, be sure the food you're reheating has been handled and stored properly. Heating may not destroy all the bacteria in food that was left out of refrigeration or stored too long. Heat cannot destroy toxins produced by some types of bacteria. If you are in doubt about the safety of the food—it is always best to throw it out.

Use the same techniques for reheating that are recommended above for microwaving raw foods safely. This goes for home-cooked leftovers, frozen or shelf-stable convenience foods, and carry-out foods.

When reheating soup, liquids and foods in sauces or gravy, always stir before as well as during and after microwaving.

Allow reheated foods to stand briefly before eating them. People have been burned by foods that appeared cooler on the surface than they turned out to be inside.

Reheated foods should reach 165 °F to ensure that bacteria are destroyed. Food should steam throughout, not just around the edges. The center bottom of the plate or utensil containing the food should be very hot to the touch.

Microwave Food Safety Checks

- Microwave only properly-stored and handled foods.

- Remove store wrap before defrosting food in a microwave oven.

- Cook foods immediately after defrosting.

- Arrange food to promote even heating.

- Use only microwave-safe dishes.

- Cover dish with lid or heavy-duty plastic wrap turned back at one corner.

- Midway through cooking and as needed:

  —Turn dish.

  —Reposition dish on rotating turntable.

  —Rearrange or stir foods during cooking.

  —Turn large food items over.

- Allow food to stand after microwaving.

- Check for doneness:

  —Temperature should reach 160°F for meat, fish and eggs.

  —Poultry white meat should reach 170°F.

  —Poultry dark meat should reach 180°F.

- Look for visual signs of doneness:

  —Juices from meat and poultry not pink.

  —Poultry thigh joints move easily.

  —Fish is opaque and flakes easily.

  —Eggs are not runny.

- Refrigerate leftovers within two hours of cooking.

- Reheat leftovers to 165°F or until food steams throughout and center bottom of dish is hot.

Additional Information Sources

For more information about food safety, contact:

- USDA's Meat and Poultry Hotline, 10 a.m. to 4 p.m. EST 1-800-535-4555

- Food and Drug Administration (see address below)

- Your supermarket or their consumer affairs department

- Your local county extension home economist

- State extension service

- Poison control centers

- Local health department

- Your microwave oven's manufacturer

- Food manufacturers

Developed by:

Food Marketing Institute
800 Connecticut Ave., NW
Washington, DC 20006-2701

In cooperation with:

American Frozen Food Institute
1764 Old Meadow Lane, Suite 350
McLean, VA 22102

Food and Drug Administration
5600 Fishers Lane
Rockville, MD 20857

International Microwave Power Institute
13542 Union Village Circle
Clifton, VA 22024

U.S. Department of Agriculture
Food Safety and Inspection Service
Room 1165 South
14th & Jefferson Drive, SW
Washington, DC 20250

Section 5

What Happens if the Packaging Gets into the Food?

We've come a long way since making popcorn meant shaking a pan of oil and kernels over high heat on the stove. Now, in less time than it takes to get through a commercial on Monday night football, we can pop a package in the microwave and get popcorn ready to serve in its own container. Our breakfast muffin heats up the same way, and sometimes we even get eggs on the side.

Heating and eating popcorn or breakfast in the same wrappers that come from the grocery is a great convenience, and in this era of two-career families, convenience foods are in great demand. But is some of the wrap getting cooked into our food?

And what about packaged food—like bread and cheese—that's not heated? The wrap is pressed directly against the food, often for a long time. Sometimes, especially with cheese, we can faintly taste or smell the plastic wrap on the end pieces. Does that mean that we're eating more than cheese?

Food packaging is big business. A consultant for the Institute of Packaging Professionals says that 55 percent of all packaging made in the United States is for food. And the market is growing, especially for microwavable packaging. For popcorn alone, about 1.4 billion bags were sold in 1989, and FDA projects sales to nearly double to 2.6 billion bags by 1994.

Manufacturers are vigilant about the materials that go into their food packages. It's not good business if their packaging material makes

DHHS Publication No. (FDA) 92-2250

someone sick— and they know that the Food and Drug Administration is watching, too.

FDA monitors packaging that comes in contact with food, whether it is used for transport from the food processor to the grocery, or from the grocery to the home—or while it is being stored in the pantry or cooked in the microwave. Manufacturers are required by law to obtain approval from FDA for all the materials used in food packages before they can be marketed. Components that have been shown to cause cancer in humans or animals cannot be used.

After evaluating the migration and safety data, FDA writes a regulation for each new component, specifying its conditions for use in food packaging and approving it as an "indirect" food additive. Packaging components that already are on FDA's "generally recognized as safe" (GRAS) list for use in food or in food packages do not need a separate regulation.

The GRAS list was established with the 1958 Food Additives Amendment to the Federal Food, Drug, and Cosmetic Act. The only other components of packaging that do not require a regulation are those that have a "prior sanction"—that is, those that were determined safe for use before 1958.

Bread Bags

Sometimes people use—or reuse—food packages for other than their intended uses. For example, an article in the June 1991 American *Journal of Public Health* by the University of Medicine and Dentistry of New Jersey-Robert Wood Johnson Medical School told about people turning bread bags inside out and reusing them to store food or pack lunches. The article noted with concern that lead-based ink was used on the labels of many bread bags. Right side out, the ink would not come in contact with the bread, but when the bags were turned inside out, the ink could have contaminated food stored in them.

However, since publication of the journal article, FDA has learned that lead-based inks are no longer used on bread bags. Neil Sass, Ph.D., of FDA's Center for Food Safety and Applied Nutrition, says it is now highly unlikely that consumers would come in contact with lead from this source.

But the risk of lead contamination was not the only problem with inverted bread wrappers. Who else handled the bag before it was turned inside out? There may have been dirty hands, insects, or microbial contaminants from other sources, none of which should be in contact with food.

Plastics

Now, about that end piece of cheese that tasted a bit like the plastic it was wrapped in. The FDA regulation that deals with indirect additives says that if a regulated food-packaging material were found in an appropriate test to impart an odor or taste to a specific food product, the food is adulterated and therefore subject to regulatory action. Sometimes when cheese is not refrigerated for a short while (such as during the trip home from the grocery), the end pieces taste a little like plastic, even though it is safe to eat. Off-odor and taste is a problem for food processors and they try not to let off-taste happen. It doesn't help sales if the package is safe but the cheese on the ends tastes a little like the package.

Flavor trading also works in reverse. For example, that plastic jug you use to mix your orange juice in the morning still smells like juice even after you've scrubbed it with soap and hot water. That problem is known in the industry as "flavor scalping." Plastic containers sometimes absorb flavors from citrus and other foods, lessening the flavor in the juice. The industry is trying to correct this. The containers are safe, but sometimes they dilute the taste of your good orange juice.

Migration of package components is rarely a problem with containers that hold dry food, such as cereal. But when a food is wet—and especially if it contains alcohol, acid or fat—chemicals from the packaging material could migrate into the food. FDA evaluates such uses and ensures that the materials are safe for the intended use before authorizing that use by regulation. (See below.)

Microwavable Packages

Regulations approving the safety of packaging materials heated with food were written before the advent of microwavable packaging. These regulations did not anticipate the development of microwave packaging components, called heat susceptors, that act like a frying pan when you crisp a waffle, brown the bottom of a pizza, and pop popcorn, for instance.

Heat susceptor layers in a microwave package reach temperatures of 400 to 500 degrees Fahrenheit, a much higher temperature than was envisioned when the regulations were written. Heat susceptor packages are multilayered, with food contacting the hot layer, usually a polyethylene terephthalate (PET) film with a thin coating of aluminum on the back. The heat susceptor layer is bound to the outer paper or paperboard by an adhesive. Popcorn bags have an additional grease-resistant paper layer between the heat susceptor and the food.

FDA's laboratory studies have shown that at high temperatures, components of the PET film migrate at levels far in excess of those that the agency anticipated when it initially regulated the PET film as an indirect additive. In addition, FDA studies show that at these high temperatures, the PET food-contact layer cracks, facilitating the migration of the adhesive components of the package, as well as their degraded products, directly into food. (Adhesives were originally approved for use in packaging where a functional barrier would be between it and the food, resulting in minimal migration.)

A third concern is that the high temperatures achieved by heat susceptors may cause the paper parts of the package to burn or char and partially decompose. These breakdown products could migrate into the food.

The aluminum component of the heat susceptor film is on the GRAS list, and FDA does not consider it a food additive problem. But because of the migration problem of the other components at high temperatures, FDA has requested additional data from manufacturers in order to reevaluate the regulations to ensure the safety of the packaging components. In September 1989, FDA published in the Federal Register an advance notice of proposed rule-making, asking manufacturers for additional safety data.

In response to this notice, the bulk of new data was submitted by the Susceptor Microwave Packaging Committee, composed of 33 member companies of the Society of Plastics Industries and the National Food Processors Association. Fifteen companies submitted a total of 42 heat susceptor packages to the committee for study.

Based on the data submitted by industry and on FDA's own data, several hundred components could migrate out of heat susceptor packages at extremely low levels at temperatures ranging from 400 to 500 degrees Fahrenheit.

One migrant chemical that has warranted special concern is benzene, which is known to cause cancer in humans. A 1988 FDA study of 11 heat susceptor packages purchased from supermarkets showed that there were detectable low levels of benzene in eight of them.

Industry data confirmed the presence of benzene in four of the committee's 42 samples. The packaging industry reports that these four package constructions have either been withdrawn from commercial use or have been reformulated.

At this stage of FDA's study, it's not clear whether the use of heat susceptor packaging represents a health hazard. Edward Machuga, Ph.D., in FDA's division of food and color additives, says that the agency is not aware of any hazard that would result from the use of heat susceptor packaging during the limited time needed by FDA to complete its review of this type of packaging.

FDA is completing its evaluation of heat susceptor packaging based on the data now in its files. This means evaluating not only the data submitted in response to the advance notice but also the data submitted years ago in petitions that led to the current regulation of these components at lower temperatures.

"If no high temperature migration data are available for a particular component," says Dr. Machuga, "we will calculate a worst-case estimate of dietary exposure based on the use level in the package. We will then determine if existing toxicological studies support this worst-case estimate of dietary exposure. If they do not, then additional data will need to be submitted in the form of a food additive petition. The manufacturer might be required to perform additional toxicological feeding studies or to carry out studies that would provide an assessment of dietary exposure under actual use conditions." (For more on microwave packaging, see "Keeping Up with the Microwave Revolution" in the March 1990 *FDA Consumer*.)

"Sous Vide"

Dry boil-in-bag foods, such as rice in plastic mesh-like packages, have been around for about 30 years, and FDA scientists have determined that the components of those packages are safe at boiling-water temperatures. But a fairly recent innovation, vacuum-packed refrigerated foods known by the French words "sous vide," a very different process, also gets dropped into boiling water in home preparation.

Processors of "sous vide" foods seal raw ingredients, often entire recipes, in plastic pouches, then vacuum out the air. They then minimally cook the pouch under precise conditions and immediately refrigerate it. Some processors replace some of the air with nitrogen or carbon dioxide. Processing food in this manner eliminates the need for the extreme cold of freezing and the intense heat of canning, thus better preserving taste.

619

The "sous vide" method of packaging can be used for most foods, including pasta, vegetables, fish, chicken, and beef. These types of food fit right into today's often hectic lifestyle, but they must be handled with care, say FDA food scientists. The danger here is not from packaging components migrating into the food—the packages are made with plastic materials that can safely be heated at boiling temperatures. The possible harm could come from the food itself spoiling because harmful bacteria that are present in most foods may not be destroyed in "sous vide" processing, and could grow in unrefrigerated conditions.

FDA recommends that "sous vide" foods be used by the expiration date printed on the package, be refrigerated constantly, and be heated according to the time and temperature of package directions. (For more on "sous vide" foods, see "The Big Chill" in the September 1989 *FDA Consumer.*)

FDA is very aware of the benefits of food packaging. Industry researches innovations constantly and works with FDA to stay within the parameters of safety that have been set for packaging materials that contact food. If FDA finds a violation, it contacts the manufacturer, and corrective action is taken. Any imminent danger to health is acted upon immediately with recall or regulatory action.

Recycled Plastics

There is a growing industry, government and consumer interest in recycling materials in the United States, including the recycling of plastics (polymers) for use in food-contact situations. FDA supports these recycling goals and is also aware of its responsibility to ensure the safety of materials that may come in contact with food.

One of the problems with recycled materials in food packaging, say FDA scientists, is that a plastic bottle may have been used (in its first life) to hold, for instance, motor oil. If that bottle were recycled, contaminants from the motor oil could remain. FDA has appointed a task force to develop a set of principles for recycled plastic food-contact materials.

Recycled glass and cans pose no problems, says Robert Testin, Ph.D., associate professor in Clemson University's Packaging Science Department. In order to melt them for recycling, temperatures must be very high—so high that most contaminants are removed.

But paper and plastics are recycled at much lower temperatures, and contaminants could remain. Some recycled products could be made of newspaper. Newspaper may contain dioxins and furans, a complex mixture of related compounds that are formed in trace amounts when chlorine or chlorine derivatives are used as the primary bleaching agents in making white paper products. The most toxic dioxin is 2,3,7,8-tetrachlorodibenzo-p-dioxin (TCDD), which has been shown to cause cancer in laboratory test animals.

The paper industry is participating in a voluntary program to reduce TCDD levels in all food-contact paper products to 2 parts per trillion (ppt) or less. Industry representatives have informed FDA that 82 percent of food-contact bleached paper products met the 2 ppt or less TCDD standard as of Dec. 31, 1990, and that all of these products are expected to meet this standard by the end of 1992. In milk cartons, the TCDD level is even lower—it averages 0.4 ppt. (See "Deciding About Dioxins" in the February 1990 issue of *FDA Consumer*.)

At present, the only uses for recycled plastic materials in food packaging reviewed by FDA are in egg (in the shell) cartons, berry baskets, harvesting crates, and soda bottles. Richard White, consumer safety officer in FDA's food and color additives division, explains that egg cartons made with polystyrene and berry baskets and harvesting crates made with polyethylene terephthalate (PET) are washed, ground and remolded to be recycled safely for the same uses.

The only FDA-reviewed procedure for recycling plastic soda bottles made with PET involves a regeneration process that breaks the plastic into its monomers (small molecules that are basic repeating links), which are then reprocessed into PET again. Other approaches to recycling plastic bottles are currently being evaluated by FDA.

Industry has technology to separate out components during recycling from packages that contain more than one material, such as both plastic and paper. It is also investigating the possibility of using recycled plastic as a buried layer in multilayered packages so that the recycled layer will not be in direct contact with food.

FDA realizes that recycling packaging for food contact use is a complex issue, and problems posed by recycled materials are currently under review.

by Judith Foulke

Judith Foulke is a staff writer for *FDA Consumer*.

Appendix C

Sources of Additional Information

Section 1

Getting Information From FDA

A woman called the Food and Drug Administration's office in Orlando, Fla., to thank consumer affairs officer Lynne Isaacs for the nutrition and diet information Isaacs had sent a few weeks before.

"She told me that she was ready for a serious well-balanced diet," Isaacs said. "She had tried all the fad diets and knew they didn't work. Then she admitted there was one fad she had never tried—a product that claims to burn the fat off while you sleep. She said that because she was an insomniac she figured the product would never get a chance to work. Of course that product doesn't work anyway, but I think her reason for not trying it may have been unique."

Thousands of people call or write FDA each year wanting information on a gamut of FDA-regulated items, from aspirin, tongue depressors, and canned green beans to cancer drugs, heart pacemakers, and infant formula.

Exactly what information does FDA have for consumers, and how can they get it?

Consumer Affairs Officers

FDA has consumer affairs officers (also known as public affairs specialists) throughout the country who can respond to questions about the agency and what it regulates.

"Every time there's something in the news about infant formula or baby food, mothers start calling," says Marie Ekvall, FDA's consumer affairs officer in Chicago. "I can hear the baby crying; sometimes the mother's crying, too."

Ekvall can usually give enough information over the phone to help the mother determine if there is any risk for her baby. As a follow-up, Ekvall then sends a reprint from FDA Consumer that will give the mother detailed information on infant nutrition.

In addition to reprints of articles from FDA Consumer, CAOs also have brochures, posters, teacher kits, press releases, and background papers on all kinds of FDA-related topics.

Consumers interested in audiovisuals can borrow or buy agency-produced slide shows, videotapes and films. CAOs have information on the titles available, prices, and how to order audiovisuals.

CAO's arc also available to speak to consumer and other groups on specific topics such as food labeling, health fraud, or AIDS.

To get in touch with your area's CAO, look for the Food and Drug Administration entry under the Department of Health and Human Services in the U.S. Government section of your local phone book.

Consumer Inquiries Staff

FDA's Consumer Inquiries Staff, located at agency headquarters in metropolitan Washington, D.C., is devoted solely to answering consumers' questions. The staff often consults various other FDA offices to find answers to detailed or complicated questions. last year, Consumer Inquiries received an average of 2,400 requests per month for information.

Send requests for information to FDA, Consumer Inquiries Staff, HFE-88, Room 16-63, 5600 Fishers Lane, Rockville, Md. 208S7, telephone (301) 443-3170.

Bulletin Boards

Most people would describe a bulletin board as a piece of cork, some thumb-tacks, and lots of papers with important information and announcements. But tacks and cork have been replaced by computers and modems on FDA's electronic bulletin board, which contains:

- press releases

- the FDA *Enforcement Report's* listing of recalls and litigations

626

- drug and device approvals

- congressional testimony

- speeches by FDA's commissioner

- FDA *Federal Register* summaries

- current information on AIDS, including published information on experimental drugs

- articles from *FDA Consumer*

- articles from the *FDA Drug Bulletin.*

Consumers who have computers with modems can subscribe to FDA's bulletin board by contacting BT Tymnet, 6120 Executive Blvd., Rockville, Md. 20852; telephone 800-872-7654.

For more details on the types of information "posted" on the bulletin board, contact FDA Press Office, HFI-20, Rockville, Md. 20857; telephone (301) 443-3285.

Freedom of Information Staff

The Freedom of Information Act makes most unpublished documents concerning FDA's regulatory activities available to the public. These include:

- enforcement records, including product notifications

- summaries of safety and effectiveness data from approved new drug applications

- regulatory letters telling companies to correct violations found during FDA inspections.

An FOI request for agency records can be denied only under set guidelines. Documents that may be exempt from public disclosure under the Freedom of Information Act include:

- trade secrets and confidential commercial or financial information

- certain interagency or intra-agency memos or letters

- personnel, medical and similar files that, if released, would constitute an invasion of privacy

- certain records compiled for law enforcement purposes

All FOI- requests should be in writing. For consumers, there is a copying fee of 10 cents per page and a search fee of $10 per hour. No fee is charged if the total is less than $10.

For more information or to make an FOI request, contact the Freedom of Information Staff, HFI-35, FDA. Room 12A-16, 5600 Fishers Lance, Rockville, Md. 20857.

What Does FDA Regulate?

FDA's responsibilities include foods, drugs, cosmetics, biological products, medical devices, radiological devices, and veterinary products sold in interstate commerce. (For information about what FDA does not regulate, see below.)

Some of the agency's specific responsibilities include:

Drugs:

- new drug approval

- good manufacturing practices for all prescription and non-prescription drug manufacturers

- prescription drug advertising

- tamper-resistant packaging

Biologics:

- human vaccine licensing

- blood banks

- allergenic product licensing

- licensing of test kits to screen blood for the AIDS virus

Foods:

- labeling

- safety of all food products except meat and poultry (sec below)

- good manufacturing practices

- bottled water

Medical Devices:

- pre-market approval of new devices

- manufacturing controls

- medical device reporting of malfunctions or serious adverse reactions

- registration and device listing

Electronic Products:

- radiation safety performance standards for microwave ovens, television receivers, diagnostic x-ray equipment, cabinet x-ray systems (e.g., baggage x-rays at airports), laser products, ultrasonic therapy equipment, mercury vapor lamps, and sunlamps

- guidance to health professionals and consumers about recommended practices to reduce unnecessary exposure to radiation

Veterinary Products:

- livestock feeds

- pet foods

- veterinary drugs and devices

Borderline

Because the federal government only regulates products that are shipped in interstate commerce, the states enforce many of the same regulations federal agencies do on products that never cross a state's borders. Consumers with questions or complaints about those products should contact their state governments.

The states, not the federal government, are responsible for licensing physicians, pharmacists, and other health professionals. And state and local governments inspect and regulate such establishments as restaurants and health spas.

Our Lips Are Sealed

"Some of the hardest questions FDA has to deal with are ones about a specific drug," says Marie Ekvall, FDA's consumer affairs officer in Chicago. "I encourage [callers] to talk to [their] doctor or pharmacist. and I let them know about resource books like the *Physicians' Desk Reference,* but I have to be careful not to play doctor," she says. "We get a lot of calls that, by law, we simply aren't allowed to answer," says Janet McDonald, San Francisco's CAO. For example, FDA employees cannot release any confidential information on unapproved drugs, including clinical trials, unless the manufacturer gives the agency permission or has already released the information to the public.

"This is information people usually have to get from their physicians or from private, nonprofit organizations such as those that deal with Alzheimer's disease or arthritis," says McDonald.

But there are some calls that just can't be answered by FDA or anyone else. For example, there's the boy who wrote Orlando's Isaacs to find out where he could buy a "hoverboard," one of those flying skateboards in the movie "Back to the Future II."

'Those things haven't been invented yet. I'd know because my 8-year-old would be begging for one," says Isaacs. "But if they were real, I guess they'd belong to the Consumer Product Safety Commission."

Sorry, I'll Have to Refer You to . . .

FDA doesn't have all the answers. Several other government agencies have responsibilities closely related to FDA's, so it isn't unusual for consumers to be confused about who watches over what. Here's a confusion-controlling list of subjects consumers often call FDA about, but which are under the purview of another agency. (Addresses listed below are for headquarters offices in Washington, D.C. Local offices are listed in the phone book under U.S. Government.)

Alcohol

The labeling and quality of alcoholic beverages are regulated by the Treasury Department's Bureau of Alcohol, Tobacco, and Firearms. AFT's address is Room 4402, Ariel Rios Federal Building, 1200 Pennsylvania Ave., N.W., Washington, D.C. 20226; telephone (202) 566-7135.

Information on drug and alcohol abuse, including counseling information, is available from the Alcohol, Drug Abuse, and Mental Health Administration's National Clearinghouse for Alcohol and Drug Abuse, P.O. Box 2345, Rockville, Md. 20852; (301) 468-2600.

Consumer Products

While FDA keeps watch over the quality of bread, the toaster used to brown it is the responsibility of the Consumer Product Safety Commission. Household appliances (except those that emit radiation), baby furniture, and toys are some of the more common products CPSC covers. Letters can be sent to CPSC, Washington, D.C. 20207, or the commission can be called toll free on 800-638-2772.

Drugs

Drugs of Abuse: Illegal drugs with no approved medical uses, such as heroin, are the sole responsibility of the Drug Enforcement Administration. Because some medically accepted drugs have a potential for abuse (for example, amphetamines, barbiturates and morphine), FDA assists DEA in deciding how stringent DEA controls on such drugs should be. DEA also limits the amount of these drugs that can be manufactured each year. Everyone who markets controlled drugs, from manufacturers and distributors to pharmacists, must register with DEA. Questions about these responsibilities should be sent to the Drug Enforcement Administration, U.S. Department of Justice, Washington, D.C. 20537; telephone (202) 307-1000.

Nonprescription Drug Advertising: the Federal Trade Commission is the primary agency for regulating ads for nonprescription drugs. The commission's address is 6th St. and Pennsylvania Ave., N.W., Washington, D.C. 20580; telephone (202) 326-2180.

Child-Resistant Packages: CPSC is responsible for child-resistant packages. See address above.

Food Stamps

The federal food stamp program is administered by local governments, usually as part of their social service departments.

Meat and Poultry

The U.S. Department of Agriculture's Food Safety and Inspection Service is responsible for the safety, labeling, and all other issues concerning meat and poultry. Consumers with questions on these issues, as well as how to safely handle, prepare and store chicken, beef and pork, should write or call the Food Safety and Inspection Service's Meat and Poultry Hotline, Room 1163S, Washington, D.C. 20250; telephone 800 535-4555.

Pesticides

FDA, USDA, and the Environmental Protection Agency share the responsibility for regulating pesticides. EPA determines the safety and effectiveness of the chemicals and establishes tolerance levels for residues on feed crops and raw and processed foods. These tolerance levels (the amount of pesticide allowed to remain on a crop after harvesting) are normally set 100 times below the level that might cause harm to people or the environment. To ensure that pesticide residues do not exceed the allowable levels, FDA tests all foods except meat and poultry, which fall under USDA's jurisdiction. Questions for EPA can be sent to Room W311, Mail Code A-107, 401 M St., S.W., Washington, D.C. 20460; telephone (202) 382-4361.

Radiation

Environmental: EPA monitors radiation in the environment.

Nuclear Industry: Licensing and regulation of the nuclear industry is the Nuclear Regulatory Commission's responsibility. NRC also ensures that the public is protected from hazards arising from nuclear materials in power reactors, hospitals, research laboratories, or other commercial facilities. Questions for NRC should be sent to the NRC Office of Public Affairs, Washington, D.C. 20555, telephone (202)-492-7715.

Restaurants and Grocery Stores

Inspections and licensing of restaurants and grocery stores are usually handled by local health departments.

Tobacco

Collecting taxes on cigarettes and other tobacco products is ATF's responsibility. Information on the health effects of smoking is available from the Office of Smoking and Health, Centers for Disease Control, 5600 Fishers Lane, Rockville, Md. 20857; telephone (301)- 443-5287.

Veterinary Products

EPA regulates products used directly on animals to control pests. USDA's Animal and Plant Health Inspection Service handles animal vaccines. The inspection service's address is APHIS, Veterinary Services, U.S. Department of Agriculture, Washington, D.C. 20090-6464; telephone (202) 447-5193.

Water

Depending on how it gets to consumers, water is regulated by either FDA or EPA. If the water comes through the tap, it must meet EPA's national standards for drinking water. Bottled water, however, is FDA's responsibility.

by Dori Stehlin

Dori Stehlin is a staff writer for *FDA Consumer*. Monica Arcarese, a student at Towson State University, also contributed to the article while a summer intern at FDA.

Section 2

Where to Get More Nutrition Information

Do you want to know how much fat there is in your favorite ice cream? Is a family member doing a science project and are you helping with the research? Looking for a publication to hand out to your community youth or adult group? The USDA and the Land-Grant university system have professionals ready to help you find the answers and materials you need. Several electronic system and networks are also available to assist you in finding food and human nutrition information.

USDA and Land-Grant Sources

Cooperative Extension Service

The Cooperative Extension Service has State, county, city, and area staff who link research-based nutrition, food safety, and food quality information with technology to help people improve their lives. These individuals are faculty and staff of Land-Grant universities located in each State across the country.

Telephone numbers and addresses for the more than 3,000 county and city offices across the Nation can be found in the government pages of local telephone books or by calling the local telephone information service. Ask to speak with the Extension home economist or nutritionist.

Excerpt from *Nutrition: Eating for Good Health*, U.S. Department of Agriculture, Agriculture Information Bulletin 685

Food and Nutrition Information Center, National Agricultural Library

Nutritionists and registered dietitians help people find information or educational materials in the following areas of food and human nutrition: nutrition education, human nutrition, food safety, food service management, nutrition software, and food technology. For example, the staff will help locate hard-to-find answers to questions, provide literature searches from the Library's bibliographic database, AGRICOLA (see explanation below), or assist you in finding the best audio-visual materials for a lesson or presentation. The center publishes Nutri-Topics and other resource lists on a variety of specific food and human nutrition topics.

The center has a food and nutrition software demonstration center, where an individual can preview any of over 200 software programs.

Contact:

Food and Nutrition Information Center
USDA/National Agricultural Library
Room 304
10301 Baltimore Blvd.
Beltsville, MD 20705-2351
301-504-5719 (automated system available 24 hours a day)
Fax: 301-504-6409
Internet address: fnic@nalusda.gov

USDA/FDA Food Labeling Education Information Center, National Agricultural Library

Located in the Food and Nutrition Information Center at the National Agricultural Library, this center is set up to assist educators, health professionals, and nutritionists locate information about educational programs related to food labeling.

Contact:

USDA/FDA Food Labeling Education Information Center

Food and Nutrition Information Center,
Room 304
USDA/National Agricultural Library
10301 Baltimore Blvd.
Beltsville, MD 20705-2351
301-504-5719 (automated system available 24 hours a day)
Internet address: Gmcneal@nalusda.gov

Meat and Poultry Hotline, Food Safety and Inspection Service

The hotline is staffed by home economists and registered dietitians who can answer questions about food safety, storage, preparation, and labeling (including nutrition labeling), as well as nutrition questions concerning meat and poultry products. The toll-free number is 1-800-535-4555; the hotline is staffed from 10:00 a.m. to 4:00 p.m., EST. In the Washington, DC, area call 202-720-3333.

Food and Nutrition Service

The Food and Nutrition Service administers Federal food assistance programs, including food stamps; food distribution; supplemental food for women, infants, and children; school lunch; school breakfast; special milk; child care; summer feeding; and other child-nutrition and family-food-assistance programs. Information about these programs may be obtained by contacting the following FNS Regional Public Information Offices:

Northeast Regional Public Affairs Director
10 Causeway Street
Boston, MA 0222-1068
617-565-6418

Mid-Atlantic Regional Public Affairs Director
Mercer Corporation Park
CN 02150
Trenton, NJ 08650
609-259-5091

Southeast Regional Public Affairs Director
Suite 112
77 Forsyth St., S.W.
Atlanta, GA 30303
404-730-2588

Midwest Regional Public Affairs Director
77 West Jackson St., 20th Floor
Chicago, IL 60602
312-353-1044

Mountain Plains Regional Public Affairs Director
Room 903
1244 Speer Boulevard
Denver, CO 80204
303-844-0312

Southwest Regional Public Affairs Director
Room 5C30
1100 Commerce Street
Dallas, TX 75242
214-767-0256

Western Regional Public Affairs Director
Room 400
550 Kearny St.
San Francisco, CA 94108
415-705-1311

You may also contact:

Director of Public Information
Food and Nutrition Service
USDA
3101 Park Center Dr.
Room 819
Alexandria, VA 22302
703-305-2276

Human Nutrition Information Service

The Human Nutrition Information Service provides information for professionals and the general public on nutrition topics, such as the nutritive value of foods, food money management, dietary guidelines, guides for food selection and storage, and preparation of food. HNIS research includes the fields of food consumption, nutrition knowledge and attitudes, dietary survey methodology, food composition, and nutrition education. Requests for information and publications may be directed to:

Office of Governmental Affairs and Public Information
Human Nutrition Information Service/USDA
6505 Belcrest Rd., Room 344
Hyattsville, MD 20782
301-436-5196

Agricultural Research Service

ARS conducts research to ensure an adequate and safe food supply that meets the nutritional needs of American consumers. Promoting optimum health and well-being by improving the nutritive value of food is also a major objective of ARS. For information contact:

ARS Information Office
Room 450
6303 Ivy Lane
Greenbelt, MD 20770
301-344-2340

Electronic Access to Information

Human nutrition information is available through several computer-based systems. Electronic bulletin boards and databases are an important method of information exchange. They are accessible around the clock, so information is available whenever it is needed.

Internet

The National Research and Education Network (NREN), a part of Internet, is a worldwide network that can provide access to valuable information collections and services. Using Internet, you can search subject matter databases, participate in discussion groups, and send or receive electronic mail. There is a great deal of information available about using Internet. Ask a librarian, contact a computer specialist, or talk with friends, family members or colleagues who may already be using the network about where to get more of the details. Almanac, listservs, gopher, and wide area information server (WAIS) are some of the network information tools available. These networking tools allow you to explore and locate valuable resources anywhere in the world. All Land-Grant universities and many USDA agencies have computers connected to Internet.

The first step in getting access to Internet is to establish an account on a computer that is connected to the network. If you have questions about access, contact your local library or computer specialist.

Information servers called Almanac process information requests through electronic mail. Currently there are seven Almanac servers in operation. Their Internet addresses are as follows:

Location	Internet address
Oregon State University	almanac@oes.orst.edu
Purdue University	almanac@ecn.purdue.edu
Extension Service-USDA	almanac@esusda.gov
North Carolina State University	almanac@ces.ncsu.edu
Univeristy of California	almanac@silo.ucdavis.edu
University of Wisconsin	almanac@joe.uwex.edu (This is for the Journal of Extension)

To find out what information is available in Almanac, send an electronic mail (E-mail) message to one of the above addresses. In the body of the message type the command:

send catalog

Use lower case characters. Do not type any other text. For example, you can subscribe to *Food Market News* through the almanac site at Oregon State University.

To obtain a users' guide, in the body of the message type the command:

send guide

It may take only a few seconds or several minutes for your request to be honored, and the materials will be available when you read the E-mail.

Gopher allows you to locate resources from hundreds of locations worldwide. This powerful tool permits you to access a library in another country as quickly as accessing the card catalog in your own State's library system.

The Cooperative Extension System currently operates seven gopher sites. You can access a site, for example by using telenet with the address:

info.umd.edu

This connects you with the University of Maryland's gopher. The menu path to reach the Extension Service-USDA gopher is "Other Gopher Information Servers"/"North America"/"USA"/"General"/Extension Service USDA Information. You can search for food, nutrition, or other related information.

Electronic Bulletin Boards

The Human Nutrition Information Service and the National Agricultural Library both maintain electronic bulletin boards that contain human nutrition information. To access an electronic bulletin board you need the following: a computer, a modem, a telephone line, and communications software.

Agricultural Library Forum (ALF)

Produced by the National Agricultural Library, ALF contains a subboard called Food. The Food subboard provides access to information and publications from the Food and Nutrition Information Center, the FDA/USDA food labeling Education Information Center, and other federal food and nutrition activities. Subjects covered include human nutrition, nutrition education, food safety, food service management, food technology, food labeling education, and food nutrition software.

There is no registration fee for the bulletin board. You will become a registered user after you first log in. If you are unfamiliar with dialing into an electronic bulletin board system, you may get assistance by calling 301-504-5113.

Modem numbers: 301-504-6510, 301-504-5111, 301-504-5496, 301-504-5497.

Communications settings are: 8 data bits, one stop bit, no parity, full duplex. Terminal emulation should be none, ASCII, or TTY.

Internet Access: telnet fedworld.doc.gov Register on this National Technical Information Service (NTIS) bulletin board system (bbs). Then select Gateway (D command). Then select federal bbs (another D), then select 2 from the list for ALF. You will be automatically connected to ALF. When you exit ALF you will still be in the Fedworld system and will need to follow directions for exiting.

Nutrient Data Bank Bulletin Board

The Nutrient Data Bank Bulletin Board is sponsored by the Human Nutrition Information Service (HNIS) in Hyattsville, MD. It is operated as a public service to provide information about current HNIS publications and computer files on the nutrient composition of foods. There is no registration fee.

The telephone number is 301-436-5078

Internet access: telnet info.umd.edu

Communications settings are: 8 data bits, one stop bit, no parity, full duplex.

International Food and Nutrition Database (IFAN) (a computer-based information system)

IFAN is part of PENpages, a computer-based information system at Penn State's University Park campus. Penn State is one of the Land-Grant universities that are located in every State and that play key roles with USDA in conducting research and in providing education and information access for the public. IFAN is a full-text database containing documents including newsletters, fact sheets, research summaries, and other nutrition-related materials.

There is no registration fee for using IFAN. To access IFAN, you need a computer, modem, and communications software that is VT-100 or VT-102 compatible.

Modem number: 814-863-4820

Internet address: psnutrition@psupen.psu.edu

After connecting, press <enter> until the prompt psupen> is displayed. Type <connect pen>. At the prompt, type the two-letter abbreviation for your state. Press <enter> to get the PENpages menu.

For additional information, contact:

IFAN Editor
Penn State Nutrition Center
417 East Calder Way
University Park, PA 16801-5663
814-865-6323

Bibliographic Databases

AGRICOLA. AGRICOLA is a bibliographic database consisting of records for journal articles, monographs, theses, patents, software, audiovisual materials, and technical reports relating to all aspects of agriculture. The database contains information on human nutrition, nutrition education, food safety, food service management, food science, and food technology.

The database is available on-line through the commercial vendor, DIALOG Information Services. It is updated monthly. For information on subscription rates and fees, call 1-800-3-DIALOG. AGRICOLA is also on CD-ROM from SilverPlatter Information, Inc. For subscription rates for the disk, which is issued quarterly, call 1-800-343-0064.

The database is also available at university and college libraries, and at many public libraries. Ask a librarian or information specialist for assistance.

QUERRI (Questions on University Extension Regional Resource Information). QUERRI is a bibliographic database supported by the Cooperative Extension Services of Illinois, Indiana, Iowa, Kansas, Michigan, Minnesota, Missouri, Nebraska, North Dakota, Ohio, South Dakota, and Wisconsin. The food and nutrition materials listed in QUERRI are related to family and consumer issues. You will find the materials by conducting keyword searches in the database. Copies of the listed materials can be ordered from the distribution offices of the producing institutions.

There is no registration fee for using QUERRI. You will need a computer, modem, and communications software. You can connect either through a modem or Internet. When you connect to QUERRI the first time, select "How to Use QUERRI" from the main menu and go through a short tutorial.

Modem number: 515-294-(your baud speed)

Internet address: telnet isn.rdns.iastate.edu

Modem settings: 8 data bits, one stop bit, no parity, full duplex.

Sandra L. Facinoli
Coordinator, Food and Nutrition Information Center
National Agriculture Library

Section 3

Informational Sources Cited in This Book

The organizations listed below are sources of additional information that are mentioned in the various chapters and appendices of this book. They are listed alphabetically, with subordinate departments listed under the parent organizations.

Administration on Aging
330 Independence Avenue, S.W.
Washington, DC 20201
(202) 619 0774

U.S. Government agency that provides information on health and aging programs, offered through State and area agencies on aging.

Alzheimer's Association
Suite 1000
919 N. Michigan Avenue
Chicago, IL 60611
(312) 335-8700 1-(800) 272-3900 toll-free hotline

Offers a hotline that provides information and assistance for families coping with Alzheimer's disease.

American Association of Retired Persons
1909 K Street, N.W.
Washington, DC 20049
(707) 434-7777

Membership organization for people over age 50, offering publications and volunteer-run programs on a variety of economic, social, and health issues.

American Dietetic Association
Suite 800
216 West Jackson Boulevard
Chicago, IL 60606
(312) 899-0040

Professional organization offering assistance in locating a registered dietitian in your community.

American Frozen Food Institute
1764 Old Meadow Lane, Suite 350
McLean, VA 22102

American Geriatrics Society
Suite 300
770 Lexington Avenue
New York, NY 10021
(212) 308-1414

Professional organization of physicians with geriatric training, offering assistance in locating a doctor in your community with special training in treating older adults.

Arthritis Foundation
1314 Spring Street, N.W.
Atlanta, GA 30309
(404) 872-7100

Provides information and programs on arthritis, including treatment options and self-help materials for those with arthritis and their families.

Food and Drug Administration
Office of Consumer Affairs
5600 Fishers Lane, HFE 88
Rockville, MD 20857
(301) 443-3170

U.S. Government agency that answers questions about the safety of food additives, drugs, and medical devices.

Food Marketing Institute
800 Connecticut Ave., NW
Washington, DC 20006-2701

International Microwave Power Institute
13542 Union Village Circle
Clifton, VA 22024

National Cancer Institute
Office of Cancer Communications
Building 31, Room 10A24
9000 Rockville Pike
Bethesda, MD 20892
1 (800)422 6237 toll-free hotline

U.S. Government agency that provides information on cancer prevention and treatment.

National Institute on Aging
Public Information Office
9000 Rockville Pike
Bethesda, MD 20892
(301) 496-1752

U.S. Government agency that provides information on health and other issues of interest to older people.

National Institutes of Health
Room 10 A 24, Building 31
Bethesda, MD 20892

National Heart, Lung, and Blood Institute
Information Office
Building 31, Room 4A21 9000 Rockville Pike
Bethesda, MD 20892
(301) 496-4236

U.S. Government agency that conducts research and provides information about heart, lung. and blood diseases.

Office of Disease Prevention and Health Promotion
National Health Information Center
P.O. Box 1133
Washington, DC 20013-1133
1 (800) 336-4797

U.S. Government agency that operates a clearinghouse and hotline to provide health information and referrals.

U.S. Department of Agriculture
Center for Nutrition Policy and Promotion
1120 20th Street NW, Suite 200 North
Washington, DC 20036

U.S. Department of Agriculture
Food Safety and Inspection Service
Room 1165 South
14th & Jefferson Drive, SW
Washington, DC 20250

U.S. Department of Agriculture
Human Nutrition Information Service
Room 325-A
6505 Belcrest Road
Hyattsville, MD 20782.

U.S. Government agency that provides information on using the Dietary Guidelines and preparing foods.

U.S. Department of Agriculture
Meat and Poultry Hotline
1-800-535-4555
In the Washington D.C. area, call (202)-720-3333
Hours are from 10 a.m. to 4 p.m. Eastern time.

Consumers are also encouraged to contact their county extension home economist (Cooperative Extension System, found in the government pages of local telephone books) or a nutrition professional from your local Public Health Department, hospital, American Red Cross, dietetic association, diabetes association, heart association, or cancer society.

Index

Index

Italicized page numbers indicate a photo or illustration.

A

adults (older), 135-204
  Alzheimer's disease, 178
  appetite loss, 179-80
  arthritis, 181
  blood cholesterol, 138-40
  body weight, 165-66, 167-68
  constipation, 152
    see also fiber
  eating alone, 180
  fats, 137, 138, 139-40, 144, 148
  fluid intake, 152
  frozen meals, 163-65
  handling food, 165
  immune system, 406
  information on, 202-04
  labels, 158-60
  medication and food, 155-56
  memory loss, 178-79
  menus, 156-58, 162-63
  Nutrition Facts Label, 159
  physical activity, 166
  servings, 149
  shopping, 158-62
  snacks, 169
  sodium, 140-43, 145
alcohol, 34-36
  and blood cholesterol, 71-72
  and teens, 114
Alzheimer's disease, 178
anorexia nervosa
  see body weight
antioxidants, 405
artifical sweeteners
  see sweets
atherosclerosis
  see heart disease

B

babies
  see children
BMR
  see energy metabolism, basal metabolic rate
beans
  see legumes
bioavailability, 383-88
  see also individual nutrients and vitamins
  analyzing and measuring, 384
  definition of, 383, 384
body weight, 285-93

653